Food Hypersensiti

Diagnosing and managing food allergies and intolerance

Food Hypersensitivity

Diagnosing and managing food allergies and intolerance

Edited by

Isabel Skypala

BSc Nutrition and Dietetics, PG Dip Allergy, RD
Specialist Allergy Dietitian, Director of Rehabilitation
and Therapies,
Royal Brompton & Harefield NHS Trust,
and Honorary Senior Lecturer, Imperial College London

Carina Venter

BSc Dietetics, PG Dip Allergy, PhD, RD
Senior Allergy Dietitian, David Hide Asthma and Allergy
Research Centre, Isle of Wight,
and Senior Research Fellow, University of Portsmouth

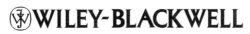

A John Wiley & Sons, Ltd., Publication

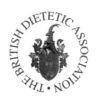

Blackwell Publishing was acquired by John Wiley & Sons in February 2007. Blackwell's publishing
programme has been merged with Wiley's global Scientific, Technical, and Medical business to form
Wiley-Blackwell.

Registered office
John Wiley & Sons Ltd, The Atrium, Southern Gate, Chichester, West Sussex, PO19 8SQ,
United Kingdom

Editorial offices
9600 Garsington Road, Oxford, OX4 2DQ, United Kingdom
2121 State Avenue, Ames, Iowa 50014-8300, USA

For details of our global editorial offices, for customer services and for information about how
to apply for permission to reuse the copyright material in this book please see our website at
www.wiley.com/wiley-blackwell.

Library of Congress Cataloging-in-Publication Data
Food hypersensitivity : diagnosing and managing food allergies and intolerance / edited
by Isabel Skypala, Carina Venter.
        p. cm.
    Includes bibliographical references and index.
    ISBN 978-1-4051-7036-9 (pbk. : alk. paper)   1. Food allergy—Diagnosis.
2. Food allergy—Diet therapy.   I. Skypala, Isabel.   II. Venter, Carina.

    RC596.F668 2009
    616.97′50654—dc22

                                                        2008047431

A catalogue record for this book is available from the British Library.

Set in 10/12.5pt Sabon by Graphicraft Limited, Hong Kong
Printed in Singapore by Utopia Press Pte Ltd

1   2009

Contents

List of contributors   ix
Foreword   xi

PART 1:   DIAGNOSIS

1   Classification and Prevalence of Food Hypersensitivity   3
Carina Venter

    1.1   Introduction   3
    1.2   Nomenclature and classification   3
    1.3   Immunological basis of food allergy   6
    1.4   Symptoms associated with food hypersensitivity   9
    1.5   Prevalence   9
    1.6   Conclusion   17

2   The Role of Food Hypersensitivity in Different Disorders   22

    2.1   The role of food hypersensitivity in skin disorders   22
        Rosan Meyer and George Du Toit
    2.2   The role of food hypersensitivity in respiratory disorders   31
        Isabel Skypala
    2.3   The role of food hypersensitivity in gastrointestinal disorders   37
        Miranda Lomer
    2.4   The role of food hypersensitivity in behavioural disorders   58
        Donna C. McCann, Zoe Connor
    2.5   The role of food hypersensitivity in neurological disorders   68
        Sue Luscombe, Susan Thurgood
    2.6   The role of food hypersensitivity in musculoskeletal disorders   81
        Anna Carling

3   The Diagnosis of Food Hypersensitivity   85
Carina Venter, Berber Vlieg-Boerstra and Anna Carling

    3.1   Introduction   85
    3.2   Clinical history   85
    3.3   Diagnostic tests   86
    3.4   Complementary and alternative medicine   90
    3.5   Diagnostic exclusion diets   92
    3.6   Oral food challenges   94
    3.7   Conclusion   103

4   Triggers of Food Hypersensitivity   107
     Isabel Skypala

     4.1 Introduction   107
     4.2 Allergens and the immune system   107
     4.3 Food allergen classes and nomenclature   108
     4.4 How does a food allergen induce allergy?   108
     4.5 Classification of food allergens   109
     4.6 Advances in food allergen technology   110
     4.7 Peanut allergens   111
     4.8 Food labelling   112

PART 2:   DIETARY MANAGEMENT

5   Milk and Eggs   117
     Tanya Wright and Rosan Meyer

     5.1 Introduction   117
     5.2 Cow's milk   117
     5.3 Egg allergy   128

6   Seafood   136
     Isabel Skypala

     6.1 Introduction   136
     6.2 Prevalence and natural history   136
     6.3 Foods involved   137
     6.4 Diagnosis   139
     6.5 Avoidance   142

7   Fruits and Vegetables   147
     Isabel Skypala

     7.1 Introduction   147
     7.2 Prevalence and natural history   147
     7.3 Foods involved   149
     7.4 Presenting symptoms and diagnosis   157
     7.5 Management   160

8   Peanuts, Legumes, Seeds and Tree Nuts   166
     Ruth Towell

     8.1 Peanuts   166
     8.2 Other legumes   171
     8.3 Seeds   174
     8.4 Tree nuts   176

9   Food Hypersensitivity Involving Cereals   183

     9.1 Coeliac disease   183
          Norma McGough, Emma Merrikin and Emily Kirk
     9.2 Allergy to wheat and other cereals   203
          Isabel Skypala

10   Other Causes of Food Hypersensitivity   210
     Isabel Skypala

     10.1   Reactions to food additives   210
     10.2   Pharmacologic food reactions   221
     10.3   Food-dependent exercise-induced anaphylaxis   229

PART 3:   OTHER ASPECTS OF MANAGEMENT, ALLERGY PREVENTION AND
NUTRITIONAL CONSIDERATIONS

11   Nutritional Consequences of Avoidance, and Practical Approaches to
     Nutritional Management   243
     Ruth Kershaw

     11.1   Introduction   243
     11.2   Assessment of dietary adequacy   243
     11.3   Factors affecting nutritional status   245
     11.4   Ensuring optimal nutritional status while following a
            food-avoidance diet   246
     11.5   The nutritional consequences of avoiding a number of common
            food allergens   247
     11.6   Vitamin and mineral supplements   257
     11.7   Other common nutritional issues encountered when implementing
            food-avoidance diets   260
     11.8   Conclusion   262

12   Lifestyle Issues   265
     Tanya Wright

     12.1   Introduction   265
     12.2   The burden of anaphylaxis and food allergy   265
     12.3   The importance of reintroduction of foods   265
     12.4   Cross-contamination   266
     12.5   Items on prescription   266
     12.6   Recipe information   267
     12.7   Product information   267
     12.8   Awareness products   268
     12.9   Nurseries, childminders and carers   268
     12.10   Managing food allergy at school   269
     12.11   Managing food allergy at home   270
     12.12   Managing food allergy at work   271
     12.13   Eating out   271
     12.14   Going on holiday   272
     12.15   Support and resources   273

13   Allergy Prevention and the Effect of Nutrition on the Immune System   278
     Carina Venter

     13.1   Introduction   278
     13.2   Introduction to the immune system   279
     13.3   Supporting the immune system through nutrition   282
     13.4   Conclusions   294

viii   Contents

14   Management of Allergic Disease   303

    14.1   Allergic rhinitis   303
           Samantha Walker
    14.2   Asthma   309
           Jane Leyshon
    14.3   Atopic eczema   315
           Helen Cox
    14.4   Anaphylaxis   322
           Samantha Walker

Appendix 1:   Patient information literature for a food challenge   329
Appendix 2:   Food challenge protocol for adults   331
Appendix 3:   Food challenge procedures   335
Appendix 4:   Prolonged open food challenge procedures   337
Appendix 5:   Food challenge form   339
Appendix 6:   Food challenge symptom score chart   342
Appendix 7:   Dietary management summaries   345

Index   355

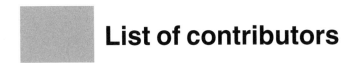

List of contributors

Anna Carling, BSc, PG Dip Allergy, RD
Senior Dietitian, Royal United Hospital, Bath NHS Trust

Zoe Connor, BSc, RD, MSc
Dietitian and Freelance Nutrition Consultant, www.nutritionnutrition.com

Helen Cox, MBChB, FRCP, FRCPCH, MD
Consultant in Paediatric Allergy and Immunology, Imperial College Healthcare NHS Trust

George Du Toit, MBBCh, DCH, FCP, M Med, Dip Allergy, FRCPCH, FAAAAI
Consultant in Paediatric Allergy, Evelina Children's Hospital, Guy's & St Thomas' NHS Foundation Trust and King's College London

Ruth Kershaw, BSc, RD
Specialist Paediatric Allergy Dietitian, Lecturer in Human Nutrition and Dietetics (Placement Support), London Metropolitan University Trust

Emily Kirk, MNutr, RD
Coeliac Disease Specialist Dietitian, Coeliac UK

Jane Leyshon, RGN, BA(Hons) Community Health Studies, PGCE
Head of Academic Studies, Education for Health Respiratory Nurse Specialist in General Practice

Miranda Lomer, PhD, RD
Consultant Dietitian in Gastroenterology, Guy's and St Thomas' NHS Foundation Trust and King's College London

Sue Luscombe, Dip Allergy, RD
Specialist Dietitian, Bedford Hospital NHS Trust

Donna C. McCann, PhD, MA, PGCE
Visiting Research Fellow, School of Psychology, University of Southampton

Norma McGough, BSc, RD
Head of Diet & Health, Coeliac UK

Emma Merrikin, BSc, RD
Coeliac Disease Specialist Dietitian, Coeliac UK

Rosan Meyer, B Dietetics, M Nutrition, PhD, RD
Paediatric Research Dietitian, Department of Paediatrics, Imperial College London

Isabel Skypala, BSc Nutrition and Dietetics, PG Dip Allergy, RD
Specialist Allergy Dietitian, Director of Rehabilitation and Therapies, Royal Brompton & Harefield NHS Trust and Honorary Senior Lecturer, Imperial College London

Susan Thurgood, BSc, RD, Cert Nut Med
Senior Specialist Dietitian, Royal London Homoeopathic Hospital

Ruth Towell, BSc (Hons) Nutrition, MSc Teaching and Learning, RD
Clinical Research Dietitian, Paediatric Allergy, King's College London and Guy's and St Thomas' NHS Foundation Trust

Carina Venter, BSc Dietetics, PG Dip Allergy, PhD, RD
Senior Allergy Dietitian, David Hide Asthma and Allergy Research Centre, Isle of Wight and Senior Research Fellow, University of Portsmouth

Berber Vlieg-Boerstra, PhD, RD
Clinical Research Dietician, Paediatric Allergy, University Medical Centre, Groningen, The Netherlands and Specialist Allergy Dietician , Vlieg & Melse Dieticians, Arnhem, The Netherlands

Samantha Walker, RGN, PhD
Director of Education & Research, Education for Health, Warwick and Honorary Senior Lecturer (non-clinical), Division of Community Health Sciences, University of Edinburgh

Tanya Wright, BSc, RD, MSc
Allergy Specialist Dietitian and Allergy Services Coordinator, Buckinghamshire Hospitals NHS Trust

Foreword

The diagnosis of food hypersensitivity (FHS) represents a challenge to all who work in the field; this is predominantly due to the paucity of good diagnostic tests and the wide variability of the conditions involved. Estimates vary as to the number of people afflicted with symptoms which they perceive are triggered by particular foods, but this could be more than 20% of the UK population. Although only a much smaller percentage of these people actually have FHS, the burden of diagnosis is considerable. It is essential that all those who suspect they have FHS receive the correct diagnosis.

There is no shortage of weighty and authoritative reference books on FHS, and a wealth of books for the lay public. This book is different; the editors and contributors to the book have focussed on using their extensive expertise in the clinical setting to provide a well-referenced but very practical guide to the diagnosis and management of FHS. The spectrum of conditions covered is extensive including not only well-characterised conditions such as IgE-mediated food allergy and coeliac disease, but also the putative role of FHS in other entities such as Attention-Deficit Hyperactivity Disorder and Irritable Bowel Syndrome.

In addition to guiding the reader through the prevalence and diagnosis of FHS, including oral food challenge, the middle section provides chapters devoted to those foods or food groups involved in FHS reactions. The last section covers important wider issues such as nutritional management, prevention, living with FHS and an overview of the associated atopic conditions including asthma, eczema and rhinitis.

FHS diagnosis and management involves clinicians of many different professional backgrounds, principally doctors, dietitians and nurses. These clinicians can be working in primary, secondary or tertiary care, in general practice or a specialist allergy service. This book, with contributions from professionals from all of these disciplines, illustrates the collaborative nature of good FHS management. A large number of the contributors are dietitians, who have shared the benefit of their many years of practical expertise, illustrating how important dietitians are to the specialty of allergy and to FHS in particular.

FHS diagnosis can be highly contentious. This book has been written by professionals all of whom are well-recognised within their individual fields and are members of the British Society of Allergy and Clinical Immunology and/or the Food Allergy and Intolerance Specialist Group of the British Dietetic Association. The book will be a useful addition to the bookshelf for those working in both the general or specialist sector, and for those who are studying the topic at either undergraduate or post graduate level.

Stephen R. Durham
Professor of Allergy and Respiratory Medicine
Imperial College and Royal Brompton Hospital, London

Part 1
Diagnosis

1 Classification and Prevalence of Food Hypersensitivity

Carina Venter

1.1 Introduction

Adverse reactions to food have been reported for the last 2,000 years. Writings from ancient Rome indicate that the Romans understood that foods consumed safely by most people could provoke adverse reactions in others. Prausnitz and Kustner[1] were the first to discover that the 'substance', now known as immunoglobulin E (IgE), responsible for Kustner's allergic reaction to fish, was present in his blood serum. However, despite the long history of food allergies and intolerances, it still remains a very controversial subject.

Many people believe that they are allergic or intolerant to a food, although in the majority of cases this will not be confirmed by the necessary tests, food exclusion and food challenges/reintroduction. For some of them, however, these allergies or intolerances could be life-threatening or have a huge impact on their quality of life, and extreme avoidance of the culprit food may be the only way to avoid severe symptoms. For others, such stringent avoidance measures may not be applicable, but they may nonetheless lead to an unnecessary reduction in their quality of life.

This chapter sets out to explain the different terminology and mechanisms involved in food allergy. It also looks critically at the true prevalence of allergies and intolerances, and at the foods and symptoms involved.

1.2 Nomenclature and classification

'Adverse food reactions' is the umbrella term referring to any untoward reaction following the ingestion of a food (or food additive). These can be divided into *toxic* and *non-toxic* reactions. Toxic substances may occur naturally in foods (e.g. scombroid fish poisoning or aflatoxins in peanuts), or may be added during food preparation[2].

One method of classifying the non-toxic reactions is to divide them into *food allergy* (immune-mediated) and *food intolerance* (non-immune-mediated) (Figure 1.1). However, in the clinical practice of allergy it is often unclear whether the problem is an allergy or an intolerance, due to the time delay between ingestion and symptoms and insufficient diagnostic tools[2,3]. There is a popular practice of calling all adverse reactions 'allergies'. This is inaccurate, however, and causes confusion both for the general public and for health professionals.

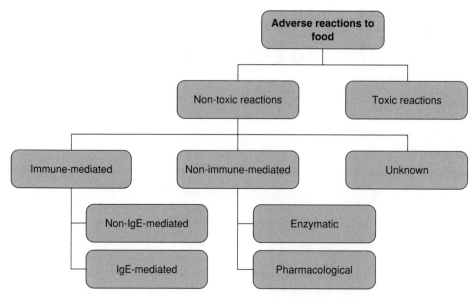

Figure 1.1   Classification of adverse reactions to food, based on the COT report[2].

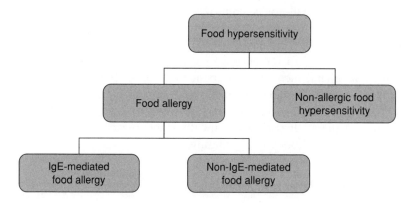

Figure 1.2   Nomenclature for food hypersensitivity[4].

A European Academy of Allergy and Clinical Immunology task force[4] has proposed that any adverse reactions to food should be called *food hypersensitivity* (Figure 1.2). When immunological mechanisms have been demonstrated, they suggest that the appropriate term is *food allergy*. If the food allergy involves IgE, then it will be known as *IgE-mediated food allergy*. Other reactions, previously sometimes referred to as 'food intolerance', should be referred to as *non-allergic food hypersensitivity*. Severe, generalised allergic reactions to food are classified as *anaphylaxis*[4]. See Table 1.1 for examples of the different food hypersensitivity presentations[5].

The term food hypersensitivity (FHS) will be used throughout this book, following the above nomenclature.

Table 1.1 Presentations of different types of food hypersensitivity (FHS)[5].

	Gastrointestinal	Cutaneous	Respiratory	Generalised
IgE-mediated food allergy	Oral allergy syndrome Gastrointestinal anaphylaxis	Urticaria Angioedema Morbilliform rashes Red flushes	Acute rhinoconjunctivitis Acute asthma	Anaphylaxis Food-dependent exercise-induced anaphylaxis (FDEIA)
Non-IgE-mediated food allergy (cell-mediated FHS)	Food protein-induced proctocolitis Food protein-induced enterocolitis Food protein-induced enteropathy Coeliac disease	Contact dermatitis Dermatitis herpetiformis	Heiner's syndrome (food-induced pulmonary haemosiderosis)	
IgE- and/or non-IgE-mediated (cell-mediated)	Allergic eosinophilic esophagitis Allergic eosinophilic gastroenteritis	Atopic dermatitis	Asthma	
Non-allergic food hypersensitivity	Lactose intolerance, galactosemia, alcohol intolerance Pharmacological reactions caused by caffeine (jitteriness), tyramine in aged cheeses (migraine), alcohol, histamine			

1.3   Immunological basis of food allergy

Food proteins are broken down into small peptides and amino acids by digestive enzymes. In a normal situation, these food particles are prevented from entering the tissues by physiological and immunological barriers in the gut. However, sometimes small amounts of intact food proteins may be absorbed through the gastrointestinal tract and elicit an immunological response when presented to T cells. This could either lead to stimulation of Th1 cells (non-IgE-mediated allergies) or Th2 cells (IgE-mediated allergies), depending on a number of factors such as the genetic make-up of the host, the characteristics of the food protein and the effect of the microenvironment. These interactions lead to the development of food tolerance in most subjects, and the development of new allergies in some subjects[6].

The Gell–Coombs classification[7] recognises four distinct types of hypersensitivity reactions (types I, II, III, IV), and each type involves different components of the immune system. The type I (IgE-mediated) response is the classic allergic response and manifests as urticaria, angio-oedema and anaphylaxis. The type II response, or immune-complex-mediated response, is one where the antigen binds to the cell surface and the presence of antibodies disrupts the membrane, leading to cell death, e.g. neutropenia and thrombocytopenia. Type III is a response involving IgG antibodies, where antigen-antibody-complement immune complexes get trapped in small blood vessels or glomeruli causing vasculitis and nephropathy. An exaggerated response can cause allergic symptoms. Finally, the type IV response is a delayed hypersensitivity response caused by the T cells, and it can manifest as a variety of clinical symptoms such as food protein-induced enterocolitis and eczema[8,9]. In many patients, more than one process may be involved at the same time; however, there is very little evidence to suggest that type II and III reactions play a role in food-related reactions.

1.3.1   IgE-mediated food allergy

During a classic IgE-mediated allergic response, food proteins (antigens) enter the body through the gastrointestinal mucosa or lung mucosa. Antigen-presenting cells (dendritic cells) engulf the antigens and present them to Th0 cells. In atopic individuals, the process stimulates the production of Th2 cells, which stimulate B cells to produce IgE food-specific antibodies to the protein encountered. Those IgE antibodies then bind to mast cells in tissues or basophils circulating in the blood via a special high-affinity receptor on the cells. IgE antibodies in plasma have a very short life, but once bound to cells (mainly mast cells) they can remain in the tissues for months waiting to come into contact with the allergen. This is called sensitisation[9].

On subsequent exposure to the allergen, the specific IgE antibodies recognise certain areas on the food protein called epitopes, which allows the protein to bind with the antibody, leading to degranulation of these cells, release of the histamine, prostaglandins, leukotrienes, platelet activation factors and bradikynin. These mediators cause vascular dilation and increased permeability, and attract cells into the tissues, leading to inflammation.

A few hours after the initial reaction a more pronounced reaction (late-phase reaction) may be experienced. This is mainly initiated by the eosinophils, but mononuclear cells, other lymphocytes and neutrophils are also involved.

1.3.2   Non-IgE-mediated food allergy

Although the mechanisms involved in food-induced reactions are not always clear, the absence of IgE production has been clearly established. A number of research studies have particularly investigated the immunological basis of gastrointestinal non-IgE-mediated allergies, and have clearly indicated involvement of T cells (mainly Th1 cells, but Th2 cells could also be involved) and cells such as eosinophils. T cells become sensitised at the initial exposure. On the subsequent contact the protein (epitope) combines with the sensitised T cells and releases their cytokines, which leads to chronic inflammation[10]. In most cases, biopsies will be needed for a formal diagnosis. However, diagnostic difficulties in non-IgE-mediated food allergies still remain, and many more basic scientific studies are needed[11,12].

There has been some interest in the role of IgG tests for the diagnosis of FHS. One study evaluated IgG tests in the diagnosis of FHS in patients suffering from irritable bowel syndrome (IBS)[13]. It is thought, however, that IgG levels to a particular food indicate the level of food consumption rather than a hypersensitivity[14]. Zuo *et al.*[15] showed that increased levels of antigen-specific IgG antibody titres for some foods were found in IBS and functional dyspepsia patients compared with controls, but were unable to correlate the level of food-specific IgG antibodies with symptom severity in either the dyspeptic or the IBS patients. This is a very interesting area and needs further research.

1.3.3   Non-allergic food hypersensitivity

Non-allergic FHS is usually (but not always) characterised by a delayed reaction, occurring hours or even days after eating certain foods. The possible causes include pharmacological reactions, substances occurring naturally in the food, and enzyme deficiencies.

Pharmacological reactions

Monosodium glutamate[16] (MSG) is commonly used as a flavour enhancer, and large amounts of MSG are reported to cause flushing, headache and abdominal symptoms. The reaction may even mimic the features of a myocardial infarction, with chest pain radiating to both arms and the back together with general weakness and palpitations[17]. The role of MSG in non-allergic FHS, and also that of food additives[18] such as artificial colours, preservatives etc., is discussed in Chapter 10.

Biogenic amines such as histamine, tyramine, phenylethylamine, serotonin and tryptamine can produce symptoms including headache, nausea and giddiness; tyramine can trigger migraine in some people. Urticaria and angio-oedema symptoms can also result primarily from the physiological actions of histamine[17]. Some individuals with urticaria have a decreased ability to degrade dietary histamine before it enters the circulation. This is determined by genetic factors, disease and medication. Excess histamine levels would cause symptoms similar to those experienced in IgE-mediated allergy. Adverse reactions depend not only on the presence of the problem food component, but also on the amount of the food component ingested and the sensitive person's efficiency in metabolising it.

Excess histamine could be caused by several factors:

1   amount of histamine produced and release intrinsically;
2   histamine production by gut bacteria;
3   dietary intake of foods containing or releasing histamine;
4   catabolic enzymes not able to reduce excess histamine within the body.

The only factor that can easily be manipulated is the amount of histamine in food. Foods high in histamine, such as fermented foods, may exacerbate urticaria and angio-oedema in these individuals (see Chapter 10).

Zuberbier et al.[19] have shown that foods naturally high in histamines and salicylates (tomato, wine and spices) cause symptoms of urticaria during food challenges. However, analysis of these foods, or components of these foods, showed that it was the aromatic volatile ingredients (ketones, alcohol and aldehydes) that were involved in the development of urticaria, rather than the histamine and/or salicylate content.

Substances naturally occurring in foods

Non-immunological reactions may also be provoked by food constituents such as benzoates, salicylates, nickel and caffeine[20]. High levels of benzoic acid in some citrus fruits may cause a harmless flare reaction around the mouth, especially in children. This is often misinterpreted as allergy, and a child may be unnecessarily stopped from consuming all citrus fruits[21] (see Chapter 10).

Enzyme deficiencies

Partial or total deficiency of one or more enzymes in the digestive tract (e.g. lactase, disaccharidase deficiency) may result in symptoms of malabsorption when foods containing certain components are consumed. Apart from lactose, intolerances are very rarely seen in young children. For more information on lactose intolerance, see Chapter 5.

The main difference between food allergy and non-allergic FHS is that food allergy is caused by a protein interacting with the immune system and non-allergic FHS is caused by substances in food other than food proteins, with no involvement of the immune system.

1.4   Symptoms associated with food hypersensitivity

Symptoms that are most commonly associated with FHS can broadly be divided into symptoms associated with the systemic system, gastrointestinal tract, skin, respiratory system or other symptoms. Symptoms experienced upon ingestion of a specific food may occur within minutes, hours or days of ingestion.

Ultimately, one would like to map the symptoms specifically against either immediate or delayed reactions, or IgE-mediated and non-IgE-mediated reactions. This is not easy, however, as many manifested symptoms (e.g. eczema) can occur either as IgE-mediated or as non-IgE-mediated reactions, or as a mixed pattern of both. Furthermore, previous research utilising either open food challenges (OFC) or double-blind, placebo-controlled food challenges (DBPCFC) has clearly shown that some symptoms can be both immediate and delayed in nature[22]. Tables 1.2 to 1.6 highlight the reported symptoms most often associated with FHS in the literature.

Non-allergic FHS typically presents with symptoms similar to those of food allergy, either IgE-mediated or non-IgE-mediated. Symptoms of non-allergic FHS, however, tend to develop more slowly, larger amounts of foods are needed, and these amounts can vary greatly from patient to patient. Anaphylactic reactions are not seen with non-allergic FHS.

1.5   Prevalence

It is important to have accurate national data on the prevalence of FHS in order to meet the needs of the allergic community, particularly as the prevalence of food allergies varies depending on the diet and exposure to food allergens. Geographical variation in the prevalence of self-reported FHS, and differences in the foods reported to cause hypersensitivity, have been well documented[64-66].

Examples include fish allergy, which is frequently seen in Spain[67], and peanut allergy, which is common in the USA[68]. Cow's milk, eggs, peanuts and tree nuts, soya and wheat are among the most common food allergens in infants and children[67,69-74]. Peanuts and tree nuts[75] as well as fish and shellfish[76] are reported to be the most common food allergens in teenagers and adults. Oral allergy syndrome is also frequently reported in this older group[77].

FHS is the most common cause of anaphylaxis in children in Western countries, and more specifically the United Kingdom[78,79]. Of these foods, peanuts and tree

Table 1.2   Systemic manifestations of FHS: nomenclature and characteristics.

Disorder	Characteristics
Anaphylaxis Exercise-induced anaphylaxis	Occurs only when the patient exercises within 2–4 hours of ingesting the food. In the absence of exercise, the person can safely ingest the food. Most common in females 15–35 years[23].

Table 1.3 Gastrointestinal allergies (IgE- and non-IgE-mediated): nomenclature, characteristics and symptoms.

Disorder	Characteristics	Symptoms
Oral allergy syndrome	Caused by sensitisation to aero-allergens (birch, ragweed and mugwort) which cross-react with fruit/vegetable/nut proteins.	Mild itch, tingling and/or angioedema of the lips, tongue, mouth, throat – systemic symptoms very rare[24].
Gastrointestinal anaphylaxis		Quick onset of nausea/vomiting, abdominal pain/cramps, with or without diarrhoea. Skin or respiratory symptoms often present[8].
Allergic eosinophilic oesophagitis	Infiltration of the oesophagus by eosinophils, basal zone hyperplasia, papillary elongation, absence of vasculitis and peripheral eosinophilia in up to 50% of patients[25]. Most frequently seen during infancy through adolescence. Prevalence of other allergic diseases common amongst those with AEE, but food allergy mostly non-IgE-mediated. Seasonal oesophageal symptoms also often seen[26]. If patients are not treated they may develop Barrett's oesophagitis.	Gastro-oesophageal reflux, nausea and vomiting, dysphagia, intermittent abdominal pain, irritability, sleep disturbance, does not respond to conventional reflux treatment[27].
Allergic eosinophilic gastroenteritis	May present in any age group, even infants. Often presents as pyloric stenosis, with outlet obstruction. Characterised by inflammation of the stomach and intestines. Clinical manifestations depend on location and extent of the inflammation. 50% are atopic and 50% will have peripheral blood eosinophilia. Endoscopy and biopsy remains the gold standard of diagnosis. Milk, soya, egg, wheat and fish allergies most commonly implicated. Resolution of symptoms upon removal of the foods within 6 weeks. Does respond to steroids as well[28,29].	
Food protein-induced proctocolitis	Usually presents in first year of life, especially first few months. Usually caused by cow's or soya milk formula or these proteins passed from mother to infant via breast milk. Infants thriving and look well. Lesions are confined to distal bowel and consist of mucosal oedema, with eosinophil infiltration in the epithelium and lamina propriety[26]. Up to 60% of cases are breastfed and reacting to cow's milk/soya milk in breast milk.	Occult blood in stool; occasionally anaemic; hypoalbuminaemia very rare; may have peripheral eosinophilia and elevated serum IgE (with a family history of allergy)[32].

Condition	Description	Clinical features / management
	More than 80% of cases will resolve on extensively hydrolysed formula (eHF), and amino-acid-based formula is rarely needed[30]. Symptoms should disappear within 48–72 hours. Important to exclude infection, necrotising enterocolitis, anal fissure and intussusceptions. If no improvement on milk and soya exclusion, could be due to allergen being missed or factors inherent to breast milk[31]. Usually become tolerant by 1 year.	
Food protein-induced enterocolitis	Most commonly seen in infants under 3 months of age, but can be delayed in breast fed infants[33]. Most commonly caused by cow's milk and soya (50% CMPA react to soya), but other foods such as oat, rice, chicken and turkey[34] can be involved. Breast-fed babies not symptomatic, but might be sensitised via breast milk. eHF suitable, amino-acid-based formula rarely needed[35]. Food challenges should be done in hospital. Usually become tolerant by 3 years. Similar syndrome seen in adults after consumption of shellfish.	Protracted vomiting and diarrhoea, often gets dehydrated (followed by hypotension)[34,36] abdominal distension, growth faltering, typical vomiting 1–3 hours after meal. On admission give IV fluids (corticosteroids may be needed) – adrenaline/antihistamine only needed if other IgE-mediated food allergies are involved.
Food protein-induced enteropathy	Presents in first few months of life. Gut shows patchy villous atrophy, infiltration of mononuclear cells and a few eosinophils[36].	Diarrhoea, mild to moderate steatorrhoea and weight loss.
Coeliac disease	Coeliac disease leads to a more extensive enteropathy than above. It is associated with HLA-DQ2, present in more than 90% of coeliacs[37].	Occasionally nausea and vomiting, mouth ulcers, weight loss or growth faltering, abdominal distension and flatulence, diarrhoea and steatorrhea.
Gastro-oesophageal reflux (GOR)	Milk allergy could be the cause in some children[38,39].	
Diarrhoea, nausea and vomiting, abdominal pain	Commonly associated with both IgE- and non-IgE-mediated allergies[38,40–44].	
Constipation	Could be caused my cow's milk or multiple food allergies. Mucosal erosion, increased intraepithelial lymphocyte counts and reduced rectal mucous production is seen[12,45,46].	

Table 1.4   Skin-related food allergies (IgE- and non-IgE-mediated): nomenclature, characteristics and symptoms.

Disorder	Characteristics	Symptoms
Acute urticaria and angioedema		Itch, hives, swelling[38,41,43,47,48]
Chronic urticaria and angioedema		Itch, hives, swelling of more than 6 weeks' duration[17,49]
Atopic dermatitis	Starts early in life, characterised by a typical distribution, extreme itch, chronic and relapsing[50]. Gastrointestinal and respiratory symptoms are also often seen in infants and children	Dry itchy skin – with classic eczema distribution[38,41,43,47]
Contact dermatitis	Often seen in those who handle raw foods, e.g. fish, shellfish, meat and egg[51]	Dry itchy skin
Dermatitis herpetiformis	Chronic blistering skin condition associated with coeliac disease	Itchy, papulovesicular rash over extensor surfaces and buttocks[52]

Table 1.5   Respiratory food allergies: nomenclature, characteristics and symptoms.

Disorder	Characteristics	Symptoms
Allergic rhinoconjuctivitis	Isolated rhinoconjuctivitis is rarely caused by food ingestion, but it can occur with other symptoms.	Itchy, red eyes and runny nose, nasal congestion, sneezing[44]
Asthma	Asthma is rarely caused by food ingestion, but acute bronchospasm is often seen with other symptoms caused by IgE-mediated food allergies[53]. However, ingestion of food allergen (in sensitised individuals) can lead to worsening of asthma in the absence of bronchospasms[54]. Food allergy is also considered to be a major risk factor for severe life-threatening asthma[55]. Inhalation of food proteins[56], as opposed to just inhaling vapours[57], can also cause asthmatic reactions, even anaphylaxis.	Wheeze, shortness of breath, dry cough (in the absence of a cold)
Heiner's syndrome	Characterised by recurrent episodes of pneumonia associated with lung infiltrates, haemosiderosis, and blood in stools, in young children. The offending foods reported most often are cow's milk, and also egg and pork. Peripheral blood eosinophilia and IgG precipitating antibodies to cow's milk have been described in this syndrome, but the underlying immunological mechanisms are not clear[58].	Recurrent pneumonia, iron-deficiency anaemia, growth faltering[59]

Table 1.6   Other manifestations of FHS: nomenclature and characteristics.

System type	Disorder	Characteristics
Other	Controversial symptoms	Otitis media[60] Enuresis[61] Colic: ill-defined syndrome characterised by inconsolable agonised crying that generally develops within the first 2–4 weeks of life and persists through the third to fourth month[62]
	Other	Irritability[38] Listlessness with other symptoms[63]

nuts are reported as the most common food causing severe IgE-mediated reactions in children and adolescents in the USA and Europe[80,81], including the UK[82].

It is well known that the reported prevalence of FHS overestimates FHS as diagnosed by food challenges and other tests. Very few population-based studies looking at FHS based on food challenges are available in the literature.

1.5.1   Prevalence of FHS in adults

Reported

In Portugal[83], self-reported food allergy in adults($\geq$ 40 years) was 4.8% (95% CI 3.4–6.9%). Most people (67.6%) reported food allergy to only one food, with fresh fruits being the most frequently reported problem (25%). Approximately 90% of those who reported a food-related problem avoided the food, but 53% reported accidental ingestion of the food during the previous year.

Vierk et al.[84] investigated the prevalence of self-reported FHS in adults in the USA by analysing questions from the US Food and Drug Administration's 2001 Food Safety Survey. The prevalence of self-reported food allergy was 9.1% among all survey respondents, with 5.3% of all respondents reporting a doctor-diagnosed food allergy. The prevalence of food allergy to the eight most common allergens (peanuts, tree nuts, egg, milk, wheat, soya, fish, and crustacean shellfish) is self-reported as 2.7% among respondents with doctors' diagnoses.

However, in a recent meta-analysis Rona et al. concluded that the prevalence of self-reported food allergy was very high compared with that obtained by objective measures[66].

Diagnosed

Woods et al.[85] established the rate of IgE-mediated food allergy to peanut, shrimp, cow's milk, wheat, and egg as defined by a positive skin prick test result and relevant clinical history in 1,140 randomly selected young adults (aged 20–45 years) in Europe to be 1.3% ($n = 15$). The prevalence of probable IgE food allergy was < 0.27% for wheat, 0.09% (95% CI 0.0–0.49%) each for cow's milk and egg,

0.53% (95% CI 0.21–1.09%) for shrimp, and 0.61% (95% CI 0.25–1.26%) for peanut.

The prevalence studies using food challenges in adults comprise information from Dutch, United Kingdom, German and Danish populations. Jansen and colleagues[86] looked at the prevalence of FHS assessed by DBPCFC in a random sample ($n = 1,483$) of an adult Dutch population and estimated the true prevalence to be 2.4%. Of the 1,483 adults who completed an initial questionnaire, only 37 eventually underwent food challenges. The research team aimed to replicate the history in terms of dose needed and challenge duration. The foods or ingredients leading to adverse reactions in this study population included pork, white wine, menthol, kiwi, additives and glucose.

The main UK prevalence data quoted widely are those from the High Wycombe study conducted in the late 1980s[87]. This study reported a population prevalence rate between 1.4% and 1.8%, looking at eight different food allergens including milk, egg, wheat, soya, citrus, fish/shellfish, nuts and chocolate. Questionnaires were sent to 15,000 households (7,500 in the Wycombe Health Authority area and 7,500 nationwide). More than half (52.7%) of the individuals from Wycombe and 41.6% of the nationwide sample responded. Following an algorithm, 93 study participants were identified for food challenges, including five children under the age of 10 and ten people aged between 10 and 30 years. Although only 18 people had a positive food challenge, 71 were considered food-allergic, based on food challenge outcome or a positive skin test plus a reliable history.

A recent cross-sectional survey from Germany (1999–2000)[88] reported that 34.9% of people experienced an adverse reaction to food at some point in their lives. The point prevalence of adverse reactions to food confirmed by DBPCFC in the Berlin population was calculated as 3.6%, and in the adult population (18–79 years) 3.7%. Two and a half per cent of the reactions were IgE-mediated and 1.1% non-IgE-mediated. Females (60.6% of the affected group) were more frequently affected than men. Based on general health data for the adult German population, the estimated prevalence of FHS was calculated as 2.6%. The most common foods implicated were nuts, fruit, vegetables, ethanol, milk, flour and cocoa.

Osterballe et al.[89] investigated a cohort of 936 adults by questionnaire, skin prick test, histamine release test and specific IgE followed by oral challenge to the most common allergenic foods. The prevalence of FHS confirmed by oral challenge was 3.2%. The most common allergenic food was peanut, in 0.4% of the adults. In addition, 0.2% were allergic to codfish and 0.3% to shrimp. The prevalence of clinical reactions to pollen-related foods in pollen-sensitised adults was estimated to 32%.

1.5.2 Prevalence of FHS in children

Reported

Rancé et al.[90] conducted a questionnaire-based survey in Toulouse schools to determine the reported rate of food allergies among schoolchildren. They distributed 3,500 questionnaires among 150 classes in eight schools, and 2,716 children

(77.6%) responded. Based on these questionnaires, 182 children (6.7%) were considered to be truly food-allergic. The main foods reported as causing adverse reactions were cow's milk, eggs, kiwis, peanuts, fish, tree nuts, and shrimp.

In the Netherlands, in a cohort of 1,039 children aged 5–6 years the reported rate of FHS was 11.4%, although only 39% of the cohort was assessed. Within this cohort, 91.5% of the parents who perceived their child to have FHS restricted the child's diet[91]. Another population-based study in the Netherlands[67] demonstrated that the prevalence of self-reported adverse reactions to foods among schoolchildren (aged 5–15 years) was 7.2%, with food additives and chocolate being the commonest foods avoided.

Steinke and colleagues[92] studied parentally reported FHS in children in Europe (Austria, Belgium, Denmark, Finland, Germany, Greece, Italy, Poland, Slovenia and Switzerland) by means of a standardised questionnaire. The number of parents contacted was 40,246, and information was obtained on 8,825 children. Parentally perceived food allergy prevalence was 4.7% (90% CI 4.2–5.2%), with the highest reported rate amongst the 2- to 3-year-olds (7.2%). Reported figures were lowest in Austria (1.7%) and highest in Finland (11.7%). Milk (38.5%), fruits (29.5%), eggs (19.0%) and vegetables (13.5%) were most often implicated, although with significant age-linked variations.

Diagnosed

Prevalence studies in children are less readily available. In the USA[43], 480 consecutive children born into a paediatric clinic were recruited at a routine two-week appointment. The researchers determined that 8% (cumulative incidence) of the children (0–3 years) out of the 28% who presented with possible symptoms of food allergy were truly food-allergic as assessed by food challenges. This study utilised open challenges and/or DBPCFCs over a one-day period using a standard dose of dried, rather then fresh, food. This implies that delayed symptoms or symptoms triggered by larger dosages of food could be missed.

In the German study previously referred to[88], 4.2% of children (0–17 years) were found to suffer from FHS as assessed by DBPCFC. In this study questionnaires were sent to 2,354 children, and 739 responded. A total of 78 oral food challenges were carried out. Half of the challenges ($n = 39$) were performed as DBPCFC and the rest as a single-blind or open food challenges, depending on the patient's compliance. Forty-eight food challenges were considered positive in 31 children. The foods most commonly implicated were apple, kiwi, soya, hazelnut, and wheat, although challenges were performed to a much wider range of foods.

Osterballe et al.[89] estimated the prevalence of FHS to the most common allergenic foods in an unselected population of children (111 children < 3 years of age, 486 children 3 years of age, 301 children > 3 years of age) by questionnaire, skin prick test, histamine release test and specific IgE followed by oral challenge to the most common allergenic foods. The prevalence of FHS was 2.3% in the children aged 3 years and 1% in those older than 3 years. The most common allergenic food was hen's egg, affecting 1.6% of the children aged 3 years.

In Thailand, a total of 656 children were surveyed (188 subjects between 6 months and 3 years of age, and 468 subjects aged 3–6 years)[93]. Parents were asked to complete a food allergy questionnaire. Families with children reporting adverse food reactions were invited to participate in further investigation for food allergy with skin prick testing and food challenges. Forty-one of the 656 children (6.25%) were reported to experience food-related problems. Common foods reported to be the cause of reactions among younger children were cow's milk and eggs, whereas seafood, particularly shrimp, was the most commonly reported food for older children. Only three of the 21 children who underwent food challenge had positive challenges, producing an estimated figure for food allergy prevalence of 0.45% (CI 0.01–0.8%).

A recent study on the Isle of Wight found that, based on OFC and a good clinical history, the prevalence of FHS is 4% at 1 year[94], 2.5% at 2 years and 3.0% at 3 years[95]. Based on DBPCFC and a good clinical history, the prevalence of FHS was 3.2% at 1 year, 2.1% at 2 years and 2.9% at 3 years. Cumulatively, by 3 years of age, 6.0% of children were diagnosed with FHS based on OFC and history, and 5.0% of children based on DBPCFC and history. Overall, the foods implicated in this study were milk, egg, peanut, corn, potato, tomato, salicylates and wheat. Only 16.1% of children who were seen at 1, 2 and 3 years of age and reported a food-related problem were diagnosed with FHS by means of an OFC and history, and 12.9% by means of a DBPCFC and history.

Very importantly, in this study the authors were able to compare UK FHS incidence rates with that of Bock[43]. Using either the OFC or DBPCFC outcome, the difference in incidence was not statistically significant ($p = 0.30$ for OFC, $p = 0.06$ for DBPCFC), indicating that FHS has not increased over the past 20 years[95].

For the school cohorts, based on open food challenge and/or suggestive history and positive skin tests, the prevalence of food hypersensitivity was 2.6% in the 6-year-old cohort. Based on double blind challenges, a clinical diagnosis or suggestive history and positive skin tests, the prevalence was 1.6%. The corresponding figures were 2.3% and 1.4% for the 11-year-olds and 2.3% and 2.1% for the 15-year-olds. The foods most commonly implicated in FHS were milk and milk products, peanut, wheat, banana, sesame, tree nuts, egg, shellfish, gluten (coeliac disease), green beans, kiwi, tomato and additives. FHS was confirmed by OFC and a good clinical history in only 21% (20/94) of 6-year-olds, 20% (18/90) of 11-year-olds and 18% (17/94) of the 15-year-olds who reported a food problem[96,97]. In the light of the discrepancy between reported and diagnosed FHS, the major implication of this study is the need for accurate diagnosis to prevent children being on unnecessarily restricted diets.

1.5.3 FHS to single foods

A wide range of foods could be causing FHS, and this will differ from person to person. The following foods/ingredients are considered to be those most commonly involved in the development of FHS by the European Union: cereals containing wheat and gluten, shellfish (crustaceans), eggs, fish, peanuts, tree nuts, cow's milk, celery, mustard, sesame seeds, molluscs, soya, lupin and sulphur dioxide[98]. The prevalence of FHS to the individual foods is discussed further in Part 2 (Chapters 5–10).

1.6 Conclusion

Food hypersensitivity is an adverse reaction upon ingestion of food which can either be immune- or non-immune-mediated. Reactions experienced with FHS may be systemic, gastrointestinal, cutaneous or respiratory in nature. There are also still a number of symptoms causing controversy amongst allergists. FHS is commonly reported, but there is a large discrepancy between reported and diagnosed FHS. The true prevalence of FHS in adults still needs further investigation; in children it lies between 1.6% and 4.0%, with no apparent increase in the past 20 years. A large number of foods are reported to cause symptoms of FHS, but only 14 foods and ingredients form the core components of FHS.

References

1. Prausnitz C, Kustner H. Studies on supersensitivity. *Centralbl Bakteriol*, 2007; **86**: 160–9.
2. Committee on Toxicity of Chemicals in Food. *Adverse Reactions to Food and Food Ingredients*. London: Food Standards Agency, 2000.
3. Ortolani C, Bruijnzeel-Koomen C, Bengtsson U *et al*. Controversial aspects of adverse reactions to food. European Academy of Allergology and Clinical Immunology (EAACI) Reactions to Food Subcommittee. *Allergy* 1999; **54**: 27–45.
4. Johansson SG, Bieber T, Dahl R *et al*. Revised nomenclature for allergy for global use: Report of the Nomenclature Review Committee of the World Allergy Organization, October 2003. *J Allergy Clin Immunol* 2004; **113**: 832–6.
5. Sicherer SH, Sampson HA. 9. Food allergy. *J Allergy Clin Immunol* 2006; **117**: S470–5.
6. Strobel S. Immunity induced after a feed of antigen during early life: oral tolerance v. sensitisation. *Proc Nutr Soc* 2001; **60**: 437–42.
7. Coombs RRA, Gell PGH. The classification of allergic reactions underlying disease. In: Gell PGH, Coombs RRA, eds. *Clinical Aspects of Immunology*. Oxford: Blackwell, 1963: 317–37.
8. Sampson HA. Food allergy. Part 1: immunopathogenesis and clinical disorders. *J Allergy Clin Immunol* 1999; **103**: 717–28.
9. Arshad SH. *Allergy: an Illustrated Colour Text*. London: Churchill Livingstone, 2002.
10. Hamelmann E, Wahn U. Immune responses to allergens early in life: when and why do allergies arise? *Clin Exp Allergy* 2002; **32**: 1679–81.
11. Shek LP, Bardina L, Castro R, Sampson HA, Beyer K. Humoral and cellular responses to cow milk proteins in patients with milk-induced IgE-mediated and non-IgE-mediated disorders. *Allergy* 2005; **60**: 912–19.
12. Murch SH. Clinical manifestations of food allergy: the old and the new. *Eur J Gastroenterol Hepatol* 2005; **17**: 1287–91.
13. Atkinson W, Sheldon TA, Shaath N, Whorwell PJ. Food elimination based on IgG antibodies in irritable bowel syndrome: a randomised controlled trial. *Gut* 2004; **53**: 1459–64.
14. Vance GH, Grimshaw KE, Briggs R *et al*. Serum ovalbumin-specific immunoglobulin G responses during pregnancy reflect maternal intake of dietary egg and relate to the development of allergy in early infancy. *Clin Exp Allergy* 2004; **34**: 1855–61.
15. Zuo XL, Li YQ, Li WJ *et al*. Alterations of food antigen-specific serum immunoglobulins G and E antibodies in patients with irritable bowel syndrome and functional dyspepsia. *Clin Exp Allergy* 2007; **37**: 823–30.

16. Freeman M. Reconsidering the effects of monosodium glutamate: a literature review. *J Am Acad Nurse Pract* 2006; **18**: 482–6.
17. Vickerstaff Joneja JM, Carmona-Silva C. Outcome of a histamine-restricted diet based on chart audit. *J Nutr Envir Med* 2001; **11**: 249–62.
18. McCann D, Barrett A, Cooper A *et al*. Food additives and hyperactive behaviour in 3-year-old and 8/9-year-old children in the community: a randomised, double-blinded, placebo-controlled trial. *Lancet* 2007; **370**: 1560–7.
19. Zuberbier T, Pfrommer C, Specht K *et al*. Aromatic components of food as novel eliciting factors of pseudoallergic reactions in chronic urticaria. *J Allergy Clin Immunol* 2002; **109**: 343–8.
20. Wuthrich B. Adverse reactions to food additives. *Ann Allergy* 1993; **71**: 379–84.
21. Durham SR. *ABC of Allergies*. London: BMJ Publications, 1998.
22. Hill DJ, Duke AM, Hosking CS, Hudson IL. Clinical manifestations of cows' milk allergy in childhood. II. The diagnostic value of skin tests and RAST. *Clin Allergy* 1988; **18**: 481–90.
23. Castells MC, Horan RF, Sheffer AL. Exercise-induced anaphylaxis. *Curr Allergy Asthma Rep* 2003; **3**: 15–21.
24. Ortolani C, Ispano M, Pastorello EA, Ansaloni R, Magri GC. Comparison of results of skin prick tests (with fresh foods and commercial food extracts) and RAST in 100 patients with oral allergy syndrome. *J Allergy Clin Immunol* 1989; **83**: 683–90.
25. Rothenberg ME, Mishra A, Collins MH, Putnam PE. Pathogenesis and clinical features of eosinophilic esophagitis. *J Allergy Clin Immunol* 2001; **108**: 891–4.
26. Rothenberg ME. Eosinophilic gastrointestinal disorders (EGID). *J Allergy Clin Immunol* 2004; **113**: 11–28.
27. Spergel JM, Beausoleil JL, Mascarenhas M, Liacouras CA. The use of skin prick tests and patch tests to identify causative foods in eosinophilic esophagitis. *J Allergy Clin Immunol* 2002; **109**: 363–8.
28. Maloney J, Nowak-Wegrzyn A. Educational clinical case series for pediatric allergy and immunology: allergic proctocolitis, food protein-induced enterocolitis syndrome and allergic eosinophilic gastroenteritis with protein-losing gastroenteropathy as manifestations of non-IgE-mediated cow's milk allergy. *Pediatr Allergy Immunol* 2007; **18**: 360–7.
29. Kelly KJ. Eosinophilic gastroenteritis. *J Pediatr Gastroenterol Nutr* 2000; **30**: S28–35.
30. Sampson HA, Anderson JA. Summary and recommendations: classification of gastrointestinal manifestations due to immunologic reactions to foods in infants and young children. *J Pediatr Gastroenterol Nutr* 2000; **30**: S87–94.
31. Makinen-Kiljunen S, Plosila M. A father's IgE-mediated contact urticaria from mother's milk. *J Allergy Clin Immunol* 2004; **113**: 353–4.
32. Anveden-Hertzberg L, Finkel Y, Sandstedt B, Karpe B. Proctocolitis in exclusively breast-fed infants. *Eur J Pediatr* 1996; **155**: 464–7.
33. Sicherer SH, Eigenmann PA, Sampson HA. Clinical features of food protein-induced entero-colitis syndrome. *J Pediatr* 1998; **133**: 214–19.
34. Nowak-Wegrzyn A, Sampson HA, Wood RA, Sicherer SH. Food protein-induced enterocolitis syndrome caused by solid food proteins. *Pediatrics* 2003; **111**: 829–35.
35. Kelso JM, Sampson HA. Food protein-induced enterocolitis to casein hydrolysate formulas. *J Allergy Clin Immunol* 1993; **92**: 909–10.
36. Latcham F, Merino F, Lang A *et al*. A consistent pattern of minor immunodeficiency and subtle enteropathy in children with multiple food allergy. *J Pediatr* 2003; **143**: 39–47.
37. Bonamico M, Ballati G, Mariani P *et al*. Screening for coeliac disease: the meaning of low titers of anti-gliadin antibodies (AGA) in non-coeliac children. *Eur J Epidemiol* 1997; **13**: 55–9.
38. Hill DJ, Firer MA, Ball G, Hosking CS. Natural history of cows' milk allergy in children: immunological outcome over 2 years. *Clin Exp Allergy* 1993; **23**: 124–31.
39. Nielsen RG, Bindslev-Jensen C, Kruse-Andersen S, Husby S. Severe gastroesophageal reflux disease and cow milk hypersensitivity in infants and children: disease association and evaluation of a new challenge procedure. *J Pediatr Gastroenterol Nutr* 2004; **39**: 383–91.
40. Hourihane JO, Bedwani SJ, Dean TP, Warner JO. Randomised, double blind, crossover challenge study of allergenicity of peanut oils in subjects allergic to peanuts. *BMJ* 1997; **314**: 1084–8.

41. Fuglsang G, Madsen G, Halken S *et al*. Adverse reactions to food additives in children with atopic symptoms. *Allergy* 1994; **49**: 31–7.
42. Sampson HA, Ho DG. Relationship between food-specific IgE concentrations and the risk of positive food challenges in children and adolescents. *J Allergy Clin Immunol* 1997; **100**: 444–51.
43. Bock SA. Prospective appraisal of complaints of adverse reactions to foods in children during the first 3 years of life. *Pediatrics* 1987; **79**: 683–8.
44. Eggesbo M, Botten G, Halvorsen R, Magnus P. The prevalence of allergy to egg: a population-based study in young children. *Allergy* 2001; **56**: 403–11.
45. Majamaa H, Moisio P, Holm K, Turjanmaa K. Wheat allergy: diagnostic accuracy of skin prick and patch tests and specific IgE. *Allergy* 1999; **54**: 851–6.
46. Majamaa H, Moisio P, Holm K, Kautiainen H, Turjanmaa K. Cow's milk allergy: diagnostic accuracy of skin prick and patch tests and specific IgE. *Allergy* 1999; **54**: 346–51.
47. Niggemann B, Sielaff B, Beyer K, Binder C, Wahn U. Outcome of double-blind, placebo-controlled food challenge tests in 107 children with atopic dermatitis. *Clin Exp Allergy* 1999; **29**: 91–6.
48. Isolauri E, Turjanmaa K. Combined skin prick and patch testing enhances identification of food allergy in infants with atopic dermatitis. *J Allergy Clin Immunol* 1996; **97**: 9–15.
49. Greaves MW. Chronic urticaria in childhood. *Allergy* 2000; **55**: 309–20.
50. Sicherer SH, Sampson HA. Food hypersensitivity and atopic dermatitis: pathophysiology, epidemiology, diagnosis, and management. *J Allergy Clin Immunol* 1999; **104**: S114–22.
51. Judd L. A descriptive study of occupational skin disease. *N Z Med J* 1994; **107**: 147–9.
52. Medica I, Zmak M, Persic M. Dermatitis herpetiformis in a 30-month-old child. *Minerva Pediatr* 2003; **55**: 171–3.
53. James JM, Burks AW. Food hypersensitivity in children. *Curr Opin Pediatr* 1994; **6**: 661–7.
54. James JM, Eigenmann PA, Eggleston PA, Sampson HA. Airway reactivity changes in asthmatic patients undergoing blinded food challenges. *Am J Respir Crit Care Med* 1996; **153**: 597–603.
55. Roberts G, Patel N, Levi-Schaffer F, Habibi P, Lack G. Food allergy as a risk factor for life-threatening asthma in childhood: a case-controlled study. *J Allergy Clin Immunol* 2003; **112**: 168–74.
56. Roberts G, Golder N, Lack G. Bronchial challenges with aerosolized food in asthmatic, food-allergic children. *Allergy* 2002; **57**: 713–17.
57. Simonte SJ, Ma S, Mofidi S, Sicherer SH. Relevance of casual contact with peanut butter in children with peanut allergy. *J Allergy Clin Immunol* 2003; **112**: 180–2.
58. Host A, Halken S. Changing patterns of paediatric food allergy with age. *Eur Respir J* 2002; **7**: 131–55.
59. Fourrier E. [Allergy to cow's milk]. *Allerg Immunol (Paris)* 1997; **29**: 25–7.
60. Tikkanen S, Kokkonen J, Juntti H, Niinimaki A. Status of children with cow's milk allergy in infancy by 10 years of age. *Acta Paediatr* 2000; **89**: 1174–80.
61. Egger J, Carter CH, Soothill JF, Wilson J. Effect of diet treatment on enuresis in children with migraine or hyperkinetic behavior. *Clin Pediatr (Phila)* 1992; **31**: 302–7.
62. Hill DJ, Hosking CS. Infantile colic and food hypersensitivity. *J Pediatr Gastroenterol Nutr* 2000; **30**: S67–76.
63. Eggesbo M, Halvorsen R, Tambs K, Botten G. Prevalence of parentally perceived adverse reactions to food in young children. *Pediatr Allergy Immunol* 1999; **10**: 122–32.
64. Sandin A, Annus T, Bjorksten B *et al*. Prevalence of self-reported food allergy and IgE antibodies to food allergens in Swedish and Estonian schoolchildren. *Eur J Clin Nutr* 2005; **59**: 399–403.
65. Eriksson NE, Moller C, Werner S *et al*. Self-reported food hypersensitivity in Sweden, Denmark, Estonia, Lithuania, and Russia. *J Investig Allergol Clin Immunol* 2004; **14**: 70–9.
66. Rona RJ, Keil T, Summers C *et al*. The prevalence of food allergy: a meta-analysis. *J Allergy Clin Immunol* 2007; **120**: 638–46.
67. Crespo JF, Pascual C, Burks AW, Helm RM, Esteban MM. Frequency of food allergy in a pediatric population from Spain. *Pediatr Allergy Immunol* 1995; **6**: 39–43.

68. Sicherer SH, Furlong TJ, Muñoz-Furlong A, Burks AW, Sampson HA. A voluntary registry for peanut and tree nut allergy: characteristics of the first 5149 registrants. *J Allergy Clin Immunol* 2001; **108**: 128–32.
69. Bock SA, Atkins FM. Patterns of food hypersensitivity during sixteen years of double-blind, placebo-controlled food challenges. *J Pediatr* 1990; **117**: 561–7.
70. Hosking CS, Heine RG, Hill DJ. The Melbourne Milk Allergy Study: two decades of clinical research. *Allergy Clin Immunol Int* 2000; **12**: 198–205.
71. Burks AW, James JM, Hiegel A, Wilson G, Wheeler JG, Jones SM *et al*. Atopic dermatitis and food hypersensitivity reactions. *J Pediatr* 1998; **132**: 132–6.
72. Dalal I, Binson I, Reifen R *et al*. Food allergy is a matter of geography after all: sesame as a major cause of severe IgE-mediated food allergic reactions among infants and young children in Israel. *Allergy* 2002; **57**: 362–5.
73. Eigenmann PA, Calza AM. Diagnosis of IgE-mediated food allergy among Swiss children with atopic dermatitis. *Pediatr Allergy Immunol* 2000; **11**: 95–100.
74. Host A, Halken S. A prospective study of cow milk allergy in Danish infants during the first 3 years of life: clinical course in relation to clinical and immunological type of hypersensitivity reaction. *Allergy* 1990; **45**: 587–96.
75. Sicherer SH, Munoz-Furlong A, Sampson HA. Prevalence of peanut and tree nut allergy in the United States determined by means of a random digit dial telephone survey: a 5-year follow-up study. *J Allergy Clin Immunol* 2003; **112**: 1203–7.
76. Sicherer SH, Munoz-Furlong A, Sampson HA. Prevalence of seafood allergy in the United States determined by a random telephone survey. *J Allergy Clin Immunol* 2004; **114**: 159–65.
77. Mattila L, Kilpelainen M, Terho EO *et al*. Food hypersensitivity among Finnish university students: association with atopic diseases. *Clin Exp Allergy* 2003; **33**: 600–6.
78. Royal College of Physicians Working Party on the provision of allergy services in the UK. *Allergy: the unmet need. A blueprint for better patient care.* London: Royal College of Physicians, 2003.
79. Alves B, Sheikh A. Age specific aetiology of anaphylaxis. *Arch Dis Child* 2001; **85**: 348.
80. Bock SA, Munoz-Furlong A, Sampson HA. Further fatalities caused by anaphylactic reactions to food, 2001–2006. *J Allergy Clin Immunol* 2007; **119**: 1016–18.
81. Eigenmann PA, Zamora SA. An internet-based survey on the circumstances of food-induced reactions following the diagnosis of IgE-mediated food allergy. *Allergy* 2002; **57**: 449–53.
82. Pumphrey RS, Gowland H. Further fatal allergic reactions to food in the United Kingdom, 1999–2006. *J Allergy Clin Immunol* 2007; **119**: 1018–19.
83. Falcao H, Lunet N, Lopes C, Barros H. Food hypersensitivity in Portuguese adults. *Eur J Clin Nutr* 2004; **58**: 1621–5.
84. Vierk KA, Koehler KM, Fein SB, Street DA. Prevalence of self-reported food allergy in American adults and use of food labels. *J Allergy Clin Immunol* 2007; **119**: 1504–10.
85. Woods RK, Abramson M, Bailey M, Walters EH. International prevalences of reported food allergies and intolerances. Comparisons arising from the European Community Respiratory Health Survey (ECRHS) 1991–1994. *Eur J Clin Nutr* 2001; **55**: 298–304.
86. Jansen JJ, Kardinaal AF, Huijbers G *et al*. Prevalence of food allergy and intolerance in the adult Dutch population. *J Allergy Clin Immunol* 1994; **93**: 446–56.
87. Young E, Stoneham MD, Petruckevitch A, Barton J, Rona R. A population study of food intolerance. *Lancet* 1994; **343**: 1127–30.
88. Zuberbier T, Edenharter G, Worm M *et al*. Prevalence of adverse reactions to food in Germany: a population study. *Allergy* 2004; **59**: 338–45.
89. Osterballe M, Hansen TK, Mortz CG, Høst A, Bindslev-Jensen C. The prevalence of food hypersensitivity in an unselected population of children and adults. *Pediatr Allergy Immunol* 2005; **16**: 567–73.
90. Rancé F, Grandmottet X, Grandjean H. Prevalence and main characteristics of schoolchildren diagnosed with food allergies in France. *Clin Exp Allergy* 2005; **35**: 167–72.
91. van Bockel-Geelkerken M, Meulmeester JF. Prevalence of putative food hypersensitivity in young children. *Ned Tijdschr Geneeskd* 1992; **136**: 1351–6.
92. Steinke M, Fiocchi A, Kirchlechner V *et al*. Perceived food allergy in children in 10 European nations: a randomised telephone survey. *Int Arch Allergy Immunol* 2007; **143**: 290–5.

93. Santadusit S, Atthapaisalsarudee S, Vichyanond P. Prevalence of adverse food reactions and food allergy among Thai children. *J Med Assoc Thai* 2005; **88**: S27–32.
94. Venter C, Pereira B, Grundy J *et al.* Incidence of parentally reported and clinically diagnosed food hypersensitivity in the first year of life. *J Allergy Clin Immunol* 2006; **117**: 1118–24.
95. Venter C, Pereira B, Voigt K *et al.* Prevalence and cumulative incidence of food hypersensitivity in the first three years of life. *Allergy* 2008: **63**: 354–9.
96. Pereira B, Venter C, Grundy J *et al.* Prevalence of sensitization to food allergens, reported adverse reaction to foods, food avoidance, and food hypersensitivity among teenagers. *J Allergy Clin Immunol* 2005; **116**: 884–92.
97. Venter C, Pereira B, Grundy J *et al.* Prevalence of sensitization reported and objectively assessed food hypersensitivity amongst six-year-old children: a population-based study. *Pediatr Allergy Immunol* 2006; **17**: 356–63.
98. European Union. Commission Directive 2007/68/EC of 27 November 2007 amending Annex IIIa to Directive 2000/13/EC of the European Parliament and of the Council as regards certain food ingredients. *Official Journal of the European Union* 2007; **L310**: 11–14.

2 The Role of Food Hypersensitivity in Different Disorders

2.1 The role of food hypersensitivity in skin disorders

Rosan Meyer and George Du Toit

2.1.1 Introduction

Food-induced allergic reactions may present with symptoms and signs varying from a few transient hives to life-threatening or fatal anaphylaxis. The most commonly involved 'target organs' are the skin, gastrointestinal tract, and upper and lower respiratory tracts. The severity of allergic reactions to the same (or different) food allergens is not stereotypical. There is inter- and intra-individual variability with respect to the dose of allergen required to induce an allergic reaction[1].

The immune mechanisms which underlie food-induced skin reactions include IgE-mediated, cell-mediated (non-IgE-mediated) and mixed cellular reactions. Non-immunological reactions may occur due to irritants, toxic substances or non-specific properties of food[2]. The most common cutaneous reactions include urticaria, angio-oedema, pruritus and atopic eczema (Table 2.1). These clinical manifestations may occur in isolation or collectively as a syndrome, e.g. Stevens–Johnson syndrome[3,4]. Pruritis is the commonest skin symptom associated with food hypersensitivity. Studies over the last 20 years have shown cutaneous reactions occurring, as one of

Table 2.1 Definition of terms used to describe cutaneous reactions.

Urticaria	Transient localised areas of oedema within skin or mucus membrane: raised, erythematous, blanching, itching and well-circumscribed wheals
Angio-oedema	Transient localised oedema within deeper areas of skin or mucous membrane instead of on the surface, as urticaria. Angio-oedema is characterised by deep swelling and has a predilection for areas of loose connective tissues such as the face, eyelids or mucous membrane involving the lips and tongue
Pruritis	An intense itching sensation
Eczema	Also known as atopic dermatitis or atopic eczema/dermatitis syndrome: a chronic inflammatory itchy skin condition that is typically an episodic disease of exacerbation and remissions

the allergic manifestations, in 75% of the positive food challenges[5,6]. Isolated skin symptoms were seen in only 30% of food hypersensitivity reactions[7].

2.1.2   Food-induced IgE-mediated skin reactions

Skin reactions are common manifestations of IgE-induced food reactions, with acute onset urticaria (with or without angio-edema) being particularly common[8]. The onset of symptoms usually occurs with the ingestion of offending foods, but in many cases skin contact may be sufficient to induce a severe allergic reaction (Table 2.2.)[9]. Additional non-specific skin rashes such as erythema, pruritis and morbilliform rashes may also be observed in IgE-mediated food hypersensitivity reactions.

Urticaria and angio-oedema

It is thought that between 15% and 24% of the population will experience urticaria and angio-oedema at some time in their lives[10]. These two allergic skin manifestations commonly occur together, but may also occur separately. Kaplan *et al.* found

Table 2.2   Summary of cutaneous food hypersensitivity reactions[2,3,7,12].

Mechanism	Disorder	Onset	Examples of foods
IgE-mediated	Urticaria	Immediate	Egg, milk, wheat, soya, fish, peanuts and tree nuts
	Contact urticaria	Immediate	Raw or processed foods: fruit (especially citrus, pineapple, berry fruits and tomato), vegetables, meat, fish, chicken, spices, oatmeal, milk and egg
	Angio-oedema	Immediate	Egg, milk, wheat, soya, fish, peanuts and tree nuts
	Pruritus	Immediate	Egg, milk, wheat, soya, peanuts and tree nuts
	Flushing	Immediate	Egg, milk, wheat, soya, peanuts and tree nuts, alcohol, histamine-containing foods (e.g. Parmesan cheese)
Mixed IgE- and cell-mediated	Eczema (atopic dermatitis)	Immediate/delayed Usually chronic and recurrent	Egg, milk, wheat, soya, ground nuts and tree nuts, foods that cross-react with birch and grass pollen (apple, carrot, hazelnut, sesame seeds)
Cell-mediated	Contact dermatitis	Delayed	Various fresh fruits, vegetables and spices
	Dermatitis herpetiformis	Delayed	Wheat-, rye- and barley-induced coeliac disease

that in 50% of cases urticaria occurs in isolation, in 40% both are seen in association, whilst only 10% of patients will experience angio-oedema in isolation[11]. Familial hereditary angio-oedema should always be excluded from the differential diagnosis of patients presenting with isolated angio-oedema. Chronic urticaria (CU) is defined as wheals which occur almost daily, lasting for more than 6 weeks. Conversely, acute urticaria (AU) is a single episode, usually intermittent and lasting less than 6 weeks in total. AU is more common in children, whilst CU is more common in adults and about twice as common in women as in men[3].

Acute urticarial reactions are frequently associated with angio-oedema[12]. Mast cell degranulation initiates the release of vasoactive mediators, including histamine, which is a major mediator of urticaria and angio-oedema[13]. This in turn triggers the release of membrane-derived mediators such as leukotrienes and prostaglandins, which contribute to the reaction, including the extravasation of fluid into the superficial tissues[14]. The exact mechanism of swelling in the deeper layer of the skin is less defined and probably involves several inflammatory mediators[12].

Food-related urticaria and angio-oedema usually occur within minutes of exposure, and may be associated with symptoms such as oropharyngeal discomfort and itching, gastrointestinal pain and/or vomiting, and a change in behaviour, e.g. a feeling of impending doom[13]. The foods that most commonly induce allergic reactions change with age – a phenomenon coined the food 'allergic march'. For young infants the most common ingested foods responsible for these type of cutaneous reactions are eggs, milk, peanut and tree nuts, which can cause generalised urticaria and angio-oedema (Table 2.2.)[15,16]. Although food-related urticaria and angio-oedema in adulthood has been described, associated with wheat, milk, egg, fish and nuts, it is very common to see these types of cutaneous reactions related not to food but to medication such as non-steroidal anti-inflammatory drugs[17]. Acute contact urticaria can also be triggered by the touching of certain foods, but the urticaria develops locally and should be distinguished from general urticaria[12]. The most common foods associated with localised contact urticaria include raw fruit like citrus, pineapple, berries and tomato, spices, milk, egg, wheat and oatmeal (Table 2.2)[7]. The diagnosis of a contact-induced allergic reaction may be difficult in such patients unless a careful history is obtained, and this should include enquiry about kissing or touching someone who has eaten or touched the food. Additional diagnostic investigation, involving one or more of skin prick test (SPT), specific IgEs, oral food challenge and elimination diets, may be required to unequivocally establish – or dismiss – an association with a food, food additive, food colorant or stabiliser[18].

Chronic urticaria is diagnosed on the basis of a patient experiencing frequent wheals, with or without angio-oedema, for more than 6 weeks. It has been suggested that AU is more common in young people, whereas CU is more common in middle-aged women, but there is currently a lack of reliable evidence regarding the prevalence of CU in the UK[11]. A major advance in the understanding of CU is the finding that functional circulating autoantibodies play a part in the pathogenesis of a significant proportion of children with CU[19]. These antibodies are usually of the IgG_3 subclass and directed against either the $Fc\varepsilon RI\alpha$ receptor or the IgE receptor[20].

It is estimated that > 30% of CU is autoimmune, 50% is idiopathic and only 5–10% is provoked by an identifiable factor[21]. The frequency of food hypersensitivity reaction in patients with CU is reported with high variability. Food additives, such as acetylsalicylic acid, are assumed to induce whealing in 5% to up to 45% of adults with CU. A study by Buss *et al.* found that 11% of adults with CU demonstrated intolerance to food dyes or additives on oral provocation[22]. In children, food sensitivity (e.g. egg, milk, wheat, soya and nuts) has been found in 12% of patients with CU[23]. The diagnosis of CU is usually made on the basis of a detailed clinical history and examination. Non-food-related urticaria and angio-oedema can be distinguished from food-related by appearing overnight, being present first thing in the morning, after exercise, stress or extreme temperature (hot sunshine, hot or cold water), and by the fact that they can produce an urticarial rash lasting for several days, unlike cutaneous food reactions[7].

Depending on the clinical history and examination, SPT, specific IgEs and/or food challenge may be useful in confirming or dismissing food as a trigger for CU. In patients with non-food-related CU a full blood count and white cell differential (for instance, to detect the eosinophilia of bowel helminth infections) and erythrocyte sedimentation rate (usually normal in CU but may be raised in urticarial vasculitis) may be useful. Thyroid autoantibodies and thyroid function tests should also be considered if thyroid dysfunction is likely[14,22].

The management of urticaria and angio-oedema is dependent on the aetiology of the symptoms: food- or non-food-associated and whether it is acute or chronic. The mainstay of management in patients with these types of food hypersensitivity reactions is the avoidance of the offending food. However, despite recent advances in the field of CU, the investigation and management of the condition remains a clinical challenge[15].

2.1.3 Food-induced non-IgE-mediated skin reactions

Atopic eczema

Atopic eczema, or atopic dermatitis, is a common skin manifestation of atopic disorders and is often associated with food allergy, allergic rhinitis and asthma[7]. Prevalence studies from developed countries indicate that eczema affects 15–30% of children and 2–10% of adults[2,24]. A total of 45% of eczema begins within the first 6 months of life, 60% during the first year and 85% within the first 5 years of life[24]. A recent study by Hill *et al.* found that up to 64% of infants whose eczema commenced before 3 months of age had a high risk for IgE-mediated food sensitisation to egg and/or cow's milk and/or peanut. The risk of IgE-mediated food sensitisation increased with the severity of eczema for those infants who developed this before 12 months of age. However, in children who developed eczema after 1 year of age, the frequency of IgE-mediated food sensitisation was only 22%[25]. Epidemiological data suggest a significant genetic component in the development of eczema[26]. It is thought that 60% of children with one affected parent, and 80% of those with two affected parents, develop eczema[24,27]. This inheritance is more strongly related to atopy (especially respiratory allergy) than eczema itself[26]. The new discovery of the filaggrin gene may explain this. The gene encodes the filaggrin protein which is found in the upper layers of skin and helps to form a protective barrier that keeps moisture in and infectious organisms out. In the UK about 10% of the population carry a single defective copy, and have dry and flaky skin[28].

The most commonly used diagnostic criteria for eczema (or atopic dermatitis) come from Hanifin and Rajka[29], and rely on information compiled from a clinical history, physical examination and laboratory data (Table 2.3).

Eczema in the young usually affects the extensor surfaces, face, neck and trunk. In older age, the more commonly affected areas are the flexural surfaces, but it can be widespread and may also affect the hands, feet, face and trunk[3]. Acute flare-up of eczema is associated with erythematous papules on a background of erythematous skin and pruritus, and sometimes vesicular ooze. This results over time in excoriation, scaling and lichenification[3]. Food allergic reactions may result in eczema exacerbations; reactions may be immediate (within 2 hours) or delayed in onset (usually within 4–12 hours). The majority of patients with food allergy have past or current eczema.

Two different forms of eczema exist: eczema associated with IgE antibodies is known as atopic eczema, and that without IgE antibodies is non-atopic eczema[3].

Table 2.3 Guidelines for the diagnosis of eczema[29].

Requires	Symptoms/laboratory data
Three or more of basic features	Morphology and distribution Flexural lichenification or linearity in adults Facial and extensor involvement in infants and children Chronic or chronically relapsing dermatitis Personal or family history of atopy (asthma, allergic rhinitis, atopic dermatitis)
Three or more minor features	Xerosis Ichthyosis/palmar hyperlinearity/keratosis pilaris Elevated serum IgE level Early onset Tendency toward cutaneous infections (*Staphylococcus aureus* and herpes simplex) Tendency toward no specific hand and foot dermatitis Nipple eczema Cheilitis Dennie–Morgan infraorbital fold Keratoconus Anterior subcapsular cataracts Pityriasis alba Anterior neck folds Itch when sweating Intolerance to wool and lipid solvents Perifollicular accentuation Food intolerance Course influenced by environmental/emotional factors

Interestingly, research has found that 40–50% of children who are affected in the first 2 years of life do not have any sign of IgE sensitisation[25,30]. Over the last decade the pathophysiology of atopic dermatitis has been a source of great controversy. Two hypotheses exist: one suggests that an intrinsic defect in the epithelial cells leads to barrier dysfunction, and the immunological involvement is purely accidental. The other proposes that the primary defect lies in an immunologic disturbance that causes IgE sensitisation, and the epithelial-barrier dysfunction is seen as a consequence of local inflammation[24]. Most recent clinical studies now support the latter theory.

Epidermal-barrier dysfunction (see research on defective filaggrin gene, above) has been shown to be a prerequisite for the development of atopic dermatitis. It is thought that the initial skin inflammation is induced by neuropeptides, irritation or pruritis[3]. Once this has occurred, molecules such as those from pollen, microbes, house-dust mite and food can penetrate the epidermal layer. On antigen exposure, naive T cells are polarised into Th0, Th1 or Th2 helper cells. The Th1 cells produce interferon-γ, the Th2 cells produce interleukin-4 (IL-4), IL-5 and IL-13, and Th0 cells produce both Th1 and Th2 cytokines. There seems to be Th2 predominance in atopic eczema, with the production of IgE from B cells (Figure 2.1). The Langerhans cells are then activated on binding with IgE and FcεRI (high affinity receptor to IgE). Allergen-derived peptides are presented to the T cells by the Langerhans cells to induce a Th2 profile and the release of IL-4, IL-5, IL-13 and IL-31. The binding of IgE to the Langerhans cells also leads to the production of monocyte chemotactic protein-1 (MCP-1) and IL-16, which facilitates the release of monocytes that differentiate into inflammatory dendritic epidermal cells (IDEC) and produce IL-1, IL-6 and tumor necrosis factor-α (TNF-α). The IDEC releases IL-12 and IL-18, leading to the switch from Th2 to Th1 and Th0, which then signals the change from acute eczema to chronic eczema (Figure 2.1)[24].

Infants with eczema have a particularly high prevalence of food allergy; this association becomes less common with increasing age. The prevalence of food allergy in eczema in childhood has been shown (through double-blind placebo-controlled challenge) to range between 33% and 56%[5,7,27,30,31]. In adults, the role of food allergens as an aggravating factor is less frequent. A study by Worm et al. indicated that only 7.4% of adults with atopic eczema reacted to the classical food allergens. In that study the most frequent food allergens associated with atopic eczema (22%) were the foods that cross-reacted with birch and grass pollen (e.g. carrots, apple, hazelnut and sesame seed), and 14.8% reacted to wheat, rye and barley[32,33]. A small number of foods account for over 90% of atopic eczema. In infants, the most common foods are eggs, milk, peanuts[25] and soya, whilst in older children the same foods, plus wheat, tree nuts, fish and shellfish, are responsible for reactions. In general, it is thought that two-thirds of atopic eczema in children is due to egg allergy. The most common foods leading to eczematous reactions in adults are peanuts, tree nuts, fish and shellfish and those foods that cross-react with birch and grass pollen (Table 2.2)[7]. It is important to note that atopic eczema is provoked not only by the ingestion of egg, milk, nuts, fish, wheat and soya, but also by the presence of the aerosolised food antigens in the environment[9,34].

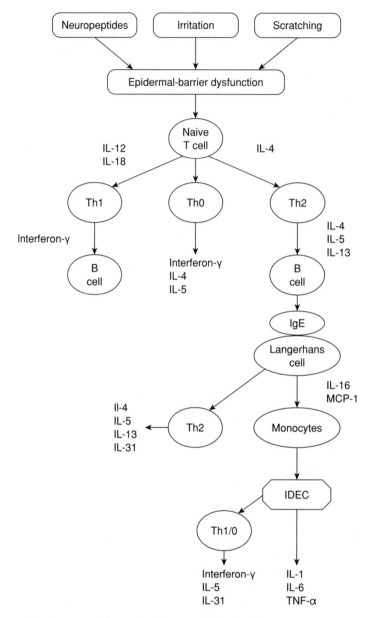

Figure 2.1 Simplified immunologic progression of atopic eczema.

2.1.4 Other cutaneous manifestations of food allergy

Dermatitis herpetiformis

This is a chronic prutitic papulovesicular cutaneous manifestation associated with gluten-sensitive enteropathy (coeliac disease). Not all people with gluten-sensitive enteropathy develop dermatitis herpetiformis. Conversely, not many patients with dermatitis herpetiformis have intestinal symptoms associated with gluten-sensitive enteropathy[2,7]. Skin lesions are usually distributed symmetrically on elbows, knees, buttocks, shoulders and scalp. Clinically it is very pruritic and polymorphic. Erythema, urticarial plaques, papules, seropapules, herpetiform vesicles, purpura and excoriations are also common, and large blisters are extremely rare[35].

Unlike other cutaneous reactions to food, dermatitis herpetiformis is not an IgE-mediated disorder, but rather characterised by granular IgA precipitates in the papillary dermis. Serum IgA in dermatitis herpetiformis has been found to bind epidermal transglutaminase. These findings may relate to the fact that dermatitis herpetiformis is associated with gluten-sensitive enteropathy, which is characterised by IgA-type autoantibodies to gliadin[35,36]. Gluten is present in wheat, rye and barley, and the avoidance of these foods in this condition usually clears the cutaneous manifestations[36].

Contact dermatitis

This is an inflammation of the epidermis and dermis that occurs as a result of direct contact between a substance and the surface of the skin. This type of cutaneous reaction is most commonly seen in occupational food handlers, involving the hands, but it can also involve the face, especially around the mouth in children[37,38]. This type of skin reaction may be either IgE- and/or cell-mediated, and symptoms therefore may be immediate (within 10 minutes to 2 hours) or delayed (2–48 hours)[2,39]. Research has reported contact dermatitis with a wide variety of foods, including raw and processed foods, spices, food additives and a variety of nuts[2].

References

1. Johansson SG, Bieber T, Dahl R *et al*. Revised nomenclature for allergy for global use: report of the Nomenclature Review Committee of the World Allergy Organization, October 2003. *J Allergy Clin Immunol* 2004; **113**: 832–6.
2. Fasano MB. Dermatologic food allergy. *Pediatr Ann* 2006; **35**: 727–31.
3. Katelaris CH, Peake JE. 5. Allergy and the skin: eczema and chronic urticaria. *Med J Aust* 2006; **185**: 517–22.
4. Werfel T. Skin manifestations in food allergy. *Allergy* 2001; **56** (Suppl 67): 98–101.
5. Sampson HA, Scanlon SM. Natural history of food hypersensitivity in children with atopic dermatitis. *J Pediatr* 1989; **115**: 23–7.
6. Falcão H, Lunet N, Lopes C, Barros H. Food hypersensitivity in Portuguese adults. *Eur J Clin Nutr* 2004; **58**: 1621–5.
7. Burks W. Skin manifestations of food allergy. *Pediatrics* 2003; **111**: 1617–24.
8. Sicherer SH, Leung DY. Advances in allergic skin disease, anaphylaxis, and hypersensitivity reactions to foods, drugs, and insects in 2007. *J Allergy Clin Immunol* 2008; **121**: 1352–8.
9. Liccardi G, De FF, Gilder JA, D'Amato M, D'Amato G. Severe systemic allergic reaction induced by accidental skin contact with cow milk in a 16-year-old boy: a case report. *J Investig Allergol Clin Immunol* 2004; **14**: 168–71.
10. Kaplan AP. Diagnostic tests for urticaria and angioedema. *Clin Allergy Immunol* 2000; **15**: 111–26.
11. Kaplan AP. Clinical practice: chronic urticaria and angioedema. *N Engl J Med* 2002; **346**: 175–9.

12. Powell RJ, Du Toit GL, Siddique N *et al*. BSACI guidelines for the management of chronic urticaria and angio-oedema. *Clin Exp Allergy* 2007; **37**: 631–50.
13. Dibbern DA Jr, Dreskin SC. Urticaria and angioedema: an overview. *Immunol Allergy Clin North Am* 2004; **24**: 141–62, v.
14. Baxi S, Dinakar C. Urticaria and angioedema. *Immunol Allergy Clin North Am* 2005; **25**: 353–67, vii.
15. Thomas P, Perkin MR, Rayner N *et al*. The investigation of chronic urticaria in childhood: which investigations are being performed and which are recommended? *Clin Exp Allergy* 2008; **38**: 1061–2.
16. Sicherer SH. Food allergy. *Lancet* 2002; **360**: 701–10.
17. Kulthanan K, Jiamton S, Boochangkool K, Jongjarearnprasert K. Angioedema: clinical and etiological aspects. *Clin Dev Immunol* 2007; **2007**: 26438.
18. Asero R, Ballmer-Weber BK, Beyer K *et al*. IgE-mediated food allergy diagnosis: Current status and new perspectives. *Mol Nutr Food Res* 2007; **51**: 135–47.
19. Scheindlin S. Chronic urticaria and angioedema. *N Engl J Med* 2002; **347**: 1724.
20. Pfeiffer C. Chronic urticaria and angioedema. *N Engl J Med* 2002; **347**: 220–2.
21. Khalaf AT, Li W, Jinquan T. Current advances in the management of urticaria. *Arch Immunol Ther Exp (Warsz)* 2008; **56**: 103–14.
22. Buss YA, Garrelfs UC, Sticherling M. Chronic urticaria: which clinical parameters are pathogenetically relevant? A retrospective investigation of 339 patients. *J Dtsch Dermatol Ges* 2007; **5**: 22–9.
23. Sackesen C, Sekerel BE, Orhan F *et al*. The etiology of different forms of urticaria in childhood. *Pediatr Dermatol* 2004; **21**: 102–8.
24. Bieber T. Atopic dermatitis. *N Engl J Med* 2008; **358**: 1483–94.
25. Hill DJ, Hosking CS, de Benedictis FM *et al*. Confirmation of the association between high levels of immunoglobulin E food sensitization and eczema in infancy: an international study. *Clin Exp Allergy* 2008; **38**: 161–8.
26. Kang K, Stevens SR. Pathophysiology of atopic dermatitis. *Clin Dermatol* 2003; **21**: 116–21.
27. Eigenmann PA, Sicherer SH, Borkowski TA, Cohen BA, Sampson HA. Prevalence of IgE-mediated food allergy among children with atopic dermatitis. *Pediatrics* 1998; **101**: E8.
28. Rogers AJ, Celedon JC, Lasky-Su JA, Weiss ST, Raby BA. Filaggrin mutations confer susceptibility to atopic dermatitis but not to asthma. *J Allergy Clin Immunol* 2007; **120**: 1332–7.
29. Hanifin JM, Rajka G. Diagnostic features of atopic dermatitis. *Acta Derm Venereol Suppl (Stockh)* 1980; **92**: 44–7.
30. Illi S, von Mutius E, Lau S *et al*. The natural course of atopic dermatitis from birth to age 7 years and the association with asthma. *J Allergy Clin Immunol* 2004; **113**: 925–31.
31. Breuer K, Heratizadeh A, Wulf A *et al*. Late eczematous reactions to food in children with atopic dermatitis. *Clin Exp Allergy* 2004; **34**: 817–24.
32. Worm M, Forschner K, Lee HH *et al*. Frequency of atopic dermatitis and relevance of food allergy in adults in Germany. *Acta Derm Venereol* 2006; **86**: 119–22.
33. Zuberbier T, Edenharter G, Worm M *et al*. Prevalence of adverse reactions to food in Germany: a population study. *Allergy* 2004; **59**: 338–45.
34. Lopata AL, Jeebhay MF, Reese G *et al*. Detection of fish antigens aerosolized during fish processing using newly developed immunoassays. *Int Arch Allergy Immunol* 2005; **138**: 21–8.
35. Karpati S. Dermatitis herpetiformis: close to unravelling a disease. *J Dermatol Sci* 2004; **34**: 83–90.
36. Alonso-Llamazares J, Gibson LE, Rogers RS 3rd. Clinical, pathologic, and immunopathologic features of dermatitis herpetiformis: review of the Mayo Clinic experience. *Int J Dermatol* 2007; **46**: 910–19.
37. Freeman S, Rosen RH. Urticarial contact dermatitis in food handlers. *Med J Aust* 1991; **155**: 91–4.
38. Kiec-Swierczynska M, Krecisz B. Occupational allergic contact dermatitis due to curcumin food colour in a pasta factory worker. *Contact Dermatitis* 1998; **39**: 30–1.
39. Shum KW, English JS. Allergic contact dermatitis in food handlers, with patch tests positive to Compositae mix but negative to sesquiterpene lactone mix. *Contact Dermatitis* 1998; **39**: 207–8.

2.2 The role of food hypersensitivity in respiratory disorders

Isabel Skypala

2.2.1 Introduction

In the authoritative text on food allergy by Metcalfe, Sampson and Simon, John James suggests that food allergy usually involves symptoms which manifest in the skin and gastrointestinal tract, with respiratory symptoms uncommon and not occurring in isolation[1]. Respiratory manifestations of food hypersensitivity include rhinoconjunctivitis, laryngeal oedema, asthma and otitis media. These symptoms may form part of a range of symptoms experienced as part of a food allergic reaction; both upper and lower respiratory tract reactions may be a significant part of an anaphylactic reaction[2]. A joint American Academy of Allergy, Asthma and Immunology and American College of Allergy, Asthma and Immunology practice guideline published in 2006 advises that IgE-mediated reactions to foods can involve symptoms of both the upper and lower respiratory tract[3], but isolated respiratory manifestations from food exposure are rare and most often reported in an occupational setting. The best example of this is baker's asthma, a food-related occupational lung disease.

However, although isolated respiratory symptoms are an uncommon manifestation of food allergy, there is an important link between respiratory conditions and food hypersensitivity. Increased respiratory allergy is associated with egg allergy[4]; there is also a relationship between asthma, allergic rhinitis and food allergy in school-age children[5], and food allergy in adults is frequently associated with other manifestations of atopy, especially hay fever[6]. It is also known that people with food allergy and asthma are more likely to have severe reactions to foods, especially peanuts[7], and respiratory symptoms may often be observed in fatal or near-fatal food anaphylaxis, highlighting the need for asthma management in a food-allergic child[8]. For more information on the prevalence, pathogenesis and management of asthma, rhinitis and anaphylaxis see Chapter 14.

Although food hypersensitivity may be an uncommon cause of isolated respiratory symptoms, it is reported that dietary factors could affect the development of asthma, with several studies showing that maternal or early-life consumption of fish and fruits/vegetables is associated with a reduced risk of developing asthma[9,10,11].

2.2.2 Prevalence

Various population studies have shown the prevalence of respiratory symptoms in connection with reported or confirmed food allergy.

Respiratory symptoms associated with food allergy

In Young's 1994 population study of the UK, nearly 15% of the respondents had asthma and 25% had hay fever[12]; these percentages were almost identical to those reported by a French population study in 2001, which showed that 24% of those with food allergy had allergic rhinitis and 16% had asthma[13]. In 1998 Woods *et al.* concluded that there was a definite association between food allergy and respiratory symptoms in young adults[14], and Schäfer *et al.* confirmed this, showing in particular that hay fever affected 73% of those with a reported food allergy[6]. However, it is not suggested that the hay fever or asthma reported in these studies is a symptom of the food allergy, but rather a concomitant allergic condition. The hay-fever prevalence suggests that for many subjects the food allergy may be a manifestation of oral allergy syndrome associated with pollen–food cross-reactivity. Estimates suggest that 3–5% of those with birch-pollen allergy may have a food allergy which is directly related to pollen–food cross-reactivity (see Chapter 7).

Respiratory symptoms caused by food allergy

Two studies have shown that the prevalence of asthma and rhinitic symptoms actually caused by food allergy is much lower. Falcão and colleagues found that 3.8% of those reporting food allergies listed dyspnoea and 1.9% rhinitis as symptoms of their allergy[15]. A study by Zuberbier in 2004 showed that 7.4% of respondents reported allergic rhinitis as a symptom and 2.1% dyspnoea[16]. A study by Osterballe and colleagues investigating 1,834 children and adults showed that 8 subjects (0.4%) reported bronchospasm to foods and 6 subjects (0.3%) rhinoconjunctivitis[17]; of these only one subject had confirmation of reported bronchospasm, and one confirmation of reported rhinoconjunctivitis, on oral food challenge. In a 2008 review Ozol and Mete concluded that asthma may develop in about 5% of individuals who suffer from food allergy, and current asthma may be triggered by foods among 6–8% of children and 2% of adults[18]. However, the commonest group of individuals likely to develop a concomitant food allergy are those with hay fever, most specifically to tree pollen.

Otitits media

Serous otitis media has multiple causes. A role for food allergy has been considered, with one study showing that the incidence of food allergy in a group with otitis media was statistically significant when compared to controls[19]. However, two reviews of respiratory manifestations of food allergy both concluded that the association between food allergy and otitis media has been overestimated, is controversial and is probably uncommon[2,18].

2.2.3   Pathogenesis of food-induced respiratory allergies

Respiratory symptoms can manifest in both IgE- and non-IgE-mediated food allergy, and also in non-allergic food hypersensitivity. Of these, reviews suggest that an immune response involving specific IgE antibodies to foods is the commonest mechanism of food-induced respiratory symptoms[2,20]. Work from Platts-Mills shows these antibodies bind to high-affinity receptors on mast cells in the nasal and bronchial mucosa during the sensitisation process, so that on re-exposure the mast cells degranulate and precipitate symptoms in the upper and/or lower respiratory tract[21], as seen with other forms of IgE-mediated food allergy. It is most commonly oral ingestion of the food allergen that initiates respiratory symptoms, but inhalation of aerosolised food can also cause reactions, for example to fish and shellfish[22].

The main non-IgE-mediated manifestation of a food causing respiratory symptoms is seen in food-induced pulmonary haemosiderosis (Heiner's syndrome), which primarily affects infants and is mostly caused by cow's milk. The immunologic mechanisms are not clear but probably involve the formation of immune complexes in what is usually known as a Gell–Coombs type III reaction [23]. Non-allergic food hypersensitivity to some additives can also provoke respiratory symptoms. Both rhinitis and asthma have been linked to food additives such as sodium metabisulphite and monosodium benzoate[24,25]. The mechanisms for rhinitis provoked by additives are unclear; Asero suggests that they are non-immunologic, although they appear to involve histamine release[24]. For some asthmatic responses due to additives such as sodium metabisulphite hypersensitivity, both immunologic and non-immunologic mechanisms have been proposed, including sulphur dioxide inhalation and histamine release[3,24,26] (see also Chapter 10).

2.2.4   Foods involved

As with other manifestations of food hypersensitivity, it is possible that any food can cause respiratory symptoms. The common foods causing food allergy are discussed in detail in Part 2 (Chapters 5–10). There are a few foods, however, that have specific associations with respiratory symptoms.

Milk

There is a widespread belief that cow's milk induces excessive mucus production and symptoms of rhinitis, blockage and wheeze in patients with respiratory conditions[27]. A survey of parents of 333 paediatric respiratory patients showed that nearly 60% believed drinking milk increases mucus production and 50% avoided giving their children milk when they were ill[28]. Half of these parents said their physician provided them with this information. Several studies have investigated this, using structured questionnaires and also double-blind placebo-controlled oral food challenges (DBPCFC). Early studies by Pinnock et al.[29], and later studies such as those from Nguyen[30]and Woods et al.[31], involved DBPCFCs with milk on asthmatic patients. However none of the studies has shown any difference between placebo and active challenges, and claims that milk increases nasal secretions or affects peak flow in adults with asthma were not substantiated. In a review of this subject in 2005, Wuthrich and colleagues concluded that recommendations to abstain from dairy products due to the belief that they induce symptoms of asthma are not supported by the evidence from research studies[27]. It is possible that aggregation after mixing of an emulsion such as milk with saliva can partly explain the sensation experienced by those who embrace the milk–mucus belief. It is very important that milk is not unnecessarily excluded from the diet, as this can have specific nutritional implications (see Chapter 10).

Wheat

Wheat can sensitise through inhalation as well as digestion, and can therefore precipitate inhalant allergies[32]. For this reason, wheat is one of the main causes of occupational asthma in the form of baker's asthma[33]. In addition to new enzymes being added to bread that may have allergic potential, a new family of cereal allergens has been identified, including wheat thioredoxin-hB (Tri a 25)[34]. Further information on wheat can be found in Chapter 9.

Alcohol

Alcoholic drinks have often been associated with asthma[35], with nearly one-third of asthmatic outpatients reporting that their asthma symptoms worsened on consumption of alcohol[36]. Alcohol consumption has also been linked to an increased risk of developing perennial allergic rhinitis[37]. Various studies have tried to identify the components in alcoholic drinks, especially wine, to understand what the main triggers are. Several suspected triggers include sodium metabisulphite and vasoactive amines, but studies to date have been inconclusive, and in a 2008 review Vally concluded that the challenge remained to clarify the specific components of alcoholic drinks which are responsible, and to elucidate the pathophysiological mechanisms underlying these sensitivities[38]. Chapter 10 contains more information about the relationship between alcohol and FHS.

Food additives

Consumption of foods containing high levels of food additives, in particular monosodium glutamate (MSG), sodium benzoate and sodium metabisulphite, has been linked to symptoms of asthma and allergic rhinitis. All of these additives are reviewed in Chapter 10, and the evidence for their involvement in provoking asthma and rhinitis is variable. MSG is thought not to be very relevant in these conditions, but the preservatives sodium benzoate and sodium metabisulphite are more likely to play a role in provoking asthma and rhinitis in particular groups of individuals (see Chapter 10).

Other foods

A study by Huang and colleagues in Taiwan showed that asthma was associated with increased intakes of liver, butcher's meat and deep-fried foods[39]. Researchers from New Zealand investigated fast-food consumption and asthma in children, and found, after adjusting for lifestyle factors including other diet and BMI variables, a dose-dependent association between hamburger consumption and asthma symptoms, as well as between frequent takeaway consumption and exercise-induced bronchial hyperresponsiveness[40]. The authors speculated that the high salt content in hamburgers may increase the risk of wheezy illness, but also that the frequent consumption of hamburgers, takeaways and fizzy drinks may all be markers for socioeconomic or lifestyle factors which could not be controlled for.

2.2.5   Food allergy as a marker of disease severity

An important aspect of the relationship between food allergy and respiratory conditions is that food allergic sensitisation or the presence of diagnosed food allergy can provide a marker for the presence and severity of respiratory conditions. It has been demonstrated by Pénard-Morand *et al.* that reported food allergy, food sensitisation and skin-prick-tested food allergy are all positively associated with asthma and allergic rhinitis in children aged 9–11 years[5]. Schäfer and colleagues showed that food-allergic adults suffered significantly more often from asthma and rhinitis than controls[6]. A study by Bakos *et al.* showed that this association persists into old age: in a study of 101 adults in a care home with a mean age of 77 years, risk factors for sensitisation to respiratory allergens included sensitisation to food allergens[41]. Studies looking in particular at populations with asthma have shown in both children and adults that food allergen sensitisation is associated with worse outcomes for asthma. Wang and colleagues showed that in children, food allergen sensitisation was highly prevalent in the inner-city population with asthma, and associated with increased asthma healthcare and medication use[42].

Roberts and colleagues compared a group of children admitted with life-threatening asthma with two case-matched control groups[43]. After regression analysis, they found that only frequent admission with asthma and having a food allergy were independently associated with life-threatening asthma. Interestingly, half of the children in the life-threatening asthma group had a food allergy, compared to only 10% of the controls. A study by Berns *et al.* evaluated the relationship between food allergy and asthma morbidity in adults[44]. They found that patients with allergies to more than one food had a significantly increased number of asthma hospitalisations, emergency department visits, and use of oral steroids, and that allergy to fish was significantly associated with a greater risk of health resource utilisation and increased frequency of oral steroid use.

References

1. James J. The respiratory tract and food hypersensitivity. In: Metcalfe DD, Sampson HJ, Simon RA, eds. *Food Allergy: Adverse Reactions to Foods and Food Additives*, 3rd edn. Oxford: Blackwell, 2003: 183–91.
2. James J. Respiratory manifestations of food allergy. *Pediatrics* 2003; **111**: 1625–30.
3. Chapman JA, Bernstein IL, Lee RE *et al.* Food allergy: a practice parameter. *Ann Allergy Asthma Immunol* 2006; **96**: S1–68.
4. Tariq SM, Matthews SM, Hakin EA, Arshad SH. Egg allergy in infancy predicts respiratory allergic disease by 4 years of age. *Pediatr Allergy Immunol* 2000; **11**: 162–7.
5. Pénard-Morand C, Raherison C, Kopferschmitt C *et al.* Prevalence of food allergy and its relationship to asthma and allergic rhinitis in schoolchildren. *Allergy* 2005; **60**: 1165–71.

6. Schäfer T, Böhler E, Ruhdorfer S et al. Epidemiology of food allergy/food intolerance in adults: associations with other manifestations of atopy. *Allergy* 2001; **56**: 1172–79.

7. Sicherer SH, Furlong TJ, Munoz Furlong A, Burks AW, Sampson HA. A voluntary registry for peanut and tree nut allergy: characteristics of the first 5149 registrants. *J Allergy Clin Immunol* 2001; **108**: 128–32.

8. Colver AF, Nevantaus H, Macdougall CF, Cant AJ. Severe food-allergic reactions in children across the UK and Ireland 1998–2000. *Acta Paediatr* 2005; **94**: 689–95.

9. Laerum BN, Wentzel LT, Gulsvik A et al. Relationship of fish and cod oil intake with adult asthma. *Clin Exp Allergy* 2007; **37**: 1616–23.

10. Chatzi L, Torrent M, Romieu I et al. Diet, wheeze, and atopy in school children in Menorca, Spain. *Pediatr Allergy Immunol* 2007; **18**: 480–5.

11. Romieu I, Torrent M, Garcia-Esteban R et al. Maternal fish intake during pregnancy and atopy and asthma in infancy. *Clin Exp Allergy* 2007; **37**: 518–25.

12. Young E, Stoneham MD, Petuckevitch A, Barton J, Rana R. A population study of food intolerance. *Lancet* 1994; **343**: 1127–30.

13. Kanny G, Moneret-Vautrin DA, Flabbee J et al. Population study of food allergy in France. *J Allergy Clin Immunol* 2001; **108**: 133–40.

14. Woods RK, Abramson M, Raven JM et al. Reported food intolerance and respiratory symptoms in young adults. *Eur Respir J* 1998; **11**: 151–5

15. Falcão H, Lunet N, Lopes C, Barros H. Food hypersensitivity in Portuguese adults. *Eur J Clin Nutr* 2004; **58**: 1621–5.

16. Zuberbier T, Edenharter G, Worm M et al. Prevalence of adverse reactions to food in Germany: a population study. *Allergy* 2004; **59**: 338–45.

17. Osterballe M, Hansen TK, Mortz CG, Høst A, Bindslev-Jensen C. The prevalence of food hypersensitivity in an unselected population of children and adults. *Pediatr Allergy Immunol* 2005; **16**: 567–73.

18. Ozol D, Mete E. Asthma and food allergy. *Curr Opin Pulm Med* 2008; **14**: 9–12.

19. Aydogan B, Kiroglu M, Altintas D et al. The role of food allergy in otitis media with effusion. *Otolaryngol Head Neck Surg* 2004; **130**: 747–7.

20. Yehia ME, Elham MH. Respiratory food allergy. *Pediatr Ann* 2006; **35**: 733–40.

21. Platts-Mills TAE. The role of immunoglobulin E in allergy and asthma. *Am J Respir Crit Care Med* 2001; **164**: S1–5.

22. James JM, Crespo JF. Allergic reactions to foods by inhalation. *Curr Allergy Asthma Rep* 2007; **7**: 167–74.

23. Bahna SL. Pathogenesis of milk hypersensitivity. *Immunol Today* 1985; **6**: 153–4.

24. Asero R. Food additives intolerance: does it present as perennial rhinitis? *Curr Opin Allergy Clin Immunol* 2004; **4**: 25–9.

25. Simon R. Adverse reactions to food and drug additives. *Immunol Allergy Clin North Am* 1996; **16**: 1, 137–76.

26. Taylor SL, Bush RK, Nordlee JA. Sulfites. In: Metcalfe DD, Sampson HJ, Simon RA, eds. *Food Allergy: Adverse Reactions to Foods and Food Additives*, 3rd edn. Oxford: Blackwell, 2003: 324–41.

27. Wuthrich B, Schmid A, Walther B, Seiber R. Milk consumption does not lead to mucus production or occurrence of asthma. *J Am Coll Nutr* 2005; **24**: 547S–555S.

28. Lee C, Dozor AJ. Do you believe milk makes mucus? *Arch Pediatr Adolesc Med* 2004; **158**: 601–2.

29. Pinnock CB, Arney WK. The milk mucus belief: sensory analysis comparing cow's milk and a soya placebo. *Appetite* 1993; **20**: 61–70.

30. Nguyen MT. Effects of cow milk on pulmonary function in atopic asthmatic patients. *Ann Allergy Asthma Immunol* 1997; **79**: 62–4.

31. Woods RK, Weiner JM, Abramson M, Thein F, Walters EH. Do dairy products induce broncho-constriction in adults with asthma? *J Allergy Clin Immunol* 1998; **101**: 45–50.

32. Wiechal M, Glaser AG, Ballmer-Weber BK, Schmid GP, Crameri R. Wheat and maize thioredoxins: a novel cross-reactive cereal allergen family related to baker's asthma. *J Allergy Clin Immunol* 2006; **117**: 676–81.

33. Alvarez MJ, Tabar AI, Quirce S *et al*. Diversity of allergens causing occupational asthma among cereal workers as demonstrated by exposure procedures. *Clin Exp Allergy* 1996; **26**: 147–53.
34. Brant A. Baker's asthma. *Curr Opin Allergy Clin Immunol* 2007; **7**: 152–5.
35. Vally H, Thompson PJ. Allergic and asthmatic reactions to alcoholic drinks. *Addict Biol* 2003; **8**: 3–11.
36. Ayres JG, Clarke TJH. Alcoholic drinks and asthma: a survey. *Br J Dis Chest* 1983; **77**: 370–5.
37. Bendtsen P, Grønbaek M, Kjaer SK *et al*. Alcohol consumption and the risk of self-reported perennial and seasonal allergic rhinitis in young adult women in a population-based cohort study. *Clin Exp Allergy* 2008; **38**: 1179–85.
38. Vally H. Allergic and asthmatic reactions to alcoholic drinks: a significant problem in the community. *Clin Exp Allergy* 2008; **38**: 1–3.
39. Huang SL, Lin KC, Pan WH. Dietary factors associated with physician-diagnosed asthma and allergic rhinitis in teenagers: analyses of the first Nutrition and Health Survey in Taiwan. *Clin Exp Allergy* 2001; **31**: 259–64.
40. Wickens K, Barry D, Friezema A *et al*. Fast foods: are they a risk factor for asthma? *Allergy* 2005; **60**: 1537–41.
41. Bakos N, Schöll I, Szalai K *et al*. Risk assessment in elderly for sensitization to food and respiratory allergens. *Immunol Lett* 2006; **107**: 15–21.
42. Wang J, Visness CM, Sampson HA. Food allergen sensitization in inner-city children with asthma. *J Allergy Clin Immunol* 2005; **115**: 1076–80.
43. Roberts G, Patel N, Levi-Schaffer F, Habibi P, Lack G. Food allergy as a risk factor for life-threatening asthma in childhood: a case-controlled study. *J Allergy Clin Immunol* 2003; **112**: 168–74.
44. Berns SH, Halm EA, Sampson HA *et al*. Food allergy as a risk factor for asthma morbidity in adults. *J Asthma* 2007; **44**: 377–81.

2.3 The role of food hypersensitivity in gastrointestinal disorders

Miranda Lomer

2.3.1 Irritable bowel syndrome

Irritable bowel syndrome (IBS) is a chronic and relapsing functional bowel disorder that affects 12% of the UK population[1]. It is characterised by abdominal pain or discomfort associated with defecation or a change in bowel habit (constipation and/or diarrhoea) without any other bowel pathology[2,3]. IBS is usually classified into three subtypes: diarrhoea-predominant (IBS-D), constipation-predominant (IBS-C) and alternating diarrhoea and constipation (IBS-A). IBS has a significant negative impact on quality of life. Twice as many women as men are affected by IBS[3], and symptoms are often more prominent around menstruation.

The aetiology of IBS is only partly understood, and multiple factors are involved. Low-grade mucosal inflammation has been demonstrated, with up-regulation of the gut immune system and increased pro-inflammatory cytokines[4]. Prior gastro-intestinal infection occurs in 4–31% of patients, and may be important in the inflammatory changes[5–8].

IBS is managed by a combination of dietary and lifestyle changes and medical treatments such as anti-diarrhoeals, laxatives, anti-spasmodics, low-dose antidepressants and psychological therapy[9]. Recent research[10] on the use of probiotics and/or pre-biotics looks promising (see also Chapter 13). Only 7% of patients have a formal diagnosis[1], so self-help often plays a crucial role[11] and patients often turn to alternative medicine such as herbal remedies, some of which may even be harmful[12].

Food hypersensitivity in irritable bowel syndrome

Diet plays a crucial role in the maintenance of gut health, mediated by its effects on the colonic microbiota[13]. Changes to the gastrointestinal environment may alter the way the gut handles food antigens, leading to sensitisation[14]. Undigested dietary components may release bioactive substances that trigger motor and sensory changes, making it difficult to identify which aspects of the diet and eating patterns exacerbate symptoms. Food hypersensitivity in IBS is difficult to detect and has been associated with immunological, allergic, toxic and psychiatric mechanisms. Whether food hypersensitivity in IBS is due to food allergy or food intolerance is a matter of much debate[14]. Up-regulation of mast cells, as in food allergy, occurs in the gastrointestinal mucosa of patients with IBS. However, there is currently insufficient evidence, due to limitations in diagnostic methodology in clinical practice, to suggest that this is due to local hypersensitivity to food antigens[15].

Traditionally, food allergy has been associated with an immediate IgE-mediated immune response to a specific dietary allergen, but there is no evidence to indicate that this kind of food hypersensitivity has a role to play in IBS[14,16]. A delayed IgG-mediated immune response to specific dietary allergens may be more useful in detecting delayed food hypersensitivity, and several studies in IBS suggest there is increased food hypersensitivity compared to controls[14,16–18]. Interestingly, the food antigens causing an immune response have not been consistent between studies due to differences in study design and populations studied with very different diets. In one study from coastal China the most common food antigens were crab, shrimp and soya, whereas milk and wheat were the most common in a UK study[17,18]. Symptoms do not always improve when the offending food antigens are removed from the diet, suggesting non-allergic food sensitivities. A raised IgG level may be secondary to mild inflammation, and it is likely that other factors, including psychological aspects, gastrointestinal microbiota and oral tolerance, are important determinants of food hypersensitivity in IBS[14,16].

Two-thirds of IBS patients perceive that their symptoms are related to food[19] and complain that they are worse postprandially[20,21]. Even the cephalic response to eating may be enhanced in IBS[20,22]. Patients are ready to seek advice from any source in a desperate attempt to alleviate symptoms, which may prove costly and often unsuccessful.

Unlike a typical food allergy, where a minute amount of food allergen will lead to an immediate reaction, in IBS the offending food is usually eaten on a regular basis and in normal portion sizes. Furthermore, food-related reactions tend to occur hours or even days after the food has been consumed, making the use of a double-blind food challenge more difficult to interpret, but still possible if carefully planned (see Chapter 3).

Management of food intolerance

In clinical practice, exclusion diets are often used to help identify specific food hypersensitivities in IBS, although the evidence is generally of poor quality because most studies have not been randomised. Burden reviewed dietary interventions in IBS from 1980 to 1999[23] and evaluated eight studies on food intolerance[24-31]. Of these, only five identified food intolerance, and differences may have been due to varying study design. The National Institute for Health and Clinical Excellence (NICE) has recently published guidelines for the diagnosis and management of IBS in primary care[32], drawing on two randomised controlled trials[17,33] and 13 other studies on food intolerance[25-28,30,34-41]. They concluded that there are differing levels of response to exclusion diets, and recommend that if food intolerance is suspected patients should be referred to a dietitian for specialist advice and monitoring. In IBS, the most frequently avoided foods are dairy products and wheat. The percentages of patients who have reported intolerance to these and other foods are: milk 42–44%, cheese 14–39%, wheat 14–60%, corn 40%, yeast 20%, eggs 26%, rye 30%, potatoes 20%, onions 22–36%, cocoa 22–25%, citrus 24%, coffee 26–33%, tea 16–25%, alcohol 10–17%, peas 17%, banana 11% and preservatives 20%[17,25-28,30,33-41].

Dietary fibre

Dietary fibre is defined as food material that is not hydrolysed by enzymes secreted by the human gastrointestinal tract[42]. Soluble fibre dissolves in water to form a gel and may be digested by the colonic microbiota, increasing bacterial numbers and thus faecal bulk. It includes β-glucans, pectins, gums, mucilages and some hemicelluloses. Dietary sources include oats, psyllium, ispaghula, nuts and seeds, some fruit and vegetables and pectins. Insoluble fibre is not readily broken down by the gastrointestinal microbiota and it increases faecal bulk, shortening colonic transit. It includes celluloses, some hemicelluloses and lignin and is chiefly found in corn (maize) and wheat bran, and in some fruit and vegetables[42].

For many years an increase in dietary fibre was recommended for IBS patients, although evidence indicates that the benefit is limited and many patients have enhanced symptoms, particularly from insoluble fibre[43]. Bloating and flatulence may be reduced by decreasing the level of dietary fibre[44]. Recent NICE guidance recommends that patients should be discouraged from taking additional insoluble fibre, and if a diet history indicates a low dietary fibre intake then an increase should be from soluble fibre[32].

Resistant starch is included as dietary fibre; this comprises starch polymers that are not readily digested in the stomach or small intestine[45]. The extent of resistance is influenced by the structure of naturally occurring starch polymers and by the food processing methods employed, e.g. how starch changes during cooking and cooling (Table 2.4)[45]. In healthy volunteers, high doses of resistant starch given over prolonged periods of time increase flatulence and bowel movement frequency[46]. No studies have been carried out in IBS, but whether regular consumption of

Table 2.4 Resistant starch classification[48,49].

Resistant starch type	Properties	Dietary sources
RS1	Physically protected starch. Resistance can be reduced by milling and chewing	Legumes, partly milled grains and seeds
RS2	Starch resistant to enzymatic hydrolysis when uncooked	Raw potatoes, green bananas, some legumes and high amylase starches
RS3	Retrograded starch, present in most starchy foods that have been cooked and cooled and dependent on processing conditions	Potato salad, bread, cornflakes and food products that are reheated prior to eating
RS4	Chemically modified starch that is less susceptible to small intestinal digestion	Some fibre-drinks, breads and cakes containing modified starch

resistant starch, particularly in processed foods, increases IBS symptoms warrants investigation.

Carbohydrate intolerance

In IBS, carbohydrate malabsorption (lactose, fructose and sorbitol) has been described in a number of studies[34,47–52]. Unabsorbed carbohydrate in the small bowel is delivered to the colon together with water due to the osmotic effect. The colonic microbiota ferment the unabsorbed carbohydrate to short-chain fatty acids and gases (hydrogen, carbon dioxide and methane). If sufficient unabsorbed carbohydrate reaches the colon it may increase the osmotic load and lead to rapid gas production[53]. In IBS, symptoms of carbohydrate intolerance (abdominal bloating and pain and diarrhoea) may be enhanced due to small intestinal bacterial overgrowth or increased gut sensation (visceral hypersensitivity)[54].

Lactose intolerance occurs in 24–45% of IBS patients[20,34,55]. Lactose is a disaccharide present in cow's, goat's, sheep's and human milk and dairy products. It is widely used in the food industry as an ingredient of processed foods or as a bulking agent in pharmaceuticals[56]. Patients who have lactose intolerance can generally manage up to 12 g lactose per day (240 ml milk) if spread throughout the day[57]. See Chapter 5 for the dietary management of lactose intolerance.

Fructose is a monosaccharide that is increasingly being used in the food industry. It may occur in the diet as the simple sugar in fruit and fruit juice, as part of the disaccharide sucrose or as fructans (oligosaccharides), present in some vegetables and wheat (Table 2.5)[58]. At least a third of IBS patients are unable to absorb 25–50 g load of fructose without developing symptoms of intolerance[61,62], and it may be the fructose-to-glucose ratio that is an important determinant of fructose malabsorption[51]. The average intake of fructans has been reported to be as high as 12 g per

Table 2.5 Foods high in fructose or fructans[48,51,59,60].

Food group	Dietary sources
Fruit	Apple, blackcurrants, cherries, dates, dried fruit (apricots, currants, figs, prunes, raisins, sultanas), grapes, guava, lychees, mango, melon, papaya, pear, watermelon
Sugars	Honey, golden syrup , treacle, honeycomb
Ingredients	High fructose corn syrup, fructose, fruit juice concentrate, corn syrup solids
Vegetables	Garlic, leek, onion, artichoke
Cereals and cereal products	Wheat flour*, white bread*, pasta*, wholegrain breakfast cereal*, crumpet*, English muffin*, crackers*, crispbread*, plain biscuit* Bread pudding, Eccles cakes, fruit cake, jam tarts, treacle tart, dried fruit snack bars, malt bread
Sauces	Barbeque sauce, brown sauce, chilli sauce, sweet pickle and chutney, jam, marmalade, plum sauce, relish (e.g. corn, cucumber or onion), sweet and sour sauce, tomato ketchup, tomato paste

* Foods with a low fructan content (0.5–10.1 g/100 g) but have been shown to lead to symptoms in irritable bowel syndrome[54].

day[63], and they have not been the focus of any concern until recently, despite wheat intolerance being common in IBS[18,28,39,64].

A diet reduced in fructose and fructans has been shown to be effective in minimising symptoms in 85% of compliant patients. Wheat tends to cause symptoms when eaten in large amounts as in the typical Western diet (e.g. bread, pasta, wheat-based breakfast cereals, biscuits and crackers), but in small amounts wheat is generally well tolerated[51]. This new dietary approach may help to explain why patients' symptoms improve when they eat less wheat.

Sorbitol is a poorly absorbed osmotically active sugar alcohol that occurs naturally in some fruit, particularly peaches, pears, plums and apple juice, but which is also added to reduced-sugar or sugar-free products, e.g. slimming products, soft drinks, chewing gum and foods aimed at people with diabetes[58]. Ingestion of 10 g of sorbitol is enough to lead to bloating, flatulence and osmotic diarrhoea in healthy subjects[65–67].

Yeast

Candida is single-cell yeast that thrives on a sugar-rich environment and is present in the skin, vagina, mouth and lower gastrointestinal tract. Following a course of antibiotics, *Candida* numbers can increase significantly[68], and effective treatment for excessive growth is with nystatin. However, this is only a short-term option, and fungal infections can reoccur. A low-carbohydrate diet has been suggested as a supplementary treatment for gastrointestinal *Candida* overgrowth[69]. The rationale for this is based on *Candida* needing sugar to grow despite most carbohydrate being absorbed proximally. There is no evidence to suggest that a low-carbohydrate diet helps the symptoms of IBS, and hypersensitivity to *Candida* in IBS is controversial[70].

Caffeine

Caffeine is a plant-derived stimulant, and the most common dietary sources are coffee, tea, sports drinks and gels, some soft drinks (e.g. cola and stimulant/energy drinks) and cocoa. Caffeine is also added to some pharmacological products, e.g. cold and flu remedies, pain killers, anti-histamine preparations, diuretics, energy boosting supplements and weight-loss products (Table 2.6).

The effect of caffeine varies from one person to the next[73], and gastrointestinal effects include increased colonic motor activity, but evidence in the literature for the effects of caffeine in IBS are lacking. Coffee stimulates the desire to defecate in 29% of individuals[74] and increases colonic motility[75] whether or not it contains caffeine. Thus, in subjects with sensitivity to coffee drinking, decaffeinated beverages may not decrease symptoms.

Summary

Food hypersensitivity is difficult to identify in IBS, but food intolerance is common and response to exclusion diets is variable (Table 2.7). Dietary management of food intolerance should be carried out with specialist advice from a dietitian. High intake of dietary fibre, particularly insoluble fibre, exacerbates symptoms, and patients should be advised to moderate intake. Carbohydrate intolerance may contribute to IBS symptoms. An increasing intake of processed foods in the modern Western diet may be increasing the exposure to lactose, fructose and sorbitol. Other dietary considerations include caffeine and yeast. The gastrointestinal environment and colonic microbiota are likely to have a role in the management of food hypersensitivity in IBS.

Table 2.6   Caffeine content of foods and beverages[71,72].

Food	Portion size	Caffeine content per serving (mg)
Coffee (instant)	250 ml	22–128
Coffee (ground)	250 ml	17–295
Cola and diet cola	330 ml	11–70
Chocolate bars	30 g	3–21
Powdered chocolate drink	250 ml	1–10
Chocolate milk drink	250 ml	2–5
Stimulant drinks	250 ml	28–87
Tea	250 ml	< 1–98
Cold and flu treatments, headache tablets and weight-control tablets	Per tablet or dose	15–200

Table 2.7 Practical guidelines for food intolerance in irritable bowel syndrome.

Dietary assessment and eating habits	Assess dietary intake and symptoms Encourage a regular meal pattern and 1.5–2 litres fluid per day (non-alcoholic and non-caffeine-based) Encourage a wide variety of foods Take time over meals and chew food thoroughly
Dietary fibre	Assess dietary fibre intake An increase in insoluble fibre (e.g. wheat) may exacerbate symptoms If an increase in dietary fibre is warranted, use soluble fibre and encourage a wide variety of dietary sources (e.g. oats, fruit and vegetables, nuts and seeds, psyllium, ipaghula)
Carbohydrate intolerance	Assess dietary intake for a high intake of lactose, fructose and/or sorbitol, as malabsorption of these carbohydrates can exacerbate symptoms
Exclusion diets	Response to exclusion diets is extremely variable, and they should only be carried out with specialist dietetic expertise and monitoring

References

1. Hungin AP, Whorwell PJ, Tack J, Mearin F. The prevalence, patterns and impact of irritable bowel syndrome: an international survey of 40,000 subjects. *Aliment Pharmacol Ther* 2003; **17**: 643–50.
2. Camilleri M. Management of the irritable bowel syndrome. *Gastroenterology* 2001; **120**: 652–68.
3. Chang L, Toner BB, Fukudo S *et al*. Gender, age, society, culture, and the patient's perspective in the functional gastrointestinal disorders. *Gastroenterology* 2006; **130**: 1435–46.
4. Drossman DA, Camilleri M, Mayer EA, Whitehead WE. AGA technical review on irritable bowel syndrome. *Gastroenterology* 2002; **123**: 2108–31.
5. Ji S, Park H, Lee D *et al*. Post-infectious irritable bowel syndrome in patients with Shigella infection. *J Gastroenterol Hepatol* 2005; **20**: 381–6.
6. McKendrick MW, Read NW. Irritable bowel syndrome: post salmonella infection. *J Infect* 1994; **29**: 1–3.
7. Neal KR, Barker L, Spiller RC. Prognosis in post-infective irritable bowel syndrome: a six year follow up study. *Gut* 2002; **51**: 410–13.
8. Parry S, Forgacs I. Intestinal infection and irritable bowel syndrome. *Eur J Gastroenterol Hepatol* 2005; **17**: 5–9.
9. Tack J, Fried M, Houghton LA, Spicak J, Fisher G. Systematic review: the efficacy of treatments for irritable bowel syndrome: a European perspective. *Aliment Pharmacol Ther* 2006; **24**: 183–205.
10. Quigley EM, Flourie B. Probiotics and irritable bowel syndrome: a rationale for their use and an assessment of the evidence to date. *Neurogastroenterol Motil* 2007; **19**: 166–72.
11. Robinson A, Lee V, Kennedy A *et al*. A randomised controlled trial of self-help interventions in patients with a primary care diagnosis of irritable bowel syndrome. *Gut* 2006; **55**: 643–8.
12. Hussain Z, Quigley EM. Systematic review: complementary and alternative medicine in the irritable bowel syndrome. *Aliment Pharmacol Ther* 2006; **23**: 465–71.
13. Gill CI, Rowland IR. Diet and cancer: assessing the risk. *Br J Nutr* 2002; **88** (Suppl 1): S73–87.
14. Park MI, Camilleri M. Is there a role of food allergy in irritable bowel syndrome and functional dyspepsia? A systematic review. *Neurogastroenterol Motil* 2006; **18**: 595–607.
15. Bischoff S, Crowe SE. Gastrointestinal food allergy: new insights into pathophysiology and clinical perspectives. *Gastroenterology* 2005; **128**: 1089–113.

16. Zar S, Kumar D, Benson MJ. Food hypersensitivity and irritable bowel syndrome. *Aliment Pharmacol Ther* 2001; **15**: 439–49.
17. Atkinson W, Sheldon TA, Shaath N, Whorwell PJ. Food elimination based on IgG antibodies in irritable bowel syndrome: a randomised controlled trial. *Gut* 2004; **53**: 1459–64.
18. Zuo XL, Li YQ, Li WJ *et al.* Alterations of food antigen-specific serum immunoglobulins G and E antibodies in patients with irritable bowel syndrome and functional dyspepsia. *Clin Exp Allergy* 2007; **37**: 823–30.
19. Simren M, Mansson A, Langkilde AM *et al.* Food-related gastrointestinal symptoms in the irritable bowel syndrome. *Digestion* 2001; **63**: 108–15.
20. Alpers DH. Diet and irritable bowel syndrome. *Curr Opin Gastroenterol* 2006; **22**: 136–9.
21. Ragnarsson G, Bodemar G. Pain is temporally related to eating but not to defaecation in the irritable bowel syndrome (IBS): patients' description of diarrhea, constipation and symptom variation during a prospective 6-week study. *Eur J Gastroenterol Hepatol* 1998; **10**: 415–21.
22. Whorwell PJ. The growing case for an immunological component to irritable bowel syndrome. *Clin Exp Allergy* 2007; **37**: 805–7.
23. Burden S. Dietary treatment of irritable bowel syndrome: current evidence and guidelines for future practice. *J Hum Nutr Diet* 2001; **14**: 231–41.
24. Bentley SJ, Pearson DJ, Rix KJ. Food hypersensitivity in irritable bowel syndrome. *Lancet* 1983; **2**: 295–7.
25. Jones VA, McLaughlan P, Shorthouse M, Workman E, Hunter JO. Food intolerance: a major factor in the pathogenesis of irritable bowel syndrome. *Lancet* 1982; **2**: 1115–17.
26. McKee AM, Prior A, Whorwell PJ. Exclusion diets in irritable bowel syndrome: are they worthwhile? *J Clin Gastroenterol* 1987; **9**: 526–8.
27. Nanda R, James R, Smith H, Dudley CR, Jewell DP. Food intolerance and the irritable bowel syndrome. *Gut* 1989; **30**: 1099–104.
28. Parker TJ, Naylor SJ, Riordan AM, Hunter JO. Management of patients with food intolerance in irritable-bowel-syndrome: the development and use of an exclusion diet. *J Hum Nutr Diet* 1995; **8**: 159–66.
29. Farah DA, Calder I, Benson L, MacKenzie JF. Specific food intolerance: its place as a cause of gastrointestinal symptoms. *Gut* 1985; **26**: 164–8.
30. Hawthorn B, Lamber S, Scott D, Scott B. Food intolerance and the irritable bowel syndrome. *J Hum Nutr Diet* 1991; **3**: 19–23.
31. Hunter JO, Workman EM, Jones AV. Dietary studies. In: Gibson PR, Jewell DP, eds. *Topics in Gastroenterology 12*. Oxford: Blackwell, 1985: 305–13.
32. National Institute for Health and Clinical Excellence. *Irritable Bowel Syndrome in Adults: Diagnosis and Management of Irritable Bowel Syndrome in Primary Care*. London: NICE, 2008.
33. Symons P, Jones MP, Kellow JE. Symptom provocation in irritable bowel syndrome: effects of differing doses of fructose–sorbitol. *Scand J Gastroenterol* 1992; **27**: 940–4.
34. Bohmer CJ, Tuynman HA. The clinical relevance of lactose malabsorption in irritable bowel syndrome. *Eur J Gastroenterol Hepatol* 1996; **8**: 1013–16.
35. Bentley SJ, Pearson DJ, Rix KJ. Food hypersensitivity in irritable bowel syndrome. *Lancet* 1983; **2**: 295–7.
36. Drisko J, Bischoff B, Hall M, McCallum R. Treating irritable bowel syndrome with a food elimination diet followed by food challenge and probiotics. *J Am Coll Nutr* 2006; **25**: 514–22.
37. Petitpierre M, Gumowski P, Girard JP. Irritable bowel syndrome and hypersensitivity to food. *Ann Allergy* 1985; **54**: 538–40.
38. Smith MA, Youngs GR, Finn R. Food intolerance, atopy, and irritable bowel syndrome. *Lancet* 1985; **2**: 1064.
39. Zar S, Mincher L, Benson MJ, Kumar D. Food-specific IgG4 antibody-guided exclusion diet improves symptoms and rectal compliance in irritable bowel syndrome. *Scand J Gastroenterol* 2005; **40**: 800–7.
40. Zwetchkenbaum J, Burakoff R. The irritable bowel syndrome and food hypersensitivity. *Ann Allergy* 1988; **61**: 47–9.
41. Kanazawa M, Fukudo S. Effects of fasting therapy on irritable bowel syndrome. *Int J Behav Med* 2006; **13**: 214–20.

42. Institute of Food Science & Technology Trust Fund. *Dietary Fibre*. London: IFST, 2007.
43. Bijkerk CJ, Muris JW, Knottnerus JA, Hoes AW, de Wit NJ. Systematic review: the role of different types of fibre in the treatment of irritable bowel syndrome. *Aliment Pharmacol Ther* 2004; **19**: 245–51.
44. Dear KL, Elia M, Hunter JO. Do interventions which reduce colonic bacterial fermentation improve symptoms of irritable bowel syndrome? *Dig Dis Sci* 2005; **50**: 758–66.
45. Nugent AP. Health properties of resistant starch. *Nutrition Bulletin* 2005; **30**: 27–54.
46. Storey D, Lee A, Bornet F, Brouns F. Gastrointestinal responses following acute and medium term intake of retrograded resistant maltodextrins, classified as type 3 resistant starch. *Eur J Clin Nutr* 2007; **61**: 1262–70.
47. Evans PR, Piesse C, Bak YT, Kellow JE. Fructose–sorbitol malabsorption and symptom provocation in irritable bowel syndrome: relationship to enteric hypersensitivity and dys-motility. *Scand J Gastroenterol* 1998; **33**: 1158–63.
48. Fernandez-Banares F, Esteve-Pardo M, Humbert P et al. Role of fructose–sorbitol malabsorption in the irritable bowel syndrome. *Gastroenterology* 1991; **101**: 1453–4.
49. Goldstein R, Braverman D, Stankiewicz H. Carbohydrate malabsorption and the effect of dietary restriction on symptoms of irritable bowel syndrome and functional bowel complaints. *Isr Med Assoc J* 2000; **2**: 583–7.
50. Nelis GF, Vermeeren MA, Jansen W. Role of fructose–sorbitol malabsorption in the irritable bowel syndrome. *Gastroenterology* 1990; **99**: 1016–20.
51. Shepherd SJ, Gibson PR. Fructose malabsorption and symptoms of irritable bowel syndrome: guidelines for effective dietary management. *J Am Diet Assoc* 2006; **106**: 1631–9.
52. Vernia P, Ricciardi MR, Frandina C, Bilotta T, Frieri G. Lactose malabsorption and irrit-able bowel syndrome: effect of a long-term lactose-free diet. *Ital J Gastroenterol* 1995; **27**: 117–21.
53. Cummings JH, Macfarlane GT. The control and consequences of bacterial fermentation in the human colon. *J Appl Bacteriol* 1991; **70**: 443–59.
54. Spiller R. Role of motility in chronic diarrhoea. *Neurogastroenterol Motil* 2006; **18**: 1045–55.
55. Parker TJ, Woolner JT, Prevost AT et al. Irritable bowel syndrome: is the search for lactose intolerance justified? *Eur J Gastroenterol Hepatol* 2001; **13**: 219–25.
56. Lomer MC, Parkes GC, Sanderson JD. Review article: lactose intolerance in clinical practice: myths and realities. *Aliment Pharmacol Ther* 2007; **27**: 93–103.
57. Suarez FL, Savaiano DA, Levitt MD. A comparison of symptoms after the consumption of milk or lactose-hydrolyzed milk by people with self-reported severe lactose intolerance. *N Engl J Med* 1995; **333**: 1–4.
58. Rumessen JJ. Fructose and related food carbohydrates: sources, intake, absorption, and clinical implications. *Scand J Gastroenterol* 1992; **27**: 819–28.
59. Holland B, Welch AA, Unwin ID et al. *McCance and Widdowson's The Composition of Foods*. London: Royal Society of Chemistry, 1991.
60. Muir JG, Shepherd SJ, Rosella O et al. Fructan and free fructose content of common Australian vegetables and fruit. *J Agric Food Chem* 2007; **55**: 6619–27.
61. Nelis GF, Vermeeren MA, Jansen W. Role of fructose–sorbitol malabsorption in the irritable bowel syndrome. *Gastroenterology* 1990; **99**: 1016–20.
62. Rumessen JJ, Gudmand-Hoyer E. Fructans of chicory: intestinal transport and fermentation of different chain lengths and relation to fructose and sorbitol malabsorption. *Am J Clin Nutr* 1998; **68**: 357–64.
63. Roberfroid MB, Delzenne NM. Dietary fructans. *Annu Rev Nutr* 1998; **18**: 117–43.
64. Niec AM, Frankum B, Talley NJ. Are adverse food reactions linked to irritable bowel syndrome? *Am J Gastroenterol* 1998; **93**: 2184–90.
65. Hyams JS. Sorbitol intolerance: an unappreciated cause of functional gastrointestinal com-plaints. *Gastroenterology* 1983; **84**: 30–3.
66. Jain NK, Rosenberg DB, Ulahannan MJ, Glasser MJ, Pitchumoni CS. Sorbitol intolerance in adults. *Am J Gastroenterol* 1985; **80**: 678–81.
67. McRorie J, Zorich N, Riccardi K et al. Effects of olestra and sorbitol consumption on objective measures of diarrhea: impact of stool viscosity on common gastrointestinal symptoms. *Regul Toxicol Pharmacol* 2000; **31**: 59–67.

68. Giuliano M, Barza M, Jacobus NV, Gorbach SL. Effect of broad-spectrum parenteral anti-biotics on composition of intestinal microflora of humans. *Antimicrob Agents Chemother* 1987; **31**: 202–6.
69. Santelmann H, Laerum E, Roennevig J, Fagertun HE. Effectiveness of nystatin in polysymp-tomatic patients: a randomized, double-blind trial with nystatin versus placebo in general practice. *Fam Pract* 2001; **18**: 258–65.
70. Santelmann H, Howard JM. Yeast metabolic products, yeast antigens and yeasts as possible triggers for irritable bowel syndrome. *Eur J Gastroenterol Hepatol* 2005; **17**: 21–6.
71. Food Standards Agency. Survey of caffeine levels in hot beverages. www.food.gov.uk/multimedia/pdfs/fsis5304.pdf. Accessed 3 April 2008.
72. Ministry of Agriculture, Fisheries and Food, Survey of caffeine and other methylxanthines in energy drinks and other caffeine-containing products (updated). Food surveillance informa-tion sheet no. 144 (no. 103 revised). London: MAFF, 1998.
73. Boekema PJ, Samsom M, van Berge Henegouwen GP, Smout AJ. Coffee and gastrointestinal function: facts and fiction. A review. *Scand J Gastroenterol Suppl* 1999; **230**: 35–9.
74. Brown SR, Cann PA, Read NW. Effect of coffee on distal colon function. *Gut* 1990; **31**: 450–3.
75. Rao SS, Welcher K, Zimmerman B, Stumbo P. Is coffee a colonic stimulant? *Eur J Gastro-enterol Hepatol* 1998; **10**: 113–18.

2.3.2 Crohn's disease

Crohn's disease is a chronic relapsing inflammatory bowel disease of unknown aetiology affecting approximately 0.1% of the UK population[1]. The pathogenesis involves a complex interaction of genetic predisposition, environmental triggers and immune dysfunction[2].

Crohn's disease is typically a transmural inflammation. Although it can affect any part of the gastrointestinal tract, it predominates as ileocolitis in 50% of cases[3]. It is characterised by discontinuous regions of inflamed bowel with normal areas in between. Presentation is usually with diarrhoea or a change in bowel habit, weight loss, abdominal pain and bloating, pyrexia and general malaise. Symptoms vary enormously, depending on the site of inflammation and the type of lesions that have developed. The severity of the disease also varies, but it commonly presents with periods of active disease and remission, although exacerbating factors are not clear.

For many years corticosteroids have been used to induce disease remission, but these are not without side effects and do not alter the course of disease. Immunosuppressive agents (azathioprine and methotrexate) induce mucosal heal-ing and are useful to maintain disease remission, although they may take several months to be effective. Biological therapy modulates cytokines involved in the inflammatory process (e.g. infliximab). It also induces mucosal healing, probably more quickly than immunosuppressive agents, and reduces the need for surgical intervention[4]. Enteral nutrition is a useful alternative to medical management in compliant patients and avoids serious side effects[5].

Malnutrition is common in Crohn's disease, resulting from anorexia, malab-sorption, increased fluid and electrolyte loss, drug–nutrient interactions and gastrointestinal bleeding[6,7]. Patients often restrict their diet for fear of exacerbating symptoms[6,8,9].

Food hypersensitivity in Crohn's disease

The gut wall provides an essential barrier between the luminal contents and the internal systems of the body, and it is continuously exposed to a wide variety of food components and antigens, the gastrointestinal microbiota and pathogens. Antigen sampling is a normal occurrence, and the gut is usually considered to be in a constant state of controlled inflammation known as 'oral tolerance'[10,11]. In Crohn's disease an immune dysfunction exists leading to a pro-inflammatory response and impairment of the gut barrier function. The mechanism of action is unclear, but food antigens within the luminal contents may promote inflammation in Crohn's disease[12]. Thus removal of the normal luminal contents by dietary manipulation has been widely investigated to see what effect this would have in modulating the mucosal immune response. Although true food allergy does not appear to be involved in the aetiopathogenesis of Crohn's disease, patients often feel that other forms of food hypersensitivity may require dietary intervention in order achieve symptomatic relief [10,11].

Diet as a risk factor for the development of Crohn's disease

Diet has a major influence on the gastrointestinal environment[13] and, with the adoption of Western dietary habits and a rise in the incidence of Crohn's disease in industrialised countries, an association of food hypersensitivity in Crohn's disease deserves attention. Retrospective assessment of the pre-illness diet is open to criticism, as dietary changes may occur soon after the development of symptoms, but a confirmed diagnosis of Crohn's disease may not happen until long afterwards[14,15]. In addition, foods may aggravate symptoms without having a role in the pathogenesis. Despite these methodological flaws, a high intake of refined carbohydrate, particularly sugar, has been repeatedly reported[14–31]. This suggests that there may be a true relationship, but identifying a likely mechanistic explanation has not yet been possible.

The modern Western diet

The ever-increasing consumption of highly processed foods and eating in fast food outlets may be an important contributing factor in the development of Crohn's disease[13]. The use of food additives has increased dramatically since the Industrial Revolution. Emulsifiers (e.g. carrageenan), thickeners and surface-finishing agents such as beeswax, carnauba wax and candelilla wax may all have antigenic potential[32,33]. Furthermore, microparticles of food additive titanium dioxide and aluminosilicates have been isolated from the base of Peyer's patches and may be potent adjuvants in antigen-mediated immune responses[34].

A recent hypothesis suggests that there is an increase in the dietary intake of fermentable oligo-, di- and mono-saccharides and polyols (FODMAPS)[35], which occur naturally in the diet but are increasingly being used in the food industry. Rapid fermentation of FODMAPS by the microbiota in the distal small bowel and colon may impair the gut barrier function. Clinical studies in Crohn's disease are currently lacking, but the idea that increased permeability in patients with Crohn's disease may be due to a dietary factor is an appealing concept[35].

Food hypersensitivity in the treatment of active Crohn's disease

Diet is fundamental in the management of Crohn's disease, and dietary manipulation may be helpful in inducing disease remission and in the prevention of relapse. Early nutrition studies used total parenteral nutrition[36] eliminating food antigens, but complete bowel rest caused gut atrophy and brings with it serious complications[37]. Enteral nutritional therapy was developed using chemically defined liquid diets to limit mucosal atrophy, reduce faecal output and have low antigenicity[38-40]. The original enteral diets were based on those that had been used in manned space programmes, where a reduced stool output was warranted[41], and consisted of basic food monomers made into a synthetic elemental diet. They could be assimilated without the need for pancreatic or brush border enzymes and comprised free amino acids, maltodextrins and glucose, a small amount of fat, minerals and micronutrients. By the early 1970s it was reported that elemental diets given preoperatively in malnourished patients with Crohn's disease improved outcome[42,43]. More recently, peptide and whole protein diets have been developed, and these provide a more palatable alternative to elemental diet. All three types of liquid formula have been shown to induce disease remission in 53–80% of patients[33,39,40,44,45], and a recent Cochrane review indicates that they are as efficacious as each other[46] (Table 2.8).

Although enteral nutrition is not as effective as corticosteroids in inducing disease remission, it does have a role in the primary treatment of active disease[46], particularly in children and adolescents[55,56]. Enteral nutrition improves nutritional status, reduces gastrointestinal protein loss and helps maintain intestinal permeability[57,58]. Furthermore, enteral nutrition down-regulates pro-inflammatory mucosal cytokine production[59] and will induce mucosal healing[59,60].

The mechanism of action of enteral nutrition is unknown, but nutrients can influence the gastrointestinal environment and microbiota[61] and mediate the expression of proteins involved in the immune response[59]. Differences in lipid composition may also affect the inflammatory process and thus contribute to the efficacy of enteral nutrition[62]. Increasing the ratio of omega-3 to omega-6 polyunsaturated fats in Crohn's disease may enhance intestinal anti-inflammatory responses[56], but studies to date have been disappointing, perhaps due to difficulties with enteral feed formulation[63,64].

Sensitivity to specific food additives has been assessed in Crohn's, disease and the efficacy of enteral nutrition may be due to avoidance of food additives[33,65] or potentially antigenic bacteria and food particles[66]. Microparticles, particularly the food additives titanium dioxide and aluminosilicates, may act as adjuvants, allowing luminal toxins and antigens to enter the gastrointestinal mucosa and inducing a pro-inflammatory immune response. A pilot study of a low microparticle diet appeared promising in the induction of disease remission[65], but a multicentre study failed to confirm these findings[67].

Table 2.8 Comparison of elemental versus non elemental dietary treatments for active Crohn's disease.

Study	Design	Intervention A (n/N) vs. intervention B (n/N)	Outcome measure	Odds ratio (95% CI)
Giaffer 1990[47]	RT DB	ED (12/16) vs. PD (5/14)	CDAI < 150 after 10 days	5.4 (1.12–26.04)
Kobayashi 1998[48]	RT	ED (7/10) vs. PD (6/9)	CDAI < 150 after 24 days	1.17 (0.17–8.09)
Park 1991[49]	RT DB	ED (2/7) vs. PD (5/7)	HBI < 2 after 28 days	0.16 (0.02–1.63)
Raouf 1991[33]	RT	ED (9/13) vs. PD (8/11)	HBI < 4 after 21 days	0.84 (0.14–4.97)
Rigaud 1991[50]	RT	ED (10/15) vs. PD (11/15)	CDAI < 150 after 28 days	0.73 (0.15–3.49)
Royall 1994[51]	RT DB	ED (16/19) vs. peptide diet (15/21)	CDAI < 150 after 21 days	2.13 (0.45–10.10)
Verma 2000[52]	RT DB	ED (8/10) vs. PD (6/11)	CDAI < 150 or reduced by > 100 after 42 days	3.33 (0.47–23.47)

RT, randomised trial; DB, double-blind; ED, elemental diet; PD, polymeric diet; CDAI, Crohn's disease activity index[53]; HBI, Harvey Bradshaw index[54].

Nutrition in disease remission

Patients usually achieve disease remission within 2–8 weeks, but mucosal healing takes up to 8 weeks[59]. Using enteral nutrition as a sole source of nutrition to prevent relapse is not a long-term option due to issues with compliance. Prevention of relapse is maintained at 1 year in only 31% and 40% of patients who had achieved disease remission with elemental and peptide diets, respectively[51,68]. Reintroduction of a normal diet identifies food intolerance in up to 66% of patients with Crohn's disease[9,69], so, understandably, patients are often cautious about reintroducing food. Supplementary enteral nutrition may help to maintain disease remission if it provides at least 35–50% of the patient's energy requirements[70]. The choice of feed, i.e. whole protein, peptide or elemental, will depend on the site, severity and symptoms of recent disease activity, and on patient compliance. Exclusion diets may also prolong the length of remission, indicating that food sensitivity may play a role[71]. Any foods that may be associated with symptoms of abdominal pain and/or diarrhoea are excluded[71]. Common food intolerances are wheat, cow's milk and yeast[9,71,72], similar to those found in IBS and suggesting coexisting IBS in Crohn's disease[73]. The LOFFLEX (low fat, fibre limited, exclusion) diet is as effective as other exclusion diets[74] and avoids foods that commonly lead to symptoms in patients with Crohn's disease. It is nutritionally complete and consists of a relatively wide variety of foods, enabling patients to stop enteral nutrition. The initial process

Table 2.9 Practical dietary guidelines in Crohn's disease.

Active disease	Enteral feeding as a sole source of nutrition:
	• induces disease remission and is particularly useful in children and adolescents, avoiding the use of corticosteroids • can be used as an adjunct to other medical treatments • improves nutritional status, reduces protein loss, induces mucosal healing, down-regulates pro-inflammatory cytokines and maintains intestinal permeability
	Polymeric, peptide and elemental feeds are equally efficacious Enteral feeding should be given for 2–8 weeks as a sole source of nutrition
Disease remission	Maintenance of disease remission can be prolonged with:
	• Enteral feeding providing up to 50% of nutritional requirements • Exclusion diets – common food intolerances include wheat, cow's milk and yeast
Symptom control	Some dietary components may aggravate strictures, chewing food thoroughly and avoidance of high-fibre foods and grisley meat may be helpful

of food reintroduction is faster than with other exclusion regimens, allowing more time between single food testing and enabling better detection of delayed reactions to food.

After the onset of disease, eating habits often change to avoid foods that may aggravate symptoms[75,76]. Furthermore, green vegetables and mechanically fibrous foods may cause obstructive symptoms in stricturing disease[9,33], and avoidance of high-fibre foods may be helpful to maintain disease remission[77]. Avoidance of milk and milk products may be due to lactose intolerance, which can result from chronic inflammation[78] and has been observed in 30% of patients with inflammatory bowel disease[79].

Summary

No evidence exists to suggest that food intolerance and food allergy are involved in the development of Crohn's disease. Enteral nutrition is an effective treatment to induce disease remission and offers an alternative to corticosteroids with minimal side effects. Patients often restrict their diet and nutritional intake for symptomatic relief, and specific food sensitivities are common (Table 2.9).

References

1. Loftus EV Jr. Clinical epidemiology of inflammatory bowel disease: Incidence, prevalence, and environmental influences. *Gastroenterology* 2004; **126**: 1504–17.
2. Ferguson LR, Shelling AN, Browning BL, Huebner C, Petermann I. Genes, diet and inflammatory bowel disease. *Mutat Res* 2007; **622**: 70–83.
3. Marteau P. Clinical and pathological aspects of inflammatory bowel disease. In: Bistrian BR, Walker-Smith JA, eds. *Inflammatory Bowel Diseases*. Basel: Karger, 1999.

4. Vermeire S, van AG, Rutgeerts P. Review article. Altering the natural history of Crohn's disease: evidence for and against current therapies. *Aliment Pharmacol Ther* 2007; **25**: 3–12.
5. O'Sullivan MA, O'Morain CA. Nutritional therapy in Crohn's disease. *Inflamm Bowel Dis* 1998; **4**: 45–53.
6. Sousa GC, Cravo M, Costa AR *et al*. A comprehensive approach to evaluate nutritional status in Crohn's patients in the era of biologic therapy: a case–control study. *Am J Gastroenterol* 2007; **102**: 2551–6.
7. O'Sullivan M, O'Morain C. Nutrition in inflammatory bowel disease. *Best Pract Res Clin Gastroenterol* 2006; **20**: 561–73.
8. Lomer MC, Kodjabashia K, Hutchinson C *et al*. Intake of dietary iron is low in patients with Crohn's disease: a case–control study. *Br J Nutr* 2004; **91**: 141–8.
9. Ballegaard M, Bjergstrom A, Brøndum S *et al*. Self-reported food intolerance in chronic inflammatory bowel disease. *Scand J Gastroenterol* 1997; **32**: 569–71.
10. Bischoff SC, Mayer JH, Manns MP. Allergy and the gut. *Int Arch Allergy Immunol* 2000; **121**: 270–83.
11. Seibold F. Food-induced immune responses as origin of bowel disease? *Digestion* 2005; **71**: 251–60.
12. Levi AJ. Diet in the management of Crohn's disease. *Gut* 1985; **26**: 985–8.
13. Russel MG, Engels LG, Muris JW *et al*. 'Modern life' in the epidemiology of inflammatory bowel disease: a case–control study with special emphasis on nutritional factors. *Eur J Gastroenterol Hepatol* 1998; **10**: 243–9.
14. Tragnone A, Valpiani D, Miglio F *et al*. Dietary habits as risk factors for inflammatory bowel disease. *Eur J Gastroenterol Hepatol* 1995; **7**: 47–51.
15. Thornton JR, Emmett PM, Heaton KW. Diet and Crohn's disease: characteristics of the pre-illness diet. *Br Med J* 1979; **2**: 762–4.
16. Silkoff K, Hallak A, Yegena L *et al*. Consumption of refined carbohydrate by patients with Crohn's disease in Tel-Aviv-Yafo. *Postgraduate Medical Journal* 1980; **56**: 842–6.
17. Sakamoto N, Kono S, Wakai K *et al*. Dietary risk factors for inflammatory bowel disease: a multicenter case–control study in Japan. *Inflamm Bowel Dis* 2005; **11**: 154–63.
18. Reif S, Klein I, Lubin F *et al*. Pre-illness dietary factors in inflammatory bowel disease. *Gut* 1997; **40**: 754–60.
19. Probert CS, Bhakta P, Bhamra B, Jayanthi V, Mayberry JF. Diet of South Asians with inflammatory bowel disease. *Arq Gastroenterol* 1996; **33**: 132–5.
20. Porro GB, Panza E. Smoking, sugar, and inflammatory bowel disease. *Br Med J* 1985; **291**: 971–2.
21. Persson PG, Ahlbom A, Hellers G. Diet and inflammatory bowel disease: a case–control study. *Epidemiology* 1992; **3**: 47–52.
22. Penny WJ, Mayberry JF, Aggett PJ *et al*. Relationship between trace elements, sugar consumption, and taste in Crohn's disease. *Gut* 1983; **24**: 288–92.
23. Mayberry JF, Rhodes J, Newcombe RG. Increased sugar consumption in Crohn's disease. *Digestion* 1980; **20**: 323–6.
24. Mayberry JF, Rhodes J, Allan R *et al*. Diet in Crohn's disease: two studies of current and previous habits in newly diagnosed patients. *Dig Dis Sci* 1981; **26**: 444–8.
25. Matsui T, Iida M, Fujishima M, Imai K, Yao T. Increased sugar consumption in Japanese patients with Crohn's disease. *Gastroenterol Jpn* 1990; **25**: 271.
26. Martini GA, Brandes JW. Increased consumption of refined carbohydrates in patients with Crohn's disease. *Klin Wochenschr* 1976; **54**: 367–71.
27. Katschinski B, Logan RF, Edmond M, Langman MJ. Smoking and sugar intake are separate but interactive risk factors in Crohn's disease. *Gut* 1988; **29**: 1202–6.
28. Kasper H, Sommer H. Dietary fiber and nutrient intake in Crohn's disease. *Am J Clin Nutr* 1979; **32**: 1898–901.
29. Jarnerot G, Jarnmark I, Nilsson K. Consumption of refined sugar by patients with Crohn's disease, ulcerative colitis, or irritable bowel syndrome. *Scand J Gastroenterol* 1983; **18**: 999–1002.
30. Gilat T, Hacohen D, Lilos P, Langman MJ. Childhood factors in ulcerative colitis and Crohn's disease: an international cooperative study. *Scand J Gastroenterol* 1987; **22**: 1009–24.

31. Brauer PM, Gee MI, Grace M, Thomson AB. Diet of women with Crohn's and other gastrointestinal diseases. *J Am Diet Assoc* 1983; **82**: 659–64.
32. Traunmuller F. Etiology of Crohn's disease: do certain food additives cause intestinal inflammation by molecular mimicry of mycobacterial lipids? *Med Hypotheses* 2005; **65**: 859–64.
33. Raouf AH, Hildrey V, Daniel J *et al.* Enteral feeding as sole treatment for Crohn's disease: controlled trial of whole protein v amino acid based feed and a case study of dietary challenge. *Gut* 1991; **32**: 702–7.
34. Ashwood P, Thompson RP, Powell JJ. Fine particles that adsorb lipopolysaccharide via bridging calcium cations may mimic bacterial pathogenicity towards cells. *Exp Biol Med (Maywood)* 2007; **232**: 107–17.
35. Gibson PR, Shepherd SJ. Personal view: food for thought. Western lifestyle and susceptibility to Crohn's disease: the FODMAP hypothesis. *Aliment Pharmacol Ther* 2005; **21**: 1399–409.
36. Ostro MJ, Greenberg GR, Jeejeebhoy KN. Total parenteral nutrition and complete bowel rest in the management of Crohn's disease. *JPEN J Parenter Enteral Nutr* 1985; **9**: 280–7.
37. Driscoll RH Jr, Rosenberg IH. Total parenteral nutrition in inflammatory bowel disease. *Med Clin North Am* 1978; **62**: 185–201.
38. Gorard DA, Hunt JB, Payne-James JJ *et al.* Initial response and subsequent course of Crohn's disease treated with elemental diet or prednisolone. *Gut* 1993; **34**: 1198–202.
39. Lochs H, Steinhardt HJ, Klaus-Wentz B *et al.* Comparison of enteral nutrition and drug treatment in active Crohn's disease: results of the European Cooperative Crohn's Disease Study. IV. *Gastroenterology* 1991; **101**: 881–8.
40. O'Morain C, Segal AW, Levi AJ. Elemental diet as primary treatment of acute Crohn's disease: a controlled trial. *Br Med J* 1984; **288**: 1859–62.
41. Greenstein JP, Birnbaum SM, Winitz M, Otey M. Quantitative nutritional studies with water soluble chemically defined diets. I. Growth, reproduction and lactation in rats. *Arch Biochem Biophys* 1957; **72**: 396–456.
42. Voitk AJ, Echave V, Feller JH, Brown RA, Gurd FN. Experience with elemental diet in the treatment of inflammatory bowel disease: is this primary therapy? *Arch Surg* 1973; **107**: 329–33.
43. Rocchio MA, Cha CJ, Haas KF, Randall HT. Use of chemically defined diets in the management of patients with acute inflammatory bowel disease. *Am J Surg* 1974; **127**: 469–75.
44. Gonzalez-Huix F, de Leon R, Fernandez-Banares F *et al.* Polymeric enteral diets as primary treatment of active Crohn's disease: a prospective steroid controlled trial. *Gut* 1993; **34**: 778–82.
45. Okada M, Yao T, Yammamoto K *et al.* Controlled trial comparing an elemental diet with prednisolone in the treatment of active Crohn's disease. *Hepatogastroenterology* 1990; **37**: 72–80.
46. Zachos M, Tondeur M, Griffiths AM. Enteral nutrition therapy for induction of remission in Crohn's disease. *Cochrane Database Syst Rev* 2007; (1): CD000542.
47. Giaffer MH, North G, Holdsworth CD. Controlled trial of polymeric versus elemental diet in treatment of active Crohn's disease. *Lancet* 1990; **335**: 816–19.
48. Kobayashi K, Katsumata T, Yokoyama K *et al.* A randomized controlled study of total parenteral nutrition and enteral nutrition by elemental and polymeric diet as primary therapy in active phase of Crohn's disease. *Nippon Shokakibyo Gakkai Zasshi* 1998; **95**: 1212–21.
49. Park RH, Galloway A, Danesh BJ, Russell RI. Double-blind controlled trial of elemental and polymeric diets as primary therapy in active Crohn's disease. *Eur J Gastroenterol Hepatol* 1991; **3**: 483–9.
50. Rigaud D, Cosnes J, Le Quintrec Y *et al.* Controlled trial comparing two types of enteral nutrition in treatment of active Crohn's disease: elemental versus polymeric diet. *Gut* 1991; **32**: 1492–7.
51. Royall D, Jeejeebhoy KN, Baker JP *et al.* Comparison of amino acid v peptide based enteral diets in active Crohn's disease: clinical and nutritional outcome. *Gut* 1994; **35**: 783–7.
52. Verma S, Brown S, Kirkwood B, Giaffer MH. Polymeric versus elemental diet as primary treatment in active Crohn's disease: a randomized, double-blind trial. *Am J Gastroenterol* 2000; **95**: 735–9.

53. Best WR, Becktel JM, Singleton JW, Kern F, Jr. Development of a Crohn's disease activity index. National Cooperative Crohn's Disease Study. *Gastroenterology* 1976; **70**: 439–44.
54. Harvey RF, Bradshaw JM. A simple index of Crohn's-disease activity. *Lancet* 1980; **1**: 514.
55. Fernandez-Banares F, Cabre E, Esteve-Comas M, Gassull MA. How effective is enteral nutrition in inducing clinical remission in active Crohn's disease? A meta-analysis of the randomized clinical trials. *JPEN J Parenter Enteral Nutr* 1995; **19**: 356–64.
56. Griffiths AM, Ohlsson A, Sherman PM, Sutherland LR. Meta-analysis of enteral nutrition as a primary treatment of active Crohn's disease. *Gastroenterology* 1995; **108**: 1056–67.
57. Sanderson IR, Boulton P, Menzies I, Walker-Smith JA. Improvement of abnormal lactulose/rhamnose permeability in active Crohn's disease of the small bowel by an elemental diet. *Gut* 1987; **28**: 1073–6.
58. Teahon K, Smethurst P, Pearson M, Levi AJ, Bjarnason I. The effect of elemental diet on intestinal permeability and inflammation in Crohn's disease. *Gastroenterology* 1991; **101**: 84–9.
59. Fell JM, Paintin M, Arnaud-Battandier F *et al.* Mucosal healing and a fall in mucosal pro-inflammatory cytokine mRNA induced by a specific oral polymeric diet in paediatric Crohn's disease. *Aliment Pharmacol Ther* 2000; **14**: 281–9.
60. Borrelli O, Cordischi L, Cirulli M *et al.* Polymeric diet alone versus corticosteroids in the treatment of active pediatric Crohn's disease: a randomized controlled open-label trial. *Clin Gastroenterol Hepatol* 2006; **4**: 744–53.
61. Lionetti P, Callegari ML, Ferrari S *et al.* Enteral nutrition and microflora in pediatric Crohn's disease. *JPEN J Parenter Enteral Nutr* 2005; **29**: S173–5.
62. Grimble RF. Dietary lipids and the inflammatory response. *Proc Nutr Soc* 1998; **57**: 535–42.
63. Gassull MA, Fernandez-Banares F, Cabre E *et al.* Fat composition may be a clue to explain the primary therapeutic effect of enteral nutrition in Crohn's disease: results of a double blind randomised multicentre European trial. *Gut* 2002; **51**: 164–8.
64. Leiper K, Woolner J, Mullan MMC *et al.* A randomised controlled trial of high versus low long chain triglyceride whole protein feed in active Crohn's disease. *Gut* 2001; **49**: 790–4.
65. Lomer MC, Harvey RS, Evans SM, Thompson RP, Powell JJ. Efficacy and tolerability of a low microparticle diet in a double blind, randomized, pilot study in Crohn's disease. *Eur J Gastroenterol Hepatol* 2001; **13**: 101–6.
66. King TS, Woolner JT, Hunter JO. Review article: the dietary management of Crohn's disease. *Aliment Pharmacol Ther* 1997; **11**: 17–31.
67. Lomer MC, Grainger SL, Ede R *et al.* Lack of efficacy of a reduced microparticle diet in a multi-centred trial of patients with active Crohn's disease. *Eur J Gastroenterol Hepatol* 2005; **17**: 377–84.
68. Mansfield JC, Giaffer MH, Holdsworth CD. Controlled trial of oligopeptide versus amino acid diet in treatment of active Crohn's disease. *Gut* 1995; **36**: 60–6.
69. Pearson M, Teahon K, Levi AJ, Bjarnason I. Food intolerance and Crohn's disease. *Gut* 1993; **34**: 783–7.
70. Akobeng AK, Thomas AG. Enteral nutrition for maintenance of remission in Crohn's disease. *Cochrane Database Syst Rev* 2007; (3): CD005984.
71. Riordan AM, Hunter JO, Cowan RE *et al.* Treatment of active Crohn's disease by exclusion diet: East Anglian multicentre controlled trial. *Lancet* 1993; **342**: 1131–4.
72. Hunter JO. Nutritional factors in inflammatory bowel disease. *Eur J Gastroenterol Hepatol* 1998; **10**: 235–7.
73. MacDermott RP. Treatment of irritable bowel syndrome in outpatients with inflammatory bowel disease using a food and beverage intolerance, food and beverage avoidance diet. *Inflamm Bowel Dis* 2007; **13**: 91–6.
74. Woolner JT, Parker TJ, Kirby GA, Hunter JO. The development and evaluation of a diet for maintaining remission in Crohn's disease. *J Hum Nutr Diet* 1998; **11**: 1–11.
75. Kelly DG, Fleming CR. Nutritional considerations in inflammatory bowel diseases. *Gastroenterol Clin North Am* 1995; **24**: 597–611.
76. Laiho K, Nuutinen O, Malin M, Isolauri E. Crohn's disease affects diet and growth in children. *J Hum Nutr Diet* 1998; **11**: 287–94.

77. Koga H, Iida M, Aoyagi K, Matsui T, Fujishima M. Long-term efficacy of low residue diet for the maintenance of remission in patients with Crohn's disease. *Nippon Shokakibyo Gakkai Zasshi* 1993; **90**: 2882–8.
78. O'Keefe SJD. Nutrition and gastrointestinal disease. *Scand J Gastroenterol Suppl* 1996; **220**: 52–9.
79. Issenman RM. Bone mineral metabolism in pediatric inflammatory bowel disease. *Inflamm Bowel Dis* 1999; **5**: 192–9.

2.3.3   Orofacial granulomatosis

Orofacial granulomatosis (OFG) is a rare chronic inflammatory disease that describes any non-caseating, epitheloid granulomatous inflammation associated with facial or oral tissues. Presentation of OFG is usually with lip swelling, but it also affects a number of sites within the oral cavity including the gingivae, sulcus, floor of the mouth and buccal mucosa, the latter often associated with a cobblestone appearance. It is more frequent in young adults and carries a high psychological burden. The lip swelling is not typically symmetrical and can affect either or both the upper or lower lips (Figure 2.2). There is often associated erythema and angular cheilitis (fissuring at the corners of the mouth).

Diagnosis of OFG is confirmed by histological changes in biopsies of affected sites, typically lip or buccal mucosa. From a clinical and histopathological perspective, there is substantial overlap between different granulomatous diseases, and the most common cause of OFG is Crohn's disease[1], although OFG often exists as a separate entity[2]. It may be associated with Melkersson–Rosenthal syndrome, or rarely with sarcoidosis or tuberculosis[3,4].

The prevalence of OFG is unknown, as there are no formal epidemiological data. Clusters of patients have been observed in Scotland, particularly around Glasgow,

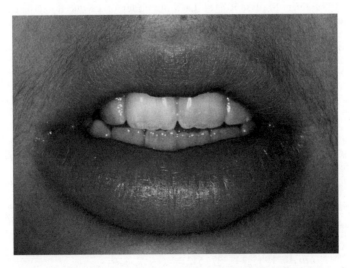

Figure 2.2   Swelling and erythema of the lower lip in a patient with orofacial granulomatosis (OFG). The upper lip shows no involvement.

and in Ireland, suggesting a Celtic predominance. Whether there is a genetic cause is still unclear[5], as there is conflicting and insufficient evidence. The pathogenesis of OFG is likely to be due to a delayed-type hypersensitivity reaction[5], which is supported by the fact that some patients with OFG are atopic[6].

Treatment is challenging but often follows a similar approach to that of Crohn's disease, using corticosteroids, immunosuppression, biological therapy and surgery. Evidence implicates a dietary antigen[7,8], and dietary manipulation may be useful, helping to avoid the use of medical therapy in many cases.

Food hypersensitivity in orofacial granulomatosis

Oral disease is often associated with contact hypersensitivity, and in OFG a delayed-type hypersensitivity reaction is recognised[5]. Between 12% and 60% of patients are atopic, which strengthens an association of OFG with food hypersensitivity[9]. Patients with OFG often report increased symptoms in response to various foods, food additives (particularly preservatives) and oral hygiene products. These reactions are predominantly delayed, and anecdotally a small number of patients report an immediate local 'tingling' reaction which precedes the typical OFG symptoms, e.g. lip swelling.

Cutaneous patch testing to evaluate symptoms in oral disease may be controversial[10]. Despite this, in patients with OFG and using the Standard European series and a few other substances, positive patch tests have been found to cinnamon, benzoic acid and benzoate salts (E210–E219), cinnamaldehyde and cocoa[11-13]. Other foods and food additives that have also been associated with OFG include wheat, dairy products, eggs, chocolate, peanuts, carbone piperitone, carvone, carmosine, tartrazine (E102), sunset yellow (E110) and monosodium glutamate (E621)[8,11,12,14-18]. Dental restorative materials have also been implicated[19-21].

There is currently insufficient evidence from *in vitro* and *in vivo* studies to suggest an immunological mechanism to the delayed hypersensitivity reaction, and no inflammatory or immunological mediators have been identified. Due to the wide range of precipitating factors, the antigen responsible for inducing symptoms may be different from one patient to the next, and may not always be dietary in origin.

Dietary management of orofacial granulomatosis

Food hypersensitivity in OFG has led to dietary treatments being used, sometimes even as first-line therapy[22]. Excluding foods identified from the results of positive patch tests led to an improvement in 'perceived' symptoms in 85% of patients[13]. Using an objective oral inflammatory activity score, a cinnamon- and benzoate-free diet (Table 2.10) followed for 12 weeks has been shown to lead to a clinical response in 68% (39/57) of patients with OFG[23].

Exclusion diets, such as a cinnamon- and benzoate-free diet, may be helpful in the management of OFG, and are often favoured over medical therapy due to the avoidance of associated side effects. Although data are limited, in patients where there has been some improvement in OFG symptoms following specific food exclusion diets,

Table 2.10 Cinnamon- and benzoate-free dietary advice

Food group	Foods to be avoided and ingredient/excipient labels to check*
Meat, poultry, fish and eggs	Dishes with a spicy sauce, ready-to-eat meals containing benzoates
Fruit and vegetables	Berries, nectarines, peaches, papaya, dried fruit, avocado, pumpkin, kidney beans, soybeans, broccoli and spinach; baked beans in tomato/spicy sauce
Cereals and cereal products	**Soya flour**; tinned spaghetti and ravioli in tomato/spicy sauce
Beverages	**Tea**, squash, cordial, carbonated drinks, milkshake syrup, ready-to-drink alcohol and mixers, spirits with added spices
Miscellaneous	Curry powder, all spice, mixed spice, **nutmeg**, **clove**, **cinnamon**, chocolate, cocoa, dry-roasted and spicy nuts, Bombay mix, crisps (except ready-salted), potato or corn snacks, ketchup, **soy sauce**, Worcestershire sauce, salad dressing, salad cream, mayonnaise
Dental care products	Tartar-control toothpastes, mouthwashes and oral hygiene products
Medicines	Tablets/capsules/liquids and vitamin/mineral supplements
Cosmetics	Make-up, lipstick, lip-gloss, cleanser, toner, moisturiser, shampoo, conditioner, shaving gel/cream, soap, body wash, shower gel, bath cream/foam, suntan lotion, aftersun, body lotion, hand cream

* Foods shown in bold may have naturally high levels of cinnamon or benzoates. Other food, beverages, dental care and cosmetic products listed should be checked and avoided if the ingredient or excipient labels contain the following: cinnamon, cinnamon oil, cinnamaldehyde, ground cinnamon, spices, spice extracts, mixed spice, E210 (benzoic acid), E211 (sodium benzoate), E212 (potassium benzoate), E213 (calcium benzoate), E214 (ethyl 4-hydroxybenzoate or ethyl para-hydroxybenzoate), E215 (ethyl 4-hydroxybenzoate, sodium salt or sodium ethyl para-hydroxybenzoate), E216 (propyl 4-hydroxybenzoate or propyl para-hydroxybenzoate), E217 (propyl 4-hydroxybenzoate, sodium salt or sodium para-hydroxybenzoate), E218 (methyl 4-hydroxybenzoate or methyl para-hydroxybenzoate), E219 (methyl 4-hydroxybenzoate, sodium salt or sodium methyl-hydroxybenzoate).

elemental or polymeric diets as a sole source of nutrition have been used with varying success[18,23]. One study demonstrated that intra-oral involvement rather than lip disease alone showed a clinical response using either a polymeric or an elemental formula for 6 weeks ($n = 8/12$)[23].

Cinnamon and benzoates in the diet

Cinnamon is a spice that has been used in cooking for thousands of years and is widely used in the food industry as a flavouring and a preservative, e.g. in breakfast cereals, desserts, chocolates and pastries. It is also often added to toothpaste and oral hygiene products. Cinnamon oil makes up 1–8% of cinnamon and provides the characteristic flavour. The pungent taste and smell comes from cinnamaldehyde, which has strong antimicrobial activity[24].

Benzoates occur naturally in some foods, particularly in berries, usually up to 0.05%[25], but in ripe fruits of the *Vaccinium* species (e.g. cranberries and bilberries) at higher concentrations of 0.03–0.13%[26] and in cinnamon at 0.3%[27]. Benzoic acid and benzoate salts are common ingredients in flavourings (e.g. chocolate) and may be used as permitted preservatives (E210–E219) up to a level of 0.1%, especially in carbonated and non-carbonated soft drinks. They are often used as flavourings in soft drinks, chewing gum, ice cream, cakes and spices. Benzoates may also be used in cosmetics, toothpaste and oral hygiene products. For more information on benzoates see Chapter 10.

Summary

A delayed-type food hypersensitivity reaction is recognised in OFG, although the immunological basis to this mechanism is not yet clear. Treatment with exclusion of dietary triggers, e.g. with a cinnamon- and benzoate-free diet, is useful in the management of symptoms but current data are based on a small numbers of cases. Due to the low numbers of OFG patients, management is ideally suited to a tertiary referral centre where there is a multidisciplinary team approach with expertise in oral medicine, gastroenterology, dietetics and psychology.

References

1. Wiesenfeld D, Ferguson MM, Mitchell DN *et al*. Oro-facial granulomatosis: a clinical and pathological analysis. *Q J Med* 1985; **54**: 101–13.
2. Sanderson J, Nunes C, Escudier M *et al*. Oro-facial granulomatosis: Crohn's disease or a new inflammatory bowel disease? *Inflamm Bowel Dis* 2005; **11**: 840–6.
3. Apaydin R, Bilen N, Bayramgurler D, Efendi H, Vahaboglu H. Detection of Mycobacterium tuberculosis DNA in a patient with Melkersson–Rosenthal syndrome using polymerase chain reaction. *Br J Dermatol* 2000; **142**: 1251–2.
4. James DG. Mimics of sarcoidosis. Oro-facial granulomatosis (Melkersson–Rosenthal syndrome). *Sarcoidosis* 1991; **8**: 84.
5. Tilakaratne WM, Freysdottir J, Fortune F. Orofacial granulomatosis: review on aetiology and pathogenesis. *J Oral Pathol Med* 2008; **37**: 191–5.
6. James J, Patton DW, Lewis CJ, Kirkwood EM, Ferguson MM. Oro-facial granulomatosis and clinical atopy. *J Oral Med* 1986; **41**: 29–30.
7. Ferguson MM, MacFadyen EE. Orofacial granulomatosis: a 10 year review. *Ann Acad Med Singapore* 1986; **15**: 370–7.
8. Reed BE, Barrett AP, Katelaris C, Bilous M. Orofacial sensitivity reactions and the role of dietary components: case reports. *Aust Dent J* 1993; **38**: 287–91.
9. Schafer T, Bohler E, Ruhdorfer S *et al*. Epidemiology of food allergy/food intolerance in adults: associations with other manifestations of atopy. *Allergy* 2001; **56**: 1172–9.
10. Torgerson RR, Davis MD, Bruce AJ, Farmer SA, Rogers RS III. Contact allergy in oral disease. *J Am Acad Dermatol* 2007; **57**: 315–21.
11. Taibjee SM, Prais L, Foulds IS. Orofacial granulomatosis worsened by chocolate: results of patch testing to ingredients of Cadbury's chocolate. *Br J Dermatol* 2004; **150**: 595.
12. Patton DW, Ferguson MM, Forsyth A, James J. Oro-facial granulomatosis: a possible allergic basis. *Br J Oral Maxillofac Surg* 1985; **23**: 235–42.
13. Wray D, Rees SR, Gibson J, Forsyth A. The role of allergy in oral mucosal diseases. *QJM* 2000; **93**: 507–11.
14. Armstrong DK, Biagioni P, Lamey PJ, Burrows D. Contact hypersensitivity in patients with orofacial granulomatosis. *Am J Contact Dermat* 1997; **8**: 35–8.
15. Oliver AJ, Rich AM, Reade PC, Varigos GA, Radden BG. Monosodium glutamate-related orofacial granulomatosis: review and case report. *Oral Surg Oral Med Oral Pathol* 1991; **71**: 560–4.

16. Pachor ML, Urbani G, Cortina P *et al*. Is the Melkersson–Rosenthal syndrome related to the exposure to food additives? A case report. *Oral Surg Oral Med Oral Pathol* 1989; **67**: 393–5.
17. Rees TD. Orofacial granulomatosis and related conditions. *Periodontol 2000* 1999; **21**: 145–57.
18. Sweatman MC, Tasker R, Warner JO, Ferguson MM, Mitchell DN. Oro-facial granulomatosis: response to elemental diet and provocation by food additives. *Clin Allergy* 1986; **16**: 331–8.
19. Guttman-Yassky E, Weltfriend S, Bergman R. Resolution of orofacial granulomatosis with amalgam removal. *J Eur Acad Dermatol Venereol* 2003; **17**: 344–7.
20. Lazarov A, Kidron D, Tulchinsky Z, Minkow B. Contact orofacial granulomatosis caused by delayed hypersensitivity to gold and mercury. *J Am Acad Dermatol* 2003; **49**: 1117–20.
21. Sciubba JJ, Said-Al-Naief N. Orofacial granulomatosis: presentation, pathology and management of 13 cases. *J Oral Pathol Med* 2003; **32**: 576–85.
22. White A, Nunes C, Escudier M *et al*. Improvement in orofacial granulomatosis on a cinnamon- and benzoate-free diet. *Inflamm Bowel Dis* 2006; **12**: 508–14.
23. Nunes C, Lomer MC, Escudier M *et al*. The dietary management of orofacial granulomatosis. *Gut* 2007; **56** (Suppl II): A117.
24. Friedman M, Kozukue N, Harden LA. Cinnamaldehyde content in foods determined by gas chromatography–mass spectrometry. *J Agric Food Chem* 2000; **48**: 5702–9.
25. Budavari S, O'Neil MJ, Smith A, Heckelman PE, Kinneary JF. *The Merck Index*, 12th edn. Rahway, NJ: Merck, 1996.
26. Hegnauer R. *Chemotaxonomie der Pflanzen*. Basel: Birkhäuser, 1966.
27. Heimhuber B, Herrmann K. Benzoe-, Phylessig-, 3-Phenylpropan- und Zimtsaure sowie Benzoylglucosen in einigen Obst- und Fruchtgemusearten. *Deutsche Lebensmittel Rundschau* 1990; **86**(7): 205–9.

2.4   The role of food hypersensitivity in behavioural disorders

2.4.1   Hyperactivity

Donna C. McCann

Introduction

One of the longest-running controversies in the area of food hypersensitivity and intolerance surrounds the question of whether modification of a child's diet has a beneficial impact on hyperactive behaviour in children. Three main dietary interventions emerged in the last century, and the most contentious of these was based on the proposal that a range of artificial food additives, such as artificial colours, flavourings and preservatives, trigger symptoms of hyperactivity or hyperkinesis in children. Benjamin Feingold, a paediatrician and allergist at the Kaiser Foundation Hospital in California, put forward this hypothesis in the 1970s on the basis of his observations of children with behavioural and learning disorders, and suggested that a diet free of such additives, the Kaiser Permanente Diet or Feingold Diet as it became more commonly known, could help in the treatment or prevention of hyperactivity in children. He claimed that about half of hyperactive children were sensitive to such additives and to natural salicylates[1].

Further diets which emerged in the wake of Feingold's diet and were also associated with beneficial effects on hyperactivity are the sugar elimination diet, for which there was shown to be little evidence in the limited research[2], and an even more restricted diet, an extension of Feingold's diet, the oligoantigenic or oligoallergenic ('few foods') diet, which eliminates not only artificial food additives but also a range of foods such as dairy products, nuts, wheat, egg, sugars and more[3,4]. This latter diet is more closely linked to the current concept of food allergy or IgE-mediated hypersensitivity than a diet free of artificial colours. However, despite evidence to the contrary, in the mind of the public there persists into the twenty-first century a link between 'allergy' to food additives and hyperactive behaviour.

History and prevalence of hyperactivity

The history of hyperactivity or hyperkinesis can be traced back to the start of the twentieth century, when a behavioural disorder was observed in children which was primarily marked by overactivity and deficits in sustained attention and inhibitory and moral control[5]. In the years that followed, however, the disorder became regarded as part of a broader syndrome encompassing a range of cognitive, behavioural and learning disorders with its basis in organic brain damage, although evidence of such damage was not always present. Hyperactivity emerged again in the late 1960s as a behavioural syndrome in its own right characterised by extreme levels of overactivity, restlessness, distractibility and short attention span relative to the normal developmental levels in children. Today more severe symptoms of overactivity, persistent impulsiveness and inattention are diagnosed as attention-deficit/hyperactivity disorder (ADHD)[6], or hyperkinetic disorder[7], a debilitating childhood psychiatric condition which can result in long-term educational and social disadvantage[8].

The worldwide pooled prevalence in young children and adolescents is 5.3%[9], and 4–10% when employing only the most recent diagnostic criteria for ADHD[10]. The strong contribution of genetic inheritance is generally acknowledged. There are also similar patterns of behaviour that may result from severe early deprivation, such as that experienced in institutional settings[11]. Current research is now focused on how both genetic and environmental influences impact on the course and development of the disorder[12]. Common treatments include behavioural therapy and pharmacotherapy with psychostimulants. However, there have been longstanding concerns surrounding the safety and use of such medication in young children.

Dietary interventions

When details of Feingold's elimination diet emerged in the mid-1970s, concern about the use of stimulant medication was already present, and growing particularly so for the parents of hyperactive children. His diet and hypothesis immediately gave rise to media interest and a flood of debate amongst the public, medical professionals and politicians. Major economic interests in the food industry, which profitably employed numerous food additives in the food manufacturing process for the purposes of colouring, flavouring, preserving, emulsifying and a range of other functions, also had a vested interest in the debate. Given the context at the time, and the presence of differing funding interests, studies and reviews relating to the issue would have been open to problems related to bias, and this, together with a range of other methodological shortcomings, may help to explain some conflicting and inconsistent findings in the early research literature.

A number of early reviews[13,14] and a 1983 meta-analysis by Kavale & Forness[15] concluded that diet modification was not an effective treatment for hyperactivity. The meta-analysis reviewed 23 studies and found non-significant treatment effects on behaviour both for diet modification and challenge with substances excluded from the diet. They quoted a range of methodological flaws in studies. However, even for a number of well-conducted double-blind placebo-controlled studies included in these reviews, negligible or questionable effects were found. The National Institutes of Health (1982) concluded that evidence from controlled trials showed a 'limited positive association' between elimination diets and decreased hyperactivity[16].

Role of food additives

From the late 1980s studies in the literature began to place more emphasis on the role played by food additives in triggering hyperactivity and its biological basis, and improved methodology was evident in the number and quality of double-blind placebo-controlled food challenge studies published. The subsequent publication of these additional relevant trials prompted further 'focused consideration of whether artificial food colours promote symptoms of hyperactivity'[17]. This meta-analysis of double-blind placebo-controlled trials focusing on the role of artificial food colours in promoting hyperactivity in children with hyperactive syndromes high-lighted a number of limitations of the earlier Kavale & Forness review[15], including the folding together in analysis of a range of studies and trials, both blind and non-blind, in hyperactive and non-hyperactive children and involving elimination and/or challenge with various foodstuffs.

Schab & Trinh's meta-analysis[17] revisited the studies included in the earlier review, omitted seven studies which did not meet their own stricter inclusion criteria, and included eight subsequently published studies together with two further studies which had been overlooked by the earlier review. Their comprehensive meta-analysis of 24 double-blind placebo-controlled trials investigating the effect of artificial food colours on behaviour in hyperactive children found a significant overall effect size of over one-quarter of a standard deviation, as opposed to the one-twentieth effect size reported by Kavale & Forness[15].

In relation to the question of whether the relationship between artificial food colours and behaviour was IgE- or pharmacologically mediated, Schab & Trinh[17] concluded that this remained unanswered. Following the publication of their review, however, a study was carried out on the Isle of Wight investigating the effects of a double-blind placebo-controlled artificial food colourings and benzoate preservative challenge on hyperactivity in a sample of children constituting 10% ($n = 277$) of the general population of 3-year-old children[18]. The researchers found a parentally reported significant effect of food colourings and the benzoate preservative on hyperactive behaviour, with subgroup analysis indicating no effect of atopy and/or prior levels of hyperactivity. The researchers concluded that if food additives have an effect, it is via a pharmacological effect best exemplified by non-IgE-dependent histamine release. This is consistent with evidence from a previous study finding no association between response and atopy[19] and studies linking responses to artificial food colours with IgE-independent histamine and other mediator release[20-22].

Following this, a further double-blind placebo-controlled food challenge was carried out on a community sample of 3-year-old ($n = 153$) and 8-year-old children ($n = 144$) in Southampton, employing an additive mix (Mix A) similar to that used in the Isle of Wight study together with another mix (Mix B) reflecting more current consumption of additives in such children[23]. The team also collected saliva samples from the children in order to investigate the role of possible genetic moderators. The main outcome measure was a global hyperactivity aggregate based on standardised scores of observed behaviours within educational settings, ratings by teachers and parents, plus, for 8/9-year-old children, a computerised test of attention. A significant effect of Mix A on behaviour was found for the 3-year-old children and of Mix B for the older children. The researchers concluded that artificial colours or a sodium benzoate preservative (or both) in the diet result in increased hyperactivity in 3-year-old and 8/9-year-old children in the general population. However, there was a wide variation in the effects of these additives on children's behaviour. Based on the proposal that the link between additives and behaviour is best characterised by non-IgE histamine release[18], the Southampton team investigated variants in genes associated with hyperactive behaviour, including genetic variants associated with the breakdown and clearance of histamine. They found that polymorphisms in the histamine N-methyltransferase gene moderated the impact of additives on behaviour[24]. This is consistent with histamine playing a mediating role in the effect of food additives on behaviour.

On the basis of the findings of the Southampton study, the accumulating evidence and various other considerations, the Foods Standards Agency (FSA) in the UK have recommended to UK Ministers that industry takes voluntary action to remove these artificial colours by 2009, and is pressing for action at a European Union level. However, the FSA acknowledged that the UK industry had already made great strides in removing such colours from food in response to consumer concerns[25].

Conclusions

The evidence suggests that food colours and possibly a preservative (sodium benzoate) can act to increase the hyperactivity level shown by some children. Across the population as a whole the effect is small (about a fifth of a standard deviation). For some children, however, the effect is more marked. It is not known what biological mechanism might mediate this effect, although it does appear that this is not an IgE-mediated allergic response. Instead, it looks as if non-IgE-mediated histamine release may play a role.

References

1. Feingold BF. Hyperkinesis and learning disabilities linked to artificial food flavors and colours. *Am J Nurs* 1975; **75**: 797–803.
2. Wolraich ML, Wilson DB, White JW. The effect of sugar on behaviour or cognition in children: a meta-analysis. *JAMA* 1995; **274**: 1617–21.
3. Kaplan BJ, McNicol J, Coute RA, Moghadam HK. Dietary replacement in preschool-aged hyperactive boys. *Pediatrics* 1989; **83**: 7–17.
4. Boris M, Mandel FS. Foods and additives are common causes of the attention deficit hyperactive disorder in children. *Ann Allergy* 1994; **72**: 462–8.
5. Still, GF. Some abnormal psychical conditions in children. *Lancet* 1902; i: 1008–12.
6. American Psychiatric Association. *Diagnostic and Statistical Manual of Mental Disorders*, 4th edn (DSM-IV). Washington, DC: APA, 1994.
7. World Health Organization. *The ICD-10 Classification of Mental and Behavioural Disorders: Diagnostic Criteria for Research*. Geneva: WHO, 1993.
8. Swanson J, Sergeant J, Taylor E *et al*. Attention deficit hyperactivity disorder and hyperkinetic disorder. *Lancet* 1998; **351**: 429–33.
9. Polanczyk G, de Lima MS, Horta BL, Biederman J, Rohde, LA. The worldwide prevalence of ADHD: a systematic review and metaregression analysis. *Am J Psychiatry* 2007; **164**: 942–8.
10. Skounti M, Philalithis A, Galanakis E. Variations in prevalence of attention deficit hyperactivity disorder worldwide. *Eur J Pediatr* 2007; **166**: 117–23.
11. Stevens SE, Sonuga-Barke EJS, Kreppner JM *et al*. Inattention/overactivity following early severe institutional deprivation: Presentation and associations in early adolescence. *J Abnorm Child Psychol* 2008; **36**: 385–98.
12. Asherson P, Kuntsi J, Taylor E. Unravelling the complexity of attention-deficit hyperactivity disorder: a behavioural genomic approach. *Br J Psychiatry* 2005; **187**: 103–5.
13. Williams JI, Cram DM. Diet in the management of hyperkinesis: a review of the tests of Feingold's hypotheses. *Can Psychiatr Assoc J* 1978; **23**: 241–8.
14. Wender EH. The food additive-free diet in the treatment of behaviour disorders: A review. *J Dev Behav Pediatr* 1986; 7: 35–42.
15. Kavale KA, Forness SR. Hyperactivity and diet treatment: a meta-analysis of the Feingold hypothesis. *J Learn Disabil* 1983; **16**: 324–30.
16. National Institutes of Health. Defined diets and childhood hyperactivity. *NIH Consensus Statement* 1982; 4: 1–11.
17. Schab DW, Trinh NT. Do artificial food colors promote hyperactivity in children with hyperactive syndromes? A meta-analysis of double-blind placebo-controlled trials. *J Dev Behav Pediatr* 2004; **25**: 423–34.
18. Bateman B, Warner JO, Hutchinson E *et al*. The effects of a double blind, placebo controlled, artificial food colourings and benzoate preservative challenge on hyperactivity in a general population sample of preschool children. *Arch Dis Child* 2004; **89**: 506–11.
19. Pollock I, Warner JO. Effect of artificial food colours on childhood behaviour. *Arch Dis Child* 1990; **65**: 74–7.
20. Supramaniam G, Warner JO. Artificial food additive intolerance in patients with angio-oedema and urticaria. *Lancet* 1986; **2**: 907–9.
21. Murdoch RD, Lessof MH, Pollock I, Young E. The effects of food additives on leukocyte histamine release in normal and urticarial subjects. *J R Coll Physicians Lond* 1987; **21**: 251–6.
22. Murdoch RD, Pollock I, Naeem S. Tartrazine induced histamine release in vivo in normal subjects. *J R Coll Physicians Lond* 1987; **21**: 257–61.
23. McCann D, Barrett A, Cooper A *et al*. Food additives and hyperactive behaviour in 3-year-old and 8/9-year-old children in the community: a randomised, double-blinded, placebo-controlled trial. *Lancet* 2007; **370**: 1560–7.
24. Food Standards Agency. Final technical report for additives and behaviour study submitted by School of Psychology, University of Southampton, 2007. www.food.gov.uk/multimedia/pdfs/additivesbehaviourfinrep.pdf.
25. Food Standards Agency. Food additives and hyperactivity: recommendation by the Executive to the Council of the FSA, 10 April 2008. www.food.gov.uk/multimedia/pdfs/board/fsa080404a.pdf.

2.4.2   Autism and autistic spectrum disorders

Zoe Connor

About autistic spectrum disorders

Autistic spectrum disorders (ASD) are common developmental disabilities that affect the way a person communicates and relates to people around them.

A diagnosis of ASD means that a person has impairments in each of the following areas, known as the 'triad of impairments':

- social interaction – difficulty with social relationships, e.g. appearing aloof and indifferent to other people and difficulty with understanding others' viewpoints and intentions;
- social communication – difficulty with verbal and non-verbal communication;
- imagination – difficulty with interpersonal play and imagination, e.g. having a limited range of imaginative activities, possibly copied and pursued rigidly and repetitively.

Autism is at the more profoundly affected end of the ASD spectrum, Asperger's syndrome is at the higher functioning end, and pervasive development disorder not otherwise specified (PDD-NOS) falls in between (this is a crude distinction; diagnosis is specified by international descriptors)[1,2]. Additionally, it is common for someone with ASD to have repetitive behaviour patterns, resistance to change in routine, and under- or oversensitivity to sensory stimuli. ASDs are lifelong conditions which are commonly managed by behavioural and educational techniques. Medical (pharmaceutical) management is usually limited to treatment of comorbidities, which may include attention-deficit/hyperactivity disorder (ADHD), motor coordination problems, anxiety and epilepsy.

Diet in the treatment of ASD

Interest in the use of dietary manipulation in the treatment of ASD dates back nearly 50 years. Dietary treatment of ASD and 'biomedical interventions' are often recommended by ASD organisations, but it is important to note that no specific diet is routinely recommended as treatment for ASD by medical and dietetic professionals, including the author of this sub-chapter. This is because there is insufficient research to prove that the benefit of trialling dietary changes outweighs the difficulty for individuals and their families in implementing these changes, and the risk to the individual's nutritional status.

Instances of biomedical interventions dramatically alleviating symptoms of ASD are commonly reported by ASD organisations, and so it is unsurprising that dietary changes are widely undertaken by parents of children diagnosed with ASD, often soon after diagnosis, and sometimes without medical or dietetic supervision. This chapter attempts to summarise the diets commonly advocated by ASD organisations, and to advise on a safe and practical way to approach them.

Overview of common food exclusions used as a 'treatment' for ASD

Gluten-free and casein-free diet (GFCF diet)

This is the most popular and best-known dietary intervention for ASD. ASD organisations often advocate strict avoidance of gluten, casein and similar proteins. Gluten is a protein contained in wheat, barley and rye, and a similar protein is found in oats. Bread, pizza, pasta, pastry, biscuits, some breakfast cereals and some processed foods contain gluten. Casein is a protein found in cow's milk, and similar proteins are found in goat's and sheep's milk. Yogurt, cheese, butter, some margarines, ice-cream, milk chocolate, biscuits and some processed products contain casein.

Some organisations recommend that casein is eliminated for a couple of weeks before gluten is additionally eliminated – due in part to reports of worsening of symptoms sometimes occurring for the first few days of eliminating a food. Organisations differ on how long elimination should last, with some saying improvements on avoiding casein are seen within 1–4 weeks, and gluten within 1–3 months, and others saying that it can take a year to see improvements in symptoms. Few organisations make the recommendation to trial the reintroduction of foods, but instead suggest long-term avoidance.

The GFCF diet is based on the theory that gluten and casein from the diet are poorly digested in the gut, are absorbed into the bloodstream through an abnormally 'leaky' gut, and then interfere with neurological processes in the brain in a way similar to opioids such as morphine[3].

No aspect of this theory has been proven, and although some studies have found that some individuals with ASD had improvements in communication and cognitive function on a GFCF diet, with regression on dietary challenge, a Cochrane review found insufficient evidence to recommend GFCF diets in the treatment of ASD[4].

Urine analyses are offered by organisations worldwide[5], with results being used as a basis for recommending a GFCF diet, based on the hypothesis that peaks found in the urine analysis of people with ASD are casein- and gluten-derived peptides. However, research by Cass *et al.* in 2008 could not corroborate this hypothesis[6].

Exclusion of phenolic compounds and foods high in salicylates

A low-salicylate and phenolic-compound diet is advocated by many ASD organisations. This involves the exclusion of a wide range of foods including cheese, chocolate, tomatoes, oranges, bananas, yeast extract, some food colourings and many other fruits and vegetables (the list of foods to avoid differs across organisations). A small sample of children with ASD have been found to have an impairment in enzymes that break down these compounds in the body[7]. This is hypothesised to lead to raised levels of neurotransmitters, which could affect symptoms of ASD. However, there is no evidence to support this, or to suggest that avoiding these foods is beneficial for ASD.

Yeast-free diet

Another approach advocated by many ASD organisations is based on the theory that yeast proliferation in the gut causes a 'leaky gut', a greater susceptibility to food allergies, and exacerbation of behavioural problems[8]. Organisations state that eating less yeast plus less sugar reduces the growth of these gut yeasts. Indeed, some individuals with ASD have been found to have higher levels of some 'unfriendly' gut bacteria[9], but there is no evidence that eating less sugar and dietary yeasts (which are not the same as gut yeasts) helps. Instead, gut bacterial overgrowth is commonly treated by prescribed medications. 'Yeast-free' diets differ across ASD organisations, but often exclude natural and refined sugars (including fruit), fermented foods such as breads, vinegar, alcohol, cheese, soya sauce, plus coffee and processed meats.

Exclusion of food additives
ASD organisations commonly advocate the avoidance of the flavour enhancer monosodium glutamate (MSG, E621) and the sweetener aspartame (E951). Some recommend the additional avoidance of all artificial colours, flavours and additives. The Feingold diet is a variation on this that involves the elimination of artificial colourings, flavourings and preservatives, as well as aspartame and salicylates[10].

It has been suggested that these additives affect the behaviour of people with ASD. This is not based on published evidence, although some artificial colours and preservatives have been linked to increased hyperactive behaviour in healthy children[11,12].

Dietary supplements
Some organisations suggest that people with ASD need particularly high 'therapeutic' doses of individual vitamins and minerals because of metabolic and biochemical abnormalities. This is not proven. Sometimes the suggested doses exceed the safe upper limit for adults, and little is known about long-term high doses in children[13].

Multiple elimination and supplementation diets
ASD organisations usually suggest a combination of the above 'biomedical interventions'. For example, a summary of recommended effective biomedical treatments based on the Defeat Autism Now! protocol[14] includes avoiding fried food, junk food, added sugar and artificial colours and preservatives, gluten, casein, corn, soya, simple carbohydrates and yeast products, plus taking multivitamin and mineral supplements including high doses of vitamins A, C, E and B vitamins, additional high doses of vitamin B6, omega-3 fatty acid supplements, digestive enzymes with each meal, antifungal medication and probiotics. This summary states that 'sometimes one treatment shows great benefit, but it is more common that each treatment helps a small amount. However the cumulative effect of multiple treatments can be substantial.' Other multiple intervention 'protocols' are the Sunderland protocol[15] and the Allergy Induced Autism Methodology[16]. Two other common ASD diets are the Body Ecology Diet (BED) and the Specific Carbohydrate Diet™ (SCD). The BED involves excluding gluten and processed foods, plus eating a number of special foods purported to 're-establish the intestinal flora and heal the body', such as fermented coconut juice and raw butter[17]. The SCD involves the elimination of grains, sucrose and lactose, with the theory that this will modify intestinal bacteria growth[18]. There is no evidence for the use of any of these interventions, or for the

cumulative effect of multiple dietary manipulations, but it is clear that diets that eliminate multiple foods put the individual at risk of a poorly balanced and nutritionally deficient diet.

Other dietary issues in ASD

It is common for children (and some adults) with ASD to have rigid eating patterns and a fear of trying unfamiliar foods. This sometimes results in faddy eating so severe that it causes nutritional deficiencies and affects growth. This can make implementing dietary changes very difficult, and increases the risk of nutrient deficiencies and growth faltering. Particular strategies for dealing with extreme faddy eating in ASD are covered in other texts[19,20], and on the author's website[21].

Gastrointestinal problems are common in ASD[22], (though possibly no more common than in the general population[23]); constipation may be under-recognised, and only fully revealed by abdominal x-ray[24]; and coeliac disease may be more common in ASD than in the general population[25].

Summary and recommendations

Summary of evidence for diet as a treatment for ASD

The professional consensus, both of a national group of UK dietitians who are experts in working with children and adults with ASD[26] and of the multi-agency guidance document the National Autism Plan[27], is that although there is insufficient evidence to recommend the use of any diet as a treatment for ASD, dietitians and other health professionals should provide support when an individual or their parents choose to try dietary changes. There are too many reports of children with ASD improving in behaviour and/or bowel habits after eliminating some foods for them to be discounted. However, the mechanism for this (until proven otherwise) is likely to be the same as for any general food intolerance, rather than any specific disorder that is particular to ASD, and so each case should be considered individually. For example, bowel problems such as diarrhoea or constipation can sometimes be caused by food intolerances, so individuals suffering from these might benefit from trying different food exclusions (medical causes should first be investigated by a doctor).

Drawbacks to implementing dietary changes

Implementing the often major changes to diet in the interventions described in this chapter can be expensive, disrupting to an individual's lifestyle, upsetting to an individual who is resistant to change (as is often the case in ASD), and without expert support from a health professional skilled in nutritional management (e.g. a registered dietitian) may lead to an insufficiently nutritious diet. Younger children and children with rigid eating preferences are particularly at risk from nutrient deficiencies and faltering growth, and this risk increases with the more foods that are excluded. Therefore biomedical interventions should be seen as short-term trials, to be pursued long-term only if medical or behavioural benefits are clearly seen for the individual.

Recommendations for trialling dietary changes

If food exclusion is to be considered, then the following may be worth a trial exclusion: caffeine, artificial colours and preservatives, mammalian milk, gluten. Before trialling food avoidances, expert advice should be sought on assessment of dietary adequacy and growth, how to avoid hidden sources of foods such as milks and gluten, and ideas of foods to replace those avoided. Advice on the need for vitamin and mineral supplements, for example calcium supplements for individuals following milk-free diets who do not like eating other good sources of calcium, should also be obtained.

Avoidance of each food or food group for 2 weeks should be long enough to see improvements in gastrointestinal problems, but individuals may prefer to wait 4 weeks to rule out any improvement in behavioural problems. It may be advisable to have a blood test for coeliac disease before undertaking a gluten-free diet, to rule out this medical cause of gluten intolerance, as the test is not reliable once gluten is being avoided.

To trial dietary changes, one food only should be excluded at a time and a diary kept of symptoms (e.g. bowel habits, behaviour, sleep pattern) before and after the change, then after reintroducing the previously excluded food. By carefully monitoring symptoms, it is then possible to identify any foods that are exacerbating symptoms. If possible, no other changes should be attempted at the same time, including introducing any therapeutic vitamin or mineral supplements or any new behavioural techniques.

Reintroduction of foods is essential to show (or rule out) that a food is responsible for exacerbating behavioural or gastrointestinal problems. If the reintroduction does cause a behavioural or gut reaction, then the food can be avoided longer-term, but it is a good idea to plan to try reintroducing it again every 3–6 months, as sometimes, particularly with children, food intolerance is grown out of. Sometimes a certain amount of a food can be tolerated, but above this amount it exacerbates symptoms, e.g. a glass of milk a day is fine, but more than this causes diarrhoea. Other people find they can tolerate particular products, e.g. goat's milk or UHT milk or yogurt, but not pasteurised cow's milk. In these cases it is fine to continue having only the tolerated amount or types of food.

If there is ever a severe reaction to a food, which involves swelling of the mouth or throat, that food should be strictly avoided and medical advice sought.

References

1. World Health Organization. *The ICD-10 Classification of Mental and Behavioural Disorders: Diagnostic Criteria for Research*. Geneva: WHO, 1993.
2. American Psychiatric Association. *Diagnostic and Statistical Manual of Mental Disorders*, 4th edn (DSM-IV). Washington, DC: APA, 1994.
3. Reichelt KL, Knivsberg AM, Lind G *et al*. The probable etiology and possible treatment of childhood autism. *Brain Dysfunct* 1991; 4: 308–19.
4. Millward C, Ferriter M, Calver S, Connell-Jones G. Gluten- and casein-free diets for autistic spectrum disorder. *Cochrane Database Syst Rev* 2008; (2): CD003498.
5. Autism Research Unit (ARU), University of Sunderland. osiris.sunderland.ac.uk/autism.
6. Cass H, Gringras P, March J *et al*. Absence of urinary opioid peptides in children with autism. *Arch Dis Child* 2008; 93: 745–50.

7. Alberti A, Pirrone P, Elia M *et al.* Sulphation deficit in 'low functioning' autistic children: a pilot study. *Biolog Psych* 1999; **46**: 420–4.
8. Shaw W. *Biological Treatments for Autism and PDD: What's Going On? What Can You Do about It?* Kansas: Great Plains Laboratory, 1998.
9. Finegold SM, Molitoris D, Song Y *et al.* Gastrointestinal microflora studies in late-onset autism. *Clin Infect Dis* 2002; **35**: S6–16.
10. Feingold Association of the United States. www.feingold.org
11. Bateman B, Warner JO, Hutchinson E *et al.* The effects of a double blind, placebo controlled, artificial food colourings and benzoate preservative challenge on hyperactivity in a general population sample of preschool children. *Arch Dis Child* 2004; **89**: 506–11.
12. McCann D, Barrett A, Cooper A *et al.* Food additives and hyperactive behaviour in 3-year-old and 8/9-year-old children in the community: a randomised, double-blinded, placebo-controlled trial. *Lancet* 2007; **370**: 1560–7.
13. Expert Group on Vitamins and Minerals Safe Upper Levels for Vitamins and Minerals. London: Food Standards Agency, 2003.
14. Adams JB. Summary of biomedical treatments for autism. ARI publication 40, April 2007. www.autism.com/treatable/adams_biomed_summary.pdf. Accessed April 2008.
15. Shattock P, Whiteley P. The Sunderland protocol: a logical sequencing of biomedical interventions for the treatment of autism and related disorders. osiris.sunderland.ac.uk/autism/durham2.htm. Accessed April 2008.
16. Autism Medical. Forum and resources. www.autismmedical.com/gateway_2/forum-and-resources (subscription-only access).
17. Body Ecology Diet. www.bodyecologydiet.com. Accessed April 2008.
18. Specific Carbohydrate Diet. www.breakingtheviciouscycle.info. Accessed April 2008.
19. Connor Z. *Diet and Autistic Spectrum Disorder.* British Dietetic Association Food Fact Sheet. www.bda.uk.com/foodfacts/0609Autism.pdf. Accessed August 2008.
20. Connor Z. Autistic spectrum disorders. In: Shaw V, Lawson M, eds. *Clinical Paediatric Dietetics*, 3rd edn. Oxford: Blackwell, 2007: 504–23.
21. Connor Z. *Nutritionnutrition: autism.* www.nutritionnutrition.com. Accessed April 2008.
22. Horvath K, Papadimitriou JC, Rabsztyn A *et al.* Gastrointestinal abnormalities in children with autistic disorder. *J Pediatr* 1999; **135**: 559–63.
23. Black C, Kaye JA, Jick H. Relation of childhood gastrointestinal disorders to autism: nested case-control study using data from the UK General Practice Research Database. *BMJ* 2002; **325**: 419–21.
24. Afzal N, Murch S, Thirrupathy K, *et al.* Constipation with acquired megarectum in children with autism. *Pediatrics* 2003; **112**: 939–42.
25. Barcia G, Posar A, Santucci M, Parmeggiani A. Autism and coeliac disease [letter]. *J Autism Dev Disord* 2008; **38**: 407–8.
26. Isherwood E, Thomas K. Professional Consensus Statement on the Dietary Management of Autism Spectrum Disorder, September 2002. Accessed from members' area at www.bda.uk.com.
27. Le Couteur A. *National Autism Plan for Children (NAPC).* National Initiative for Autism: Screening and Assessment. London: National Autistic Society, 2003. www.nas.org.uk/content/1/c4/34/54/NIASARep.pdf.

2.5   The role of food hypersensitivity in neurological disorders

2.5.1   Chronic fatigue syndrome/ME

Sue Luscombe

CFS/ME is a disabling, chronic illness classified by the World Health Organization as a neurological disorder[1]. In full, CFS/ME stands for chronic fatigue syndrome/

myalgic encephalomyelitis or encephalopathy. However, even the name is subject to disagreement and debate among medical and healthcare professionals, ME patient organisations and sufferers. Diagnosis is made by excluding other causes of the symptoms, as there is no specific diagnostic test. Despite also being recognised by many CFS/ME experts internationally as a genuine physiological illness[2,3] it is still regarded by some in the medical profession as primarily psychological in origin.

Allergy or intolerance?

Food hypersensitivities (food allergies and food intolerances) are widely reported by people with CFS/ME[4–6], and there is need for more research in this area. In one survey 73% of the people reported diet therapy (unspecified) helped with their symptoms, and also 80% were concerned about allergy issues[7]. In another survey involving 354 people with ME, 59% found dietary changes helpful[8]. The mechanisms of food hypersensitivity in this illness are poorly understood. There are contradictory results between self-reported food allergies and research studies into CFS/ME and IgE-mediated allergy. More recent research evidence suggests that IgE-mediated allergy is no more common in CFS/ME than in the normal population[9–11]. On the other hand, in one small study of 24 CFS patients it was reported that atopy coexisted in more than 50%[12]. Also, Brunet and colleagues described the detection of delayed-type hypersensitive responses to certain common environmental antigens in almost 50% of patients with CFS[13]. However, it is more likely that most adverse food reactions in CFS/ME are not IgE-mediated food allergies but rather food intolerances involving other mechanisms.

Causes of CFS/ME

No single cause has been identified to explain the development of CFS/ME. A wide variety of immune system abnormalities have been reported, but with no consistent pattern of abnormalities[14]. One study has shown reproducible alterations in gene regulation[15], and a possible association between human leucocyte antigen (HLA) class II antigens and immune dysfunction in the condition has been described[16].

Some patients report a preceding acute illness, often of an infectious nature, such as a specific influenza-like illness, streptococcal pharyngitis, gastroenteritis, glandular fever or sinusitis. In others, onset is more gradual. Patients frequently report onset at times of stressful life events in conjunction with infection, physical injury or exposure to immunisations or environmental toxins.

Prevalence of CFS/ME

Evidence suggests that[2,17]:

- the population prevalence is 0.2–0.4%;
- the most common age of onset is between the early twenties and mid-forties;

- in children, the most common age of onset is between 13 and 15 years, but cases have occurred in children of 5 or even younger;
- it is twice as common in women as in men;
- it affects all social classes to a similar extent;
- it affects all ethnic groups.

Symptoms of CFS/ME

The way in which patients describe their fatigue is very different to normal tiredness. Symptoms and their severity range greatly over time and from person to person. Those who are mildly affected can attend school or university, or go out to work, although they may need to reduce hours of work. The very severely affected can be completely bed-bound, unable to carry out any daily care such as washing and feeding, or tolerate any sensory input in the form of noise, light or strong smells such as perfumes. Symptoms include[18]:

- debilitating fatigue, both physical and mental is typically exacerbated by exercise or activity, which can have a delayed impact. Difficulties with concentration, memory and word-finding accompany the fatigue. This may mean there are limits to the time a patient can participate in a consultation;
- severe malaise, sore throat and tender lymph nodes;
- headaches, which can be severe and prolonged;
- sleep disturbances;
- myalgia (muscle pain) and/or arthralgia (joint pain), at rest and with exercise;
- irritable bowel symptoms, e.g. bloating, diarrhoea, constipation, nausea, abdominal pain.

Other symptoms can include:

- increased sensitivity to light, noise and smells;
- weight loss or weight gain;
- food intolerances;
- alcohol intolerance;
- increased sensitivity to drugs and household chemicals.

Prognosis

A systematic review of studies on the progress and prognosis of the condition suggested that patients with acute onset of illness have a better outcome than those with gradual onset[19]. Overall, the duration of illness appears to be shorter in younger people than among adults, and a higher proportion of children recover. Most people with the illness can expect some degree of improvement with time and good management of symptoms. A positive attitude towards recovery is therefore important. This involves healthy and positive food choices to ensure a good nutritional intake. Appropriate diet manipulation where IBS symptoms, food hypersensitivities or weight loss are occurring will also help. However, there is no evidence that diet interventions are primary factors in the rate of recovery.

Diet management

There are many potential difficulties in achieving adequate and balanced dietary intake in people with CFS/ME, especially in those most severely affected[20]. These arise because:

- pain and fatigue make the physical process of eating difficult;
- sensitivity to smell or taste of food may be experienced;
- nausea affects appetite;
- abnormal bowel symptoms may be experienced – diarrhoea, constipation or both, with or without bloating;
- food intolerances, especially if self-imposed or non-medically diagnosed, lead to food restrictions.

Positive nutritional management includes:

- encouraging the consumption of a healthy balanced diet (in line with the Food Standards Agency 'Eatwell' model);
- eating small frequent meals and snacks containing starchy food. This may help to improve a patient's energy levels;
- managing IBS symptoms (a significant proportion of sufferers will experience gastrointestinal symptoms such as nausea and bowel disturbances. See the section on IBS management for more guidance, although there is no research specifically on IBS treatment in CFS/ME);
- avoiding drinking fluids at meal times and instead sipping these in between meals, since there is some evidence that people with CFS/ME may have delayed gastric emptying times[21];
- assessing the diets of patients with self-reported or non-medically diagnosed food intolerance to ensure that their nutritional intake is not compromised;
- restricting caffeine intake for those who have sleep disturbances.

Popular diets

There are a number of diet theories claiming to promote recovery and relieve CFS/ME symptoms. Many of these theories in the popular press and on the internet are based on theories of food intolerances citing personal testimony/anecdotal evidence rather than scientific research, and they are medically unproven. Some of the diets exclude multiple foods and can make life even harder because of the extra effort needed to shop, and to prepare unfamiliar foods. There is also the danger that, by omitting basic food items, the diet can become nutritionally inadequate. Referral to a dietitian should be made where there is concern about weight maintenance or nutritional inadequacy.

Sometimes high-potency or mega doses of vitamin and mineral supplements are advocated, and some such supplements contain very high levels of nutrients. There is no evidence that these are useful[6,22]. It is particularly important to avoid large doses of vitamin B_6 and also fat-soluble vitamins such as vitamin A[23]. Vitamin B_6 in large doses (more than 200 mg a day) can lead to peripheral neuropathy. Too much vitamin A (over 1.5 mg a day) can make bones more likely to fracture when older, and in pregnancy may harm the unborn baby. If there is uncertainty on the adequacy of the diet, recommending a supplement of no more than 100% of the recommended daily intake would be a safer alternative.

Low-sugar, low-yeast (anti-Candida) diet

This approach is popular amongst CFS/ME sufferers, advocated in numerous articles and books. It is based on the contentious theory that colonisation of *Candida* is a major problem in CFS/ME and that recovery is aided by use of anti-fungal drugs, while at the same time cutting out foods containing yeast and sugar. The claim has been refuted by the medical profession as speculative and unproven[24,25]. The low-sugar, low-yeast (anti-*Candida*) diet has been subject to a recent controlled clinical trial, involving 52 people with CFS/ME[26]. The conclusion from this research is that the anti-*Candida* programme is of no more value in the treatment of CFS/ME than eating a healthy diet. However, there was a high drop-out from the trial (partly due to the severe diet restrictions), and with fairly small numbers further work is needed to be conclusive. There are some who report benefit with either energy levels or symptoms from following this diet. This may be because the person is avoiding highly processed and sugary foods, and eating more regularly and healthily.

Conclusions

Although there is a common belief among people with CFS/ME that food allergies and intolerances are widespread, there is a lack of epidemiological studies to confirm prevalence. Current evidence suggests that, although there is an increase in prevalence of allergies in the general population, this is no greater in people with CFS/ME. More research is needed into food hypersensitivities in CFS/ME. However, many who suffer from CFS/ME have already tried diet changes to improve symptoms. Care should be taken that the nutritional status is not compromised, and, where there are concerns, assessment by an appropriately qualified practitioner such as a dietitian is important.

References

1. World Health Organization. *International Statistical Classification of Diseases and Related Health Problems* (ICD-10). Geneva: WHO, 1994.
2. Department of Health. A report of the CFS/ME working group: report to the Chief Medical Officer of an independent working group. London: Department of Health, 2002.

3. Centers for Disease Control and Prevention. *Chronic Fatigue Syndrome Toolkit: Fact Sheets for Healthcare Professionals*. Atlanta, GA: CDC, 2006. www.cdc.gov/CFS/toolkit.htm. Accessed August 2008.

4. Loblay RH, Swain AR. The role of food intolerance in chronic fatigue syndrome. In: Hyde BM, ed. *The Clinical and Scientific Basis of Myalgic Encephalomyelitis/Chronic Fatigue Syndrome*. New York, NY: Nightingale Research Foundation, 1992.

5. Royal Australasian College of Physicians. Chronic fatigue syndrome: clinical practice guidelines. *Med J Aust* 2002; **176**: S19–55.

6. National Institute for Health and Clinical Excellence. *Chronic Fatigue Syndrome/Myalgic Encephalomyelitis (or Encephalopathy): Diagnosis and Management of CFS/ME in Adults and Children*. Clinical Guideline 53. London: NICE, 2007.

7. Cooper L. Report on survey of local ME groups (unpublished, 2000). Cited in NICE Guideline 53 (2007).

8. Action for ME members survey: your view and experiences (unpublished, 2003). Cited in NICE Guideline 53 (2007).

9. Repka-Ramirez MS, Naranch K, Park YJ, Velarde A. IgE levels are the same in chronic fatigue syndrome (CFS) and control subjects when stratified by allergy skin test results and rhinitis types. *Ann Allergy Asthma Immunol* 2001; **87**: 218–21.

10. Kowal K, Schacterele RS, Schur PH, Komaroff AL, DuBuske LM. Prevalence of allergen-specific IgE among patients with chronic fatigue syndrome. *Allergy Asthma Proc* 2002; **23**: 35–9.

11. Ferre Ybarz L, Cardona Dahl V, Cadahia Garcia A *et al*. [Prevalence of atopy in chronic fatigue syndrome]. *Allergol Immunopathol Madrid*. 2005; **33**: 42–7.

12. Straus SE, Dale JK, Wright R, Metcalfe DD. Allergy and the chronic fatigue syndrome. *J Allergy Clin Immunol* 1988; **81**: 791–5.

13. Brunet JL, Fatoohi F, Liaudet AP, Cozon GJ. The role of delayed pathology hypersensitivity in the syndrome of chronic fatigue: value of the evaluation of lymphocyte activation by flow cytometry. *Allerg Immunol (Paris)* 2002; **34** (2): 38–44.

14. Lyall M, Peakman M, Wessely S. A systematic review and critical evaluation of the immunlogy of chronic fatigue syndrome. *J Psychosom Res* 2003; **55**: 79–90.

15. Kaushik N, Fear D, Richards SCM *et al*. Gene expression in peripheral blood mononuclear cells from patients with chronic fatigue syndrome. *J Clin Pathol* 2005; **58**: 826–32.

16. Smith J, Fritz EL, Kerr JR *et al*. Association of chronic fatigue syndrome with human leucocyte antigen class II alleles. *J Clin Pathol* 2005; **58**: 860–3.

17. Royal College of Paediatrics and Child Health. *Evidence Based Guideline for the Management of CFS/ME (Chronic Fatigue Syndrome/Myalgic Encephalopathy) in Children and Young People*. London: RCPCH, 2004.

18. Fukuda K, Straus SE, Hickie I *et al*. The chronic fatigue syndrome: a comprehensive approach to its definition and study. *Ann Intern Med* 1994; **121**: 953–9.

19. Joyce J, Hotopf M, Wessely S. The prognosis of chronic fatigue and chronic fatigue syndrome: a systematic review. *QJM* 1997; **90**: 223–33.

20. Harding J. Chronic fatigue syndrome/myalgic encephalopathy. In: Thomas B, Bishop J, eds. *Manual of Dietetic Practice*, 4th edn. Oxford: Blackwell, 2007.

21. Burnet RB, Chatterton BE. Gastric emptying is slow in chronic fatigue syndrome. *Gastroenterology* 2004; **4**: 32.

22. Chambers D, Bagnall AM, Hempel S, Forbes C. Interventions for the treatment, management and rehabilitation of patients with chronic fatigue syndrome/myalgic encephalomyelitis: an updated systematic review. *J R Soc Med* 2006; **99**: 506–20.

23. Food Standards Agency. Eat well, be well: vitamin A. www.eatwell.gov.uk/healthydiet/nutritionessentials/vitaminsandminerals/vitamina. Accessed August 2008.

24. American Academy of Allergy and Immunology. Candidiasis hypersensitivity syndrome. *J Allergy Clin Immunol* 1986; **78**: 271–3.

25. Morris DH, Stare FJ Unproven diet therapies in the treatment of the chronic fatigue syndrome. *Arch Fam Med*. 1993; **2**: 181–6.

26. Hobday RA, Thomas S, O'Donovan A, Murphy M, Pinching AJ. Dietary intervention in chronic fatigue syndrome. *J Hum Nutr Diet* 2008; **21**: 141–9.

2.5.2 Migraine

Susan Thurgood

Migraine is the most common neurological disorder, affecting approximately 15% of the Western population[1]. Migraine headaches are severe and incapacitating, causing interruption to daily life. Various factors, including food, stress, menses, environmental changes, smoking and exercise, have been linked to the precipitation of migraine[2]. Unfortunately the determination of the foods that trigger migraine in an individual patient can be very time-consuming and susceptible to bias, with the added problem that spontaneous remission is common in migraine patients. Headaches in children are common, with migraine affecting 3–10% of children in the UK[3].

The pathophysiology of migraine and migraine triggers

A migraine attack is usually characterised by a severe unilateral headache accompanied by nausea, vomiting, photo- and/or phonophobia. Some people have early symptoms indicating the onset of an attack known as prodromes, which usually occur about 24 hours before the actual headache starts. Prodromes can be in the form of changes in mood, alertness or appetite. Approximately 30% of migraine sufferers have an aura: these can be visual or sensory and accompanied by speech disturbances. Mechanisms underlying migraine precipitation are largely unknown, but understanding the aura and headache components of migraine provides a basis for understanding the potential effect of possible dietary triggers. The primary event is neuronal, with sensitisation of trigeminal nerve ganglia. A secondary phase of vasoconstriction, vasodilation and vascular inflammation is mediated by chemical neurotransmitters, especially serotonin receptors. The cause of migraine in children is unknown, but a family history is common.

Dietary migraine triggers may influence the pathophysiology at one or more stages of the attack. Evaluation of the role of diet in migraine is complex because multiple triggers and variables may modify the threshold to pain in an individual[4]. In patient-based studies of adults and children the percentage of patients reporting a particular dietary trigger varied from 7%[5] to 44%[6], and a wide variety of foods was reported, the most common being chocolate, cheese, citrus fruit and alcoholic drinks[7]. Studies concluded that cheese, chocolate and red wine sensitivity, in particular, may have closely related mechanisms[8].

Migraine is commonly thought to be caused by a pharmacological adverse reaction to food[9] in which substances in a food may cause modulations in vascular tone and induce migraine in susceptible individuals.

Biogenic amines

Biogenic amines, including histamine and serotonin, are vasoactive compounds naturally found in foods, particularly in fermented products such as cheese and wine and in certain fish and meat that have been poorly stored (Table 2.11; see also

Table 2.11   Foods rich in histamine/tyramine[13].

Foods		Histamine (mg/kg)	Tyramine (mg/kg)
Fish			ND
Mackerel	(frozen)	1–20	
	(smoked or salted)	1–1788	
	(canned)	ND–210	
Herring	(frozen)	1–4	
	(smoked or salted)	5–121	
	(canned)	1–402	
Sardine	(frozen)	ND	
	(smoked or salted)	14–150	
	(canned)	3–2000	
Tuna	(frozen)	ND	
	(smoked or salted)	ND	
	(canned)	1–402	
Cheese			
Gouda		10–900	10–900
Camembert		0–1000	0–4000
Cheddar		0–2100	0–1500
Emmental		5–2500	0–700
Parmesan		10–581	0–840
Meat			
Fermented sausage		ND–650	ND–1237
Salami		1–654	
Fermented ham		38–271	123–618
Vegetables			
Sauerkraut		0–229	2–951
Spinach		30–60	
Aubergine		26	
Tomato ketchup		22	
Red wine vinegar		4	
Alcohol			
Red wine		ND–30	ND–25
Top-fermented beer		ND–14	1.1–36.4
Bottom-fermented beer		ND–17	0.5–46.8
Champagne		670	

ND, not detected

Chapter 10). Many people have reported wine as a trigger for migraine headaches[10]. Although one study found no correlation between wine intolerance and histamine level[11], it was noted that wine contains other possible triggers including tyramine, phenolic flavinoids and sulphites. Histamine is not destroyed at high temperatures (210 °C) and so may not be denatured by cooking[12].

In healthy individuals histamine, derived from the amino acid histidine, acts as a neurotransmitter and is metabolised in two ways: by amine oxidases, mainly diamine oxidase (DAO)[14], located in the jejunal mucosa, and by histamine-N-methyltransferase. Impaired histamine degradation due to reduced DAO activity causes a raised histamine level, resulting in a variety of symptoms including headache[15]. These symptoms mimic an allergic reaction, which is sometimes referred to as a pseudoallergic food reaction[16].

There are a number of studies associating histamine with migraine precipitation[17]. Histamine-induced headache is a vascular headache at least partially mediated by nitric oxide (NO)[18], and sequential infusions of histamine have been shown to provoke a dose-dependent headache in migraine patients and healthy individuals[19,20]. Migraine patients can have raised plasma histamine levels during both headaches and symptom-free periods, while some display histamine intolerance, with reduced DAO activity, and symptoms that can be triggered by histamine-rich foods (Table 2.11). A histamine-free diet[21] or antihistamines[22] can alleviate these symptoms[23]. Approximately 1% of the population has been shown to have histamine intolerance[24].

Another of the biogenic amines, serotonin, has been shown in several studies to fluctuate in migraine[25]. These amines are all substrates for the phenol sulphotransferase enzymes, and low levels of these enzymes have been found in migraine patients[26], although this may be an effect of migraine rather than a cause. However, a variety of foodstuffs has been shown to inhibit the sulphotransferases *in vitro*[27].

A review of current literature showed no relationship between consumption of biogenic amines and food intolerance reactions including migraine[28]. In patients with migraine triggered by amine-containing foods, amine intolerance should be considered, and advice on avoidance of high-amine foods should be given[13].

Trace amines

The hypothesis that trace amines such as tyramine, octopamine and synephrine, which are closely related to the classic biogenic amines, may contribute to the pathogenesis of primary headache was suggested several years ago[29]. Tyramine is, in comparison with other amines, biochemically unstable and is rapidly metabolised to octopamine or catabolised by monoamine oxidase (MAO) activity[30]. In foods, it is produced by the decarboxylation of tyrosine during fermentation or decay. Foods containing considerable amounts of tyramine include meats that are potentially spoiled or pickled, aged, smoked, fermented or marinated, and fermented foods such as cheeses. Synephrine has been found in significant levels in Seville orange juice[31], and along with octopamine has also been found in other citrus fruit.

Hannington in 1967 observed that foods high in tyramine caused a hypertensive headache response in depressed patients who were treated with monoamine oxidase inhibitors, and raised the possibility that increased sensitivity to tyramine-containing foods in migraine might be due to a deficiency of MAO activity[32]. At present this is still controversial. A recent review[26] cited six controlled studies with positive results (mostly by Hannington), and three showing negative results[33]. In 2001 a class of G-protein-coupled receptors with an affinity for trace amines, trace amine-associated receptors (TAAR), were discovered in various tissues and organs including specific brain areas, which may lead to further understanding of the mechanisms involved[34].

A recent study found that patients with primary headache had significantly elevated levels of trace amines such as octopamine and synephrine compared to a control group, while following a trace-amine-restricted diet[35].

One of the most commonly cited food triggers is chocolate[36]. Chocolate is especially rich in a variety of vasoactive amines including beta-phenylethylamine (βPEA), which can cross the blood–brain barrier and can effect cerebral flow[37]. βPEA is metabolised by MAO, and headache may be related to a deficient metabolism, but in a double-blind placebo-controlled food challenge (DBPCFC), chocolate did not appear to play a significant role in triggering headaches[38].

There are at present a number of hypotheses as to the mechanism involved, but the high circulating trace amine levels may represent an abnormal biochemical phenotypic trait accompanying migraine. An increase in brain mast cells is associated with pathological conditions such as migraine.

Aspartame

The artificial sweetener aspartame has been linked as a migraine trigger in a subpopulation[39]. In studies involving DBPCFC, headaches were significantly more frequent during aspartame consumption over a 14–24 day period[40,41]. A recent study suggested high intakes of aspartame may have neurological effects[42]. This group may benefit from advice on avoiding aspartame, including migraine medication containing aspartame[43].

Monosodium glutamate

Monosodium glutamate (MSG) has a widespread reputation for eliciting a variety of symptoms including an ability to trigger a migraine headache. There are no consistent data, however, to support this relationship. Although there have been reports of an MSG-sensitive subset of the population, this has not been demonstrated in placebo-controlled trials[44], though one study suggested that large doses of MSG given without food have precipitated migraine in susceptible individuals[45] (see also Chapter 10).

Important nutritional precipitants

Controlled trials suggest that alcohol, withdrawal of caffeine (a methylxanthine derivative) and relative hypoglycaemia[46] are the most important nutritional precipitating factors of migraine. In addition, there is some evidence that missing meals is an important factor, and dehydration deserves more attention.

Food allergy

A close association between migraine and allergic disease has been shown in a number of studies[47]. Migraine sufferers with a history of allergy have been found to have significantly higher total IgE levels, suggesting an influence of an IgE-mediated mechanism on migraine[48] in this group, but there is no real evidence for an association with serum IgE levels and migraine in non-atopic patients[4]. Also, the majority of clinical studies show no change in serum levels of immunoglobulins IgA, IgG or IgM or in complement levels in migraineurs[49]. There appears to be a decreased lymphocyte phagocytotic capacity and increased TNF-α, which may help to provide an explanation for the increased susceptibility to infection in this group[50]. It has been suggested in a prospective audit that food intolerances mediated by IgG antibodies may play a part in the development of migraine, and that changing the diet to eradicate identified foods improved migraine symptoms[51].

There has been one study in which a susceptible patient reported severe migraine 12–14 hours after DBPCFC with wheat[52]. Some studies have shown approximately 4% of patients with migraine have coeliac disease, and a gluten-free diet led to improvement in the migraine in these patients[53].

A number of studies have shown no diagnostic value for skin prick test (SPT) or measurement of total IgE in adults, although elimination diets may show a possible association between food and migraine[54]. However, studies in children seem to show a more predictive use of SPT[55]: 87% of children who had a positive SPT improved after following the resulting elimination diet[56]. In an well-conducted study in 1983, 93% of 88 children with severe, frequent migraine improved on an oligoantigenic diet, which typically consisted of one meat (lamb or chicken), one carbohydrate (rice or potato), one fruit (banana or apple) and one vegetable (a brassica)[57].

Abdominal migraine

Abdominal migraine is a form of migraine seen mainly in children. It is seen in approximately 5% of children[58], most commonly between the ages of 5 and 9 years, but it can also occur in adolescents and adults. Abdominal migraine consists primarily of abdominal pain, nausea and vomiting, but there is a lack of clear diagnostic criteria, although those criteria that are available exclude children with symptoms suggestive of food intolerance.

Not every child with abdominal pain suffers from abdominal migraine[59]. One subgroup of children with abdominal pain that is widely recognised by paediatricians is those with periodic syndrome, a term used to describe children who suffer from episodic symptoms including pallor, headache, abdominal pain and vomiting, and who experience complete resolution of these symptoms between attacks[60]. It has been noted that symptoms continued to manifest themselves in adult life in the form of vomiting, with or without migraine. More recently it has been suggested that recurrent abdominal pain should be viewed as a prodrome of migraine headache[61]. Most children who experience abdominal migraine eventually develop migraine with aura and/or migraine without aura[62]. Abdominal migraine has also been categorised as a functional gut disorder[63].

Conclusions

General dietary restrictions for all patients with migraine have not been proven to be useful[64]. Similarly, other food additives have not been proven to precipitate headache, though monosodium glutamate may cause adverse reactions including headache, but probably only when ingested in large doses on an empty stomach.

The evidence for aspartame, particularly in prolonged use, appears stronger. The possible role of biogenic or trace amines as a cause of migraine still remains unclear.

Therefore, patients should be advised that food plays a limited role as a precipitating factor of migraine, but subjective sensitivity to certain foods should be examined critically and proven precipitating factors should be avoided[65]. Where individuals report possible dietary triggers, it may be helpful for the patient to keep a careful diary of headaches and food and drink consumed, so that possible associations can be excluded. Open studies have indicated that low-fat[66] and high-carbohydrate diets could lead to improvements in migraine frequency and/or severity. As a first line a well-balanced diet is encouraged, with avoidance of dehydration, fasting or missing meals. A universal migraine diet with simultaneous elimination of all potential food triggers is generally not advised in practice. However, this may be warranted in patients with severe and frequent attacks[36].

The prevention of debilitating headaches by attention to precipitating factors may be preferable to long-term drug treatment.

References

1. Stewart WF, Shechter A, Rasmussen BK. Migraine prevalence: a review of population based studies. *Neurology* 1994; **44**: S17–23.
2. Blau JN, Thavapalan M. Preventing migraine: a study of precipitating factors. *Headache* 1988; **28**: 481–3.
3. Abu-Arefeh I, Russell G. Prevalence of headache and migraine in schoolchildren. *BMJ* 1994; **309**: 765–9.
4. Millichap JG, Yee MM, The diet factor in pediatric and adolescent migraine. *Pediatr Neurol* 2002; **28**: 9–15.
5. Stang PE, Yanagihara PA, Swanson JW *et al*. Incidence of migraine headache: a population based study in Olmstead County, Minnesota. *Neurology* 1992; **42**: 1657–62.
6. Van den Bergh V, Amery WL, Waelkens J. Trigger factors in migraine: a study conducted by the Belgian Migraine Society. *Headache* 1987; **27**: 191–6.
7. Peatfield RC, Glover V, Littlewood JT, Sandler M, Clifford Rose F. The prevalence of diet-induced migraine. *Cephalalgia* 1984; **4**: 179–83.
8. Peatfield RC. Relationships between food, wine, and beer-precipitated migrainous headaches. *Headache* 1995; **35**: 355–7.
9. Scott H, Sicherer MD, Sampson HA. Food allergy. *J Allergy Clin Immunol* 2006; **117**: S470–5.
10. Littlewood JT, Gibb C, Glover V *et al*. Red wine as a cause of migraine. *Lancet* 1988; **1**: 558–9.
11. Kanny G, Gerbaux V, Olszewski A *et al*. No correlation between wine intolerance and histamine content of wine. *J Allergy Clin Immunol* 2001; **107**: 375–8.
12. Chauchaix D, Pailler FM. Histamine in foods. *Med Armee* 1980; **8**: 455–62.
13. Maintz L, Novak N. Histamine and histamine intolerance. *Am J Clin Nutr* 2007; **85**: 1185–96.
14. Silla Santos MH. Biogenic amines: their importance in foods. *Int J Food Microbiol* 1996; **29**: 213–31.
15. Jarisch R, Wantke F. Wine and headache. *Int Arch Allergy Immunol* 1996; **110**: 7–12.
16. Hermann K, Hertenberg B, Ring J. Measurement and characterization of histamine and methylhistamine in human urine under histamine-rich and histamine-poor diets. *Int Arch Allergy Immunol* 1993; **101**: 13–19.
17. Kemper RHA, Meijler WJ, Korf J, Ter Horst GJ. Migraine and function of the immune system: a meta-analysis of clinical literature published between 1966 and 1999. *Cephalalgia* 2001; **21**: 549–57.

18. Thomsen LL, Olesen J. Nitric oxide in primary headaches. *Curr Opin Neurol* 2001; **14**: 315–21.
19. Kaliner M, Shelhamer JH, Ottesen EA. Effects of infused histamine: correlation of plasma histamine levels and symptoms. *J Allergy Clin Immunol* 1982; **69**: 283–9.
20. Lassen LH, Heinig JH, Oestergaard S, Olsen J. Histamine inhalation is a specific but insensitive laboratory test for migraine. *Cephalalgia* 1996; **16**: 550–3.
21. Steinbrecher I, Jarisch R. Histamine and headache. *Allergologie* 2005; **28**: 84–91.
22. Krabbe AA, Olesen J. Headache provocation by continuous intravenous infusion of histamine. Clinical results and receptor mechanisms. *Pain* 1980; **30**: 253–9.
23. Watke F, Gotz M, Jarisch R. Histamine free diet treatment of choice for histamine-induced food intolerance and supporting treatment for chronic headaches. *Clin Exp Allergy* 1993; **23**: 982–5.
24. Missbichler A. [Diagnostic proof of DAO activity in serum and plasma]. In: Jarisch R, ed. *Histamin-Intoleranz. Histamin und Seekrankheit* [Histamine intolerance. Histamine and motion sickness]. Stuttgart: Georg Thieme, 2004: 8–17.
25. Anthony M, Hinterberger H, Lance J. Plasma serotonin in migraine and stress. *Arch Neurol* 1967; **16**: 544–52.
26. Alam Z, Coombs N, Waring RH, Williams AC, Steventon GB. Platelet sulphotransferase activity, plasma sulphate levels and sulphation capacity in patients with migraine and tension headache. *Cephalalgia* 1997; **17**: 761–4.
27. Harris RM, Waring RH. Dietary modulation of human platelet phenolsulphotransferase activity. *Xenobiotica* 1996; **26**: 1241–7.
28. Jansen SC, van Dusseldorp M, Bottema KC, Dubois AE. Intolerance to biogenic amines: a review. *Ann Allergy Asthma Immunol* 2003; **91**: 233–40.
29. Sever PS. False transmitters and migraine. *Lancet* 1979; **1**: 33.
30. Axelrod J, Saavedra JM. Octopamine. *Nature* 1977; **265**: 501–4.
31. Penzak SR, Jann MW, Cold JA *et al.* Seville (sour) orange juice: synephrine content and cardiovascular effects in normotensive adults. *J Clin Pharmacol* 2001; **41**: 1059–63.
32. Hannington E. Preliminary report on tyramine headache. *Br Med J* 1967; **2**: 550–1.
33. Martin VT, Benbehani MM. Toward a rational understanding of migraine trigger factors. *Med Clin North Am* 2001; **85**: 911–41.
34. Borowsky B, Adham N, Jones KA *et al.* Trace amines: identification of a family of mammalian G protein-coupled receptors. *Proc Natl Acad Sci U S A* 2001; **98**: 8966–71.
35. D'Andrea G. Terrazzino S, Leon A *et al.* Elevated levels of circulating trace amines in primary headaches. *Neurology* 2004; **62**: 1701–5.
36. McCulloch J, Harper AM. Factors influencing the response of the cerebral circulation to Phenylethylamine. *Neurology* 1979; **29**: 201–7.
37. Oldendorf WH. Brain uptake of radiolabeled amino acids, amines, and hexoses after arterial injection. *Am J Physiol* 1971; **221**: 1629–39.
38. Marcus DA, Scharff L, Turk D, Gourley LM. A double-blind provocative study of chocolate as a trigger for headache. *Cephalalgia* 1997; **17**: 855–62.
39. Schiffman SS, Buckley CE, Sampson HA, *et al.* Aspartame and susceptibility to headache. *N Engl J Med* 1987; **317**: 1181–5.
40. Van den Eeden SK, Koepsell TD, Longstreth WT Jr *et al.* Aspartame ingestion and headaches: a randomized crossover trial. *Neurology* 1994; **44**: 1787–93.
41. Lipton RB, Newman LC, Cohen JS, Solomon S. Aspartame as a dietary trigger of headache. *Headache* 1989; **29**: 90–2.
42. Humphries P, Pretorius E, Naudé H. Direct and indirect cellular effects of aspartame on the brain. *Eur J Clin Nutr* 2008; **62**: 451–62.
43. Newman LC, Lipton RB. Migraine MLT-down: an unusual presentation of migraine in patients with aspartame-triggered headaches. *Headache* 2001; **41**: 899–901.
44. Feeman M. Reconsidering the effects of monosodium glutamate: a literature review. *J Am Acad Nurse Pract* 2006; **18**: 482–6.
45. Geha RS, Beiser A, Ren C *et al.* Multicenter, double-blind, placebo-controlled, multi-challenge evaluation of reported reactions to monosodium glutamate. *J Allergy Clin Immunol* 2000; **106**: 973–80.

46. Spierings ELH, Ranke AH, Hoonkoop PC. Precipitating and aggravating factors of migraine versus tension-type headache. *Headache* 2001; **41**: 554–8.
47. Aamodt AH, Stovner LJ, Langhammer A, Hagen K, Zwart JA. Is headache related to asthma, hay fever and chronic bronchitis? The head-HUNT study. *Headache* 2007; **47**: 204–12.
48. Gazzerani P, Pourpak Z, Ahmadiani A, Hemmati A, Kazemnejad A. A correlation between migraine, histamine and immunoglobulin E. *Iran J Allergy Asthma Immunol* 2003; **2**: 17–24.
49. Martelletti P, Sutherland J, Anastasi E, Di Mario U, Giacovazzo M. Evidence for an immune-mediated mechanism in food-induced migraine from a study on activated T-cells, IgG4 subclass, anti-IgG antibodies and circulating immune complexes. *Headache* 1989; **29**: 664–70.
50. Gasbarrini A, DeLuca A, Fiore G *et al.* Beneficial effects of *Helicobacter* eradication on migraine. *Hepatogastroenterology* 1998; **45**: 765–70.
51. Rees T, Watson D, Lipscombe S *et al.* A prospective audit of food intolerance among migraine patients in primary care clinical practice. *Headache Care* 2005: **2**; 105–10.
52. Scibilia J, Pastorello EA, Zisa G *et al.* Wheat allergy: a double-blind, placebo-controlled study in adults. *J Allergy Clin Immunol* 2006; **117**: 433–9.
53. Gabrielli M, Cremonini F, Fiore G *et al.* Association between migraine and celiac disease: results from a preliminary case–control and therapeutic study. *Am J Gastroenterol* 2003; **98**: 625–9.
54. Kalpaklioglu AF, Tan FU, Roc R, Tunckol M. The Role of allergy in migraine: fact or fiction *J Allergy Clin Immunol* 2005; **115**: S241.
55. Galli V, Ciccarone V, Venuta A, Ferrari P. [Hemicrania and food in the child]. *Pediatr Med Chir* 1985; 7: 17–21.
56. Lucarelli S, Lendvai D, Frediani T *et al.* [Hemicrania and food allergy in children]. *Minerva Pediatr* 1990; **42**: 215–18.
57. Egger J, Carter CM, Wilson J, Turner MW, Soothill JF. Is migraine food allergy? A double-blind controlled trial of oligoantigenic diet treatment. *Lancet* 1983; **2**: 865–9.
58. Abu-Arafeh I, Russell G. Prevalence and clinical features of abdominal migraine compared with those of migraine headache. *Arch Dis Child* 1995; **72**: 413–17.
59. Congdon P, Forsythe W. Migraine in childhood: a study of 300 children. *Dev Med Child Neurol* 1979; **21**: 209–16.
60. Symon DNK, Russell G. Abdominal migraine: a childhood syndrome defined. *Cephalalgia* 1986; **6**: 223–8.
61. Wyllie WG, Schlesinger B. The periodic group of disorders in childhood. *Br J Child Dis* 1933; **30**: 1–21.
62. Dignan F, Abu-Arafeh I, Russell G. The prognosis of childhood abdominal migraine. *Arch Dis Child* 2001; **84**: 415–18.
63. Rasquin-Webera A, Hyman PE, Cucchiara S *et al.* Childhood functional gastrointestinal disorders. *Gut* 1999; **45**: II60–8.
64. Holzhammer J, Wober C. Alimentary trigger factors that provoke migraine and tension-type headache. *Schmerz* 2006; **20**: 151–9.
65. Leira R, Rodríguez R. [Diet and migraine]. *Rev Neurol* 1996; **24**: 534–8.
66. Bic Z, Blix GG, Hopp HP, Leslie FM, Schell MJ. The influence of a low-fat diet on incidence and severity of migraine headaches. *J Womens Health Gend Based Med* 1999; **8**: 623–30.
67. Hasselmark L, Malmgren R, Hannerz J. Effect of a carbohydrate-rich diet, low in protein-tryptophan, in classic and common migraine. *Cephalalgia* 1987; 7: 87–92.

2.6   The role of food hypersensitivity in musculoskeletal disorders

Anna Carling

Musculoskeletal diseases comprise a range of disorders that affect the muscle groups and skeletal system, including rheumatoid arthritis, osteoarthritis, gout, fibromyalgia and back pain. Most of these diseases are only rarely associated with food hypersensitivity, although irritable bowel syndrome (IBS) is sometimes linked with fibromyalgia. Rheumatoid arthritis, however, is a musculoskeletal disease in which food hypersensitivity has been shown to play a part.

Rheumatoid arthritis (RA) is a chronic, systematic, inflammatory autoimmune disorder which affects the synovium of the diarthrodial joints[1]. The pathogenesis of the disease is not fully understood. Many patients think there is an association between their food intake and their symptoms of RA. Various food items, including cereals, dairy products, caffeine, yeast and citrus fruits, have been reported to cause adverse effects in RA, suggesting that food hypersensitivity may be a pathogenic factor in RA. Nevertheless, many research studies have produced conflicting results, largely as a result of poorly designed methodology. The literature shows that these studies lack controls and double-blind food challenges, the gold standard in clinical nutrition research.

In the case of IgE-mediated allergy, there is little evidence to support the idea that this mechanism is involved in RA. Pacor and colleagues reported two case histories where both patients had a known IgE-mediated allergy to milk and wheat, and their symptoms of RA were exacerbated when eating these allergens[2]. Both patients followed a 2-week elimination diet, the results of which indicated improvements in their clinical and haematological parameters. The suspected food was reintroduced as an open challenge and then as a double-blind challenge. Each challenge resulted in a deterioration of the clinical and haematological parameters. The two patients were followed up after 6 months: both had remained on their elimination diets, and were both symptom-free.

IgE-mediated food allergy is a complex immune mechanism which can cause the production TNF-α and IL-1β, from mast cells and monocytes. These pro-inflammatory cytokines are also involved in the development of RA. Karatay *et al.* set out to see if there was a relationship between food allergy and the pro-inflammatory cytokines in RA[3]. Patients attending the rheumatology clinic, with at least a 2-year history of RA, underwent skin prick test (SPT) to 31 food allergens. Beef and cow's milk allergens were not included as there was a ban on imports due to bovine spongiform encephalopathy (BSE). The study population was divided into two groups, those who had positive SPT, known as the prick positive group (PPG), and those whose SPTs were negative, known as prick negative group (PNG). Both groups followed a low allergenic diet for 12 days, after which the PPG group reintroduced the foods that had showed up positive on the SPT for 12 days. The PNG group reintroduced corn and rice diet for 12 days. (Corn was chosen as it was reported to be a 'problem' food in RA). Following this reintroduction of target foods, both groups were asked to return to a low-allergenic diet for a further 12 days. The level of TNF-α and IL-1β was recorded at baseline, at the challenge phase, and finally at the re-elimination phase. The results showed that the PNG group had no change in their TNF-α and IL-1β levels, whilst in the PPG group the TNF-α and IL-1β levels significantly increased, and 72% had an exacerbation of their symptoms after the challenge phase. Interestingly, these symptoms did not improve during the re-elimination phase, giving rise to a hypothesis that food allergy may be a triggering factor more than a causative factor. This was a small study, so further research is required to see if the levels of TNF-α and IL-1β can be regulated by exclusion of certain foods.

One dietary manipulation which patients with RA often attempt in order to control their symptoms is the initiation of a vegetarian or vegan diet. Muller and colleagues carried out a systematic review of the literature which showed that there was significant long-term benefit for some patients with RA following a vegan diet[4]. A large European epidemiological study showed a significant association between inflammatory polyarthritis (arthritis from any cause, involving two or more joints) and a high intake of red meat[5]. Kjeldsen-Kragh investigated the relationship between antibodies and a vegan diet in patients with RA[6]. The subjects first fasted for 7–10 days, then reintroduced foods following a vegan diet for 3.5 months, followed by a lactovegetarian diet for 12 months. IgE, IgA, IgG and IgM antibodies were measured against the common food allergens. At the beginning of the study, 13 subjects thought they had a food allergy, 10 of whom went on to identify foods that aggravated their symptoms through exclusion and reintroduction. However, there was no correlation between these foods and the levels of antibodies.

The American College of Rheumatology's scoring system for signs and symptoms of RA is known as ACR20. Hafström and others devised a study to assess whether a vegan diet, free of gluten, would improve the signs and symptoms of RA, using ACR20 criteria[7]. This study also examined whether the clinical effects could be associated with changes in IgG and IgA antibody levels against gliadin and β-lactoglobulin. Sixty-six patients were randomised to either a gluten-free vegan diet ($n = 38$) or a well-balanced non-vegan diet ($n = 28$). Of the 22 patients in the gluten-free vegan diet group who completed the study, nine (known as diet responders) showed an improvement in their ARC20 score, compared with only one of 25 in the non-vegan group. The levels of IgG and IgA anti-gliadin and anti-β-lactoglobulin antibodies were similar in both groups at the start of the study. However, at the end of the study there was a significant reduction in IgG anti-gliadin and anti-β-lactoglobulin antibodies in the diet responders group. The authors suggested that for a subgroup of patients with RA an improvement in signs and symptoms after following a vegan and gluten-free diet may be due to a diminished immune response to exogenous food antigens. However, further research is required.

Hvatum and colleagues reviewed previous studies which showed there was no clear link between serum antibodies, diet and RA[8]. It was thought that the intestinal immune system could be activated in patients with RA, which is not reflected in the serum antibodies. This led to a small study of 14 patients with RA and 20 healthy subjects (control group) who had their IgM, IgA and IgG to various dietary antigens including wheat, oats, soya, cow's milk, egg, pork and fish in the jejunal perfusion fluid and the blood serum measured. The results showed that there was a rise only in IgM to some food antigens in the jejunal perfusion in patients with RA as compared to the control group. The authors suggested that there may be a connection between mucosal immune activity and the pathogenesis of RA, but again further research is required.

In summary, research has shown that in the case of RA and food hypersensitivity, dietary manipulation seems to improve the symptoms of the disease, but only in some patients. The reason for this, and the mechanism involved, is not clear. Answering such questions will depend on further rigorous research.

References

1. Rayman M, Callaghan A. *Nutrition and Arthritis*. Oxford: Blackwell, 2006.
2. Pacor ML, Lunardi C, Di Lorenzo G, Biasi D, Corrocher R. Food allergy and seronegative arthritis: report of two cases. *Clin Rheumatol* 2001; **20**: 279–81.
3. Karatay S, Erdem T, Yildirim K *et al*. The effect of individualized diet challenge consisting of allergenic foods on TNF-α and IL-1β levels in patients with rheumatoid arthritis. *Rheumatology* 2004; **43**: 1429–33.
4. Muller H, de Toledo FW, Resch KL. Fasting followed by vegetarian diet in patients with rheumatoid arthritis: a systematic review. *Scand J Rheumatol* 2001; **30**: 1–10.
5. Pattison DJ, Symmons DP, Lunt M. Dietary risk factors for the development of inflammatory polyarthritis: evidence for a role of high level of red meat consumption. *Arthritis Rheum* 2004; **50**: 3804–12.
6. Kjeldsen-Kragh J. Rheumatoid arthritis treated with vegetarian diets. *Am J Clin Nutr* 1999; **70**: S594–600.
7. Hafström I, Ringertz B, Spångberg A *et al*. A vegan diet free of gluten improves the signs and symptoms of rheumatoid arthritis: the effects on arthritis correlate with a reduction in antibodies to food antigens. *Rheumatology* 2001; **40**: 1175–9.
8. Hvatum M, Kanerud L, Hällgren R, Brandtzaeg P. The gut-joint axis: cross reactive food antibodies in rheumatoid arthritis. *Gut* 2006; **55**: 1240–7.

3 The Diagnosis of Food Hypersensitivity

Carina Venter, Berber Vlieg-Boerstra and Anna Carling

3.1 Introduction

It is very important to have a diagnosis made by clinicians who have knowledge and skills in this area. The final diagnosis of any FHS should be confirmed by a clinical history, blood tests, skin tests or keeping a food and symptom diary followed by a special test diet to identify the foods causing the symptoms. Blood tests and skin prick tests will only be helpful in the diagnosis of IgE-mediated food allergy, and even then are not 100% reliable. The best method of diagnosing IgE-mediated allergy, and the only method for non-IgE-mediated allergy and food intolerances (non-allergic food hypersensitivity), is an elimination diet followed by reintroduction of the food or a food challenge.

3.2 Clinical history

Careful history taking and physical examination form the basis of diagnosis of all types of FHS.

Taking a history indicates to the clinician:

- which diagnostic tests should be used;
- whether a food and symptom diary is needed, although cause and effect cannot always be established from diet diaries alone;
- which foods should be avoided during the diagnostic test diet;
- whether a food challenge at home/hospital or gradual introduction of the food(s) may be required.

A good clinical history by itself cannot correctly identify FHS. Despite careful history taking, the correlation between suspected food allergy and food allergy as confirmed by DBPCFC is between 12% and 21% of patients[1-3]. This is important, as false negative diagnoses can lead to the risk of ongoing symptoms with further (severe) reactions. False positive diagnoses, on the other hand, can lead to unnecessary restrictions on lifestyle and possible disease from nutrient restriction[4-6].

3.3   Diagnostic tests

Figure 3.1 shows the range of diagnostic tests for FHS, grouped by category of hypersensitivity.

3.3.1   IgE-mediated food allergy

Both skin prick tests (SPT) (measures specific IgE attached to mast cells in the skin) and specific IgE tests (measures levels of circulating specific IgE to allergen in the circulation) are useful in the diagnosis of IgE-mediated FHS. However, the presence of IgE in the skin or in the blood only indicates that an individual is sensitised to an allergen, not necessarily that he or she is clinically allergic. Therefore neither a positive skin reaction nor a detectable serum IgE level is an absolute indicator of FHS.

Skin prick tests

When performing SPT (Figure 3.2), glycerinated food extracts (1:10 or 1:20 weight per volume dilutions) are placed on the skin and pricked with a lancet or needle. A positive (histamine) and negative (saline) control should always be used[7]. The positive control gives an indication of skin reactivity and the negative control can identify patients with dermatographism. The size of the wheal caused by the food allergen should be interpreted in relation to the size of the negative control in order to make a correct diagnosis. Most importantly, SPT size does not predict the severity of the reaction.

SPT can be performed using commercial allergens (which are not standardised, but improving) or using fresh foods. The latter is also known as the prick-to-prick test (PPT), and it also needs standardisation[8–10]. Fresh foods are used because food allergens, specifically those of fruit and vegetables, may be destroyed during the preparation of commercial extracts, or in some cases (e.g. spices) because no commercial allergen extract is available.

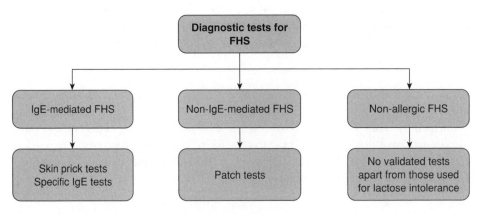

Figure 3.1   Diagnostic tests for food hypersensitivity.

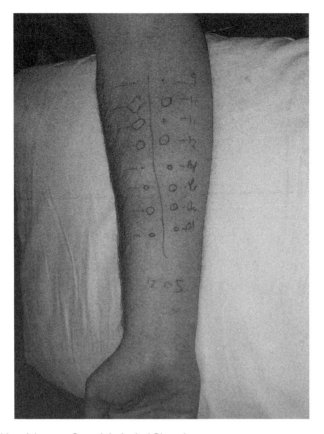

Figure 3.2   Skin prick tests. Copyright Isabel Skypala.

There is no lower age limit for performing a SPT. In general, a SPT is considered positive if the wheal diameter is at least 3 mm larger than the negative control[11–13] in children older than 2 years, and at least 2 mm larger in children younger than 2 years[14]. This is supported by the fact that the histamine-induced wheals in children increase 125% from 4 days to 2 years and 150% from 2 to 18 years, indicating that skin reactivity may increase over time, affecting SPT wheal size[15]. A positive SPT indicates with 50% positive predictive accuracy that the patient may have a true IgE-mediated allergy to the food. Negative SPTs are extremely useful (95% negative predictive value) in ruling out IgE-mediated food allergy. However, a small proportion of children may react immediately to foods to which they had a negative SPT.

There are now more specific clinical decision points available in the literature which can be used to indicate whether a food challenge is needed and how likely the challenge is to be positive (Table 3.1)[16–26]. Use of these diagnostic decision points has an economic implication, as it can greatly reduce the number of specific IgE tests and food challenges needed or even the number of patients prescribed an elimination diet for long periods of time. The decision points can therefore give a good

Table 3.1   Food hypersensitivity: expected food challenge outcomes for specific IgE and skin prick test results.

Food	Specific IgE (kU$_A$/L)	Specific IgE and skin prick test result Specific IgE grade	SPT	Expected food challenge outcome
Milk	> 15[17,19] > 50[27]	3–6	8[13] 5[18] 3–4[22] 15 using fresh cows' milk[26]	Reaction highly probable (challenge may not be needed)
	0.35–15[17]	1–2	3–8	**Reaction probable (challenge needed)**
	> 5[17,20]	3–6	6[13]	Young children under 1–2 years (reaction highly probable)
	< 0.35[17]	0	NA[13]	Reaction unlikely (home or physician challenge)
Egg	> 7[17,19] > 2 (50% positive challenge)[2,6]	3–6	7[13] 4[18] 3–4[22]	Reaction highly probable (challenge may not be needed)
	0.35–7[17]	1–2	3–7	**Reaction probable (challenge needed)**
	> 2[21]	2–6	5[23]	Young children under 1–2 years (reaction highly probable)
	< 0.35[17]	0	NA[13]	Reaction unlikely (home or physician challenge)
Peanut	> 14[17,19] > 10[23] > 2 (50% positive challenge)[24] > 15[25]	3–6	8[13,25] 6[18] ≥ 15[23]	Reaction highly probable (challenge may not be needed)
	0.35–14[17]	1–2	3–8	**Reaction probable (challenge needed)**
	NA	NA	4[13]	Young children under 1–2 years (reaction highly probable)
	< 0.35[17]	0	NA[13]	Reaction unlikely (home or physician challenge)
Fish	> 20[17,19]	4–6	NA	Reaction highly probable (challenge may not be needed)
	0.35–20[17]	1–3	> 3	**Reaction probable (challenge needed)**
	NA	NA	NA	Young children under 1–2 years (reaction highly probable)
	< 0.35[17]	0	NA[13]	Reaction unlikely (home or physician challenge)

Table 3.1   (cont'd)

Food	Specific IgE (kU$_A$/L)	Specific IgE and skin prick test result Specific IgE grade	SPT	Expected food challenge outcome
Wheat	> 26[20]–80[17]	6	NA	Reaction highly probable (challenge may not be needed)
	0.35–80[17]	1–5	> 3	**Reaction probable (challenge needed)**
	NA	NA	NA	Young children under 1–2 years (reaction highly probable)
	< 0.35[17]	0	NA[13]	Reaction unlikely (home or physician challenge)
Soya	> 30[20]–60[17]	5–6	3[18]	Reaction highly probable (challenge may not be needed)
	0.35–60[17]	1–4	> 3	**Reaction probable (challenge needed)**
	NA	NA	NA	Young children under 1–2 years (reaction highly probable)
	< 0.35[17]	0	NA[13]	Reaction unlikely (home or physician challenge)

indication of which children may not need to undergo food challenges. However, an SPT below the cut-off point with a good history does not rule out an allergy and will still need to be investigated. Caution needs to be applied in extrapolating these data to other populations, as a number of factors can affect the reliability of the SPT. There are as yet no validated clinical decision points for adults; all of the published research is on children aged up to 18 years.

Specific IgE tests

Specific IgE tests used to be conducted by employing radio-allergo-sorbent tests (RAST). Nowadays, specific IgE is measured as fluorescent enzyme-labelled IgE (CAP-RAST FEIA), which is more sensitive (89%) and specific (91%). Specific IgE levels can be monitored as specific levels of kilo-units of allergen per litre (kU$_A$/L) or as 'graded' levels (grade 1–6). Generally, level 2 and above is considered as positive in clinical practice, although this is not evidence-based. Specific IgE levels of > 15 kU$_A$/L for milk, > 7 kU$_A$/L for egg and > 14 kU$_A$/L for peanut corresponds with grade 3–6 (personal communication, Sheffield laboratories).

The preferred method of dealing with specific IgE levels is to assess the particular level of kU$_A$/L. In general, the higher the level of specific IgE the more likely the child is to be allergic, but there is no clear cut-off point between being allergic and not. Therefore, in order to establish the reliability of specific IgE tests, researchers have established cut-off points for diagnosis of FHS (Table 3.1). The same caveats apply to these cut-off points as to those validated for SPT: they should be viewed as guidelines rather than set diagnostic points.

Cut-off levels to predict challenge outcome vary between centres. Cut-off levels differ according to the test used, and this has important implications as new methods for detecting specific IgE levels are being developed; most importantly, specific IgE levels give no indication of the dose the patient may react to.

The preference for using either SPT or specific IgE tests varies between clinicians and researchers. SPT is often regarded as the method of choice due to the ease of use, low cost and immediate results. However, specific IgE tests of any type are very useful in children with severe skin disease, in cases of dermatographism, or when it is impossible to discontinue antihistamine. As with SPT, specific IgE levels do not predict the severity of the reaction.

3.3.2   Non-IgE-mediated FHS

Skin prick tests and specific IgE tests

SPTs and specific IgE tests are not useful in the diagnosis of delayed type/non-IgE-mediated food allergy or non-allergic FHS, because the production of food-specific IgE antibodies is not involved in the pathogenesis of these conditions.

Patch tests

Food allergens are applied to a healthy area of the patient's skin and the effects evaluated 48–72 hours later. It is used in the USA in the diagnosis of allergic eosinophilic disease, and in Europe, including some centres in the UK, for the diagnosis of atopic dermatitis[27,28].

3.3.3   Non-allergic FHS

No tests have been sufficiently validated to test so-called food intolerances. Lactose intolerance, however, can be diagnosed by means of the hydrogen breath test or testing the pH of the stools.

3.4   Complementary and alternative medicine

Some people believe that 'food allergies' could be a contributing factor or indeed the cause of their physical and emotional symptoms. With the growth of accessible information on the internet and easy access to complementary medicines in the high street, it is difficult for the public to decipher which food allergy diagnostic methods are reliable and scientifically sound.

The prevalence of complementary and alternative medicine (CAM) in allergic disease appears to be growing. This is supported by the work of Michaelis *et al.*, who found that 40% of patients who visited their allergy clinic had seen a CAM therapist[29], whilst Ko *et al.* reported that 22% of their referrals had used alternative food allergy testing and 18% were seeing a CAM therapist[30].

Alternative testing for food hypersensitivity can be divided into two main groups: tests which use the body's 'energy', and blood analysis tests. With regard to body energy testing, commonly used procedures to examine food hypersensitivity include Vega testing (electrodermal testing), applied kinesiology, hair analysis and the pulse test.

Vega testing

The purpose of Vega testing is to measure the electrical conductivity in the body. It is hypothesised that an offending food will alter the electrical conductivity, realised by a 'dip' in the electrical wave. Interestingly, research into the effectiveness of Vega testing showed that the results of the procedure were no better than chance in diagnosing food allergy[31].

Kinesiology

Applied kinesiology is based on the concept that certain foods cause an energy imbalance. This energy imbalance is detected by testing the response of the muscle. The client is asked to hold glass vials which contain food concentrates, and a counter force is applied to the client's arm muscle. If the muscle appears weak this would indicate that the client is to avoid that food substance. Pothmann found that applied kinesiology is again no better than chance at diagnosing food allergy[32].

Hair analysis and pulse testing

The method of hair analysis looks at the energy fields and compares them to established data to confirm or deny food allergies. The literature does not support any scientific basis for this test. A similar lack of scientific information underlies the pulse test. With this method the pulse is taken immediately before the suspect food is eaten and then taken again following a 15-minute period. An increase in pulse rate is said to indicate a food allergy.

Blood tests

Food hypersensitivity testing using the patient's blood samples includes IgG testing, the Antigen Leukocyte Cellular Antibody Test (ALCAT) and the Food Allergen Cellular Test (FAC-test). With both ALCAT and FAC-test, blood is incubated with food extracts. ALCAT then examines the size, shape and damage to the white blood cells whilst FAC-test measures the chemical mediators released by the white blood cells. Neither of these tests has a rational scientific basis, nor is there research in the literature regarding the effectiveness of such testing. With IgG testing, it is believed that an increase in IgG with certain foods could indicate food hypersensitivity.

Zuo *et al.*[33] and Atkinson *et al.*[34] both showed that there was an increase in IgG to certain foods in patients with irritable bowel syndrome, but more research is required to see if this also relates to food hypersensitivity.

Issues concerning the use of CAM

The most common result of these alternative food allergy tests is a long list of foods to be excluded from an individual's diet. The implications of unnecessarily excluding food groups from a diet are numerous, not only from a nutritional point of view, but also from the added stress caused to the individual who has to buy and prepare different foods. Many of the CAM therapists have no nutritional training and are unable to advise on the practical issues of following a restricted diet or ensuring that a restricted diet is nutritional. Frequently the concept of reintroducing foods back into the diet is ignored, resulting in very restricted diets for an unnecessary length of time. Teuber and Porch-Curren reviewed alternative and complementary medicine approaches to allergic disorders[35]. The authors report an absence of well-performed research studies supporting these approaches in the literature, but highlight studies that have refuted their utility. They go on to hypothesise that beneficial placebo effects may be responsible for the perceived clinical effectiveness in many cases of food intolerance. If supporters of alternative and complementary medicine wish to have a credible place in the diagnosis and treatment of food allergies, then rigorous research methodology should be employed, including randomised controlled trials. Only then will individuals who might suffer from genuine food allergies or intolerances be able to make a truly informed decision.

3.5   Diagnostic exclusion diets

For many patients seen in clinical practice, particularly those suffering from non-IgE-mediated allergy or non-allergic FHS, diagnosis can only be made by means of a combination of clinical history and dietary investigations (diagnostic exclusion diets).

3.5.1   Types of diagnostic exclusion diets

Single-food exclusion diet

This excludes all sources of a single food (e.g. milk) as identified from the patient's dietary history.

Multiple-food exclusion diet

A multiple exclusion diet excludes a number of foods at the same time. Foods most commonly associated with a particular disorder are usually avoided, such as milk and egg for eczema[36], and milk, egg and wheat for eosinophilic diseases[28].

Few-foods diet

A few-foods diet includes foods that are known to rarely cause allergic symptoms in the population and also not regularly eaten by the patient. It generally includes two meats, two starchy foods, two fruits, two vegetables and water to drink. If no improvement occurs it may be considered to construct a second few-foods diet not using any of the food in the first diet. If this also produces no relief, the regimen should be discontinued.

Elemental and protein hydrolysate formula diets

This diet requires the use of amino-acid-based formula in infants and children, and the elemental sip feeds in adults. It can be used in infants and children in the diagnosis of a range of diseases. In adults it is often used in the diagnosis of severe allergic symptoms or in patients claiming to suffer from a range of non-allergic FHS in order to establish if food consumption does play a role in their symptoms (just as with the few-foods diet).

For all types of exclusion diets, patients need to be clearly educated regarding the avoidance of food(s), label reading, food substitutes and following a healthy balanced diet, despite the dietary restrictions. Expertise on nutritional issues is of particular importance when dealing with children's diets. As well as foods and beverages, non-dietary sources of substances that can provoke reactions may also need to be excluded, but this is very individual and may not always be necessary. Food exclusion diets are usually followed for a period of 2–3 weeks, but in the case of fluctuating disease patterns it may be necessary to continue single and multiple exclusion diets for up to 6 weeks; few-foods diets should not be continued for more than 3 weeks.

3.5.2   Monitoring progress

Patients should keep a food and symptom diary whilst on the diet, starting one week prior to commencing the diet so that alteration in symptoms can be related to any dietary change. If improvement does not occur, the patient's food intake should be carefully reviewed to ascertain whether the procedure was followed correctly and, if so, whether other foods should be excluded or whether FHS is unlikely to exist.

3.5.3   Food reintroduction

Dietary exclusion needs to be followed by reintroduction of the food, either during a food challenge or in a reintroduction plan at home. Deciding which method to use provides another grey area in dealing with FHS. In general, patients with either a history of immediate symptoms or a positive SPT/specific IgE tests should be invited to a controlled setting for a food challenge. All other patients could undergo either a food challenge at home or a food reintroduction plan, depending on the facilities and staff available. Any patient who has experienced moderate to severe symptoms occasioning a visit to hospital should always undergo food challenge in a medical setting with appropriate facilities for resuscitation.

For the diagnosis of non-IgE-mediated food allergy or non-allergic FHS, foods could be reintroduced singly, and usually at intervals of a few days. The period between the consumption of a food and the return of symptoms can vary; there may be an immediate response, but in many chronic disorders it may take a week or more after daily ingestion of the suspect food. However, one should always take into account that this method is open to false positive observations. If parents are convinced of FHS, they will observe symptoms anyway.

There is no universally agreed order in which foods should be reintroduced. This will vary from patient to patient and according to the condition being treated.

The quantity of food reintroduced is a matter of debate. Too small a quantity of food (i.e. less than normally consumed) may be insufficient to provoke symptoms[37]. On the other hand, sensitivity to a food may be heightened after a period of withdrawal, particularly in the case of infants and children[38]. As a general guideline, foods should be reintroduced in amounts similar to that consumed prior to exclusion. Gradual reintroduction may be more appropriate in children, or if reactions may be severe.

It is important to give patients clear guidance on the form in which a food should be reintroduced. Composite dishes, ready meals and other convenience foods should only be reintroduced into the diet when all the likely suspect ingredients have been tested separately. Dietary assessment should be carried out throughout this period to determine if any nutritional supplementation is required.

The reintroduction process can be very slow, up to 9 months in some cases when a number of foods need to be reintroduced. Patients need to be highly motivated, and will require a lot of support. There is always a conflict between the desire to make the diet more acceptable to the patient and the need to ensure that foods are not introduced so quickly that no conclusions can be drawn. If carried out correctly, the potential rewards from these dietary manipulations are high: the quality of life of patients who have been chronically ill for years may be significantly improved. Conversely, patients who have undergone these procedures without identification of any food-related FHS should be reassured that the investigation has not 'failed' but simply demonstrated that their symptoms are not diet-related.

3.6   Oral food challenges

The accepted standard in objectively diagnosing FHS is the oral food challenge, and in particular the double-blind placebo-controlled food challenge (DBPCFC). Suspected food allergic reactions may need to be confirmed or refuted by food challenge tests for a reliable diagnosis and a diet which is optimally adjusted to the patient's needs. In addition, a confirmed diagnosis of FHS needs to be updated on a regular base to monitor for resolution or persistence of the food allergy. Particularly in children, the food allergy may change over time, depending on the allergenic food in question. It is known, for example, that cow's milk allergy may be outgrown, whereas allergic reactions to peanut or nuts may last for years or may not resolve at all[39]. Food challenges may also need to be performed to establish threshold values for the individual patients and to investigate the severity of the reactions[40]. The impact of intrinsic human factors (e.g. asthma and exercise) and extrinsic event factors (e.g. season, location and especially dose of allergen) need to be considered carefully when interpreting results of food challenges[41]. A food challenge will also provide useful information on the quantity of food allergen which provokes a response and may reveal that the patient has a higher level of tolerance than previously assumed. This is helpful, as it helps to remove fear and may be useful even though the patient cannot calculate the amount of allergenic protein from the label, nor can he/she assess how much allergen will be consumed when using precautionary labelled foods because of varying and unexpected amounts of allergenic protein in these kinds of products[42].

3.6.1   Types of food challenges

Open food challenges (OFC)

During an open food challenge (OFC), both the patient and the clinician performing the challenge know the ingredients of the challenge food, e.g. peanut flapjack used for a peanut challenge. For clinical, non-scientific purposes, from a practical point of view, the open food challenge may be the challenge of choice in most cases when dealing with adults or children suffering from objective symptoms (e.g. urticaria, angio-oedema etc.), although it should be borne in mind that OFC produces 27% more positive challenges than DBPCFC[43].

Single-blind placebo-controlled food challenges (SBPCFC)

For single-blind placebo-controlled food challenges (SBPCFC), the health professionals involved should be able to administer the challenge without the patient knowing which dose is active and which is placebo. Sufficient masking of the challenge food is therefore very important. During SBPCFC, foods will be masked, and, just as in a DBPCFC, an active and placebo challenge will take place.

Double blind placebo controlled food challenges (DBPCFC)

The DBPCFC is internationally recommended as the 'gold standard' for both research and clinical diagnostic evaluations[44]. One of the strengths of the DBPCFC is that neither the patient nor the investigator knows when the active or the placebo challenge is performed. It therefore rules out measurement and reporting bias from the observer and the psychological effect from the patient. For clinical purposes, the SBPCFC or DBPCFC would probably be the challenge of choice in most cases when dealing with adults or children suffering from either subjective symptoms such as stomach ache, nausea, headache, lassitude and other non-specific symptoms, or symptoms that could be difficult to assess due to the nature of the disease, e.g. eczema[43].

Which challenge type is best?

As mentioned over the years, the DBPCFC has been regarded as the gold standard for diagnosing food allergy[44,45] and should be the diagnostic procedure of choice in diagnosing food allergy. However, to date, this test is only used in a limited number of centres, probably due to its labour-intensive nature, lack of available and easy-to-use challenge materials (recipes), and a lack of uniform protocols for the performance of food challenge tests. Although several guidelines have been published on the administration of the test procedure[44–46], there have been few attempts to standardise or validate the test procedure and its parameters for clinical and scientific purposes[45,47–50].

OFCs are much easier to perform, because the food does not need to be disguised, randomisation is not necessary, and specific recipes do not need to be developed and validated. OFCs are useful to refute the diagnosis of food allergy in patients where the culprit food is not likely to elicit allergic reactions. However, open food challenge carries a considerable chance of false positive reactions[1–3,51]. Brouwer and co-workers found that DBPCFC confirmed a diagnosis of cow's milk allergy in only 4 of 14 infants recruited from a primary care setting with atopic eczema and a positive OFC, indicating a false positive rate for OFC of 71% (10/14)[51].

3.6.2   Preparation for oral food challenges

History

Patients should not undergo a food challenge if they have current symptoms of a seasonal allergy, if they are unwell on the day, or if they are taking medication that could influence the challenge result.

Patients should be well informed prior to the challenge regarding the challenge procedure, use of medication, food intake, and about what will happen after the challenge. (See Appendix 1 for an example of patient challenge information).

It is important to obtain sufficient information from the patient in order to plan a food challenge. There is a number of issues which may affect the challenge, and therefore the following information will be useful[16]:

- the age of patient, to determine how difficult it may be to perform the food challenge and to help in identifying the possible food causing the symptoms;
- the age of onset of symptoms, as well as the frequency and reproducibility of the reaction;
- the type of food or foods, e.g. raw egg or cooked egg, and the quantity of food reported to cause symptoms;
- the time of onset of symptoms, type and duration of the symptoms;
- a thorough description of the most recent reaction;
- whether more than one food or factor is needed to elicit a positive challenge outcome, e.g. more than one food eaten together, exercise-induced anaphylaxis, or a food with concomitant drug intake;

- a list of foods that are well tolerated and that could be used as placebo or vehicle.

Location

For patients with no detectable specific IgE or a negative SPT, and a history of only delayed symptoms, food challenges can be performed at home. For all other patients the food challenge should be performed in hospital. In some cases, the physician may decide that the food challenge may be performed at home if the challenge is considered as a low-risk challenge, e.g. in case of no detectable specific IgE and mild symptoms. For those patients with a history of delayed symptoms, a negative challenge in hospital may need to be continued at home. When challenges are performed in hospital, the setting for the challenge should be in close proximity to the person taking the medical responsibility, with easy access to facilities for resuscitation and drugs and, if possible, a relaxed atmosphere[52].

Application

Each patient requires a named member of staff with the appropriate resuscitation training who is in charge of the food challenge and monitoring of the patient. It is important that all clinical staff involved should be able to carry out baseline observations at regular time intervals, and that they should be able to recognise allergy-related symptoms and know how to treat these. When performing food challenges in children, play therapists may be needed to handle children who become difficult about eating the challenge food. At the start of the challenge, the supervising doctor will need to assess the patient and prescribe all drugs which may be needed to treat symptoms such as urticaria or anaphylaxis. The use of IV cannulas during food challenges differs between hospitals. It is therefore very important that doctors should know what the policy of the particular hospital is. Prior to the challenge commencing, informed verbal or written consent should be obtained and documented according to local policies. Other considerations will include whether a latex-free area is required, and the length of time patients should be kept following the last dose of food. The observation period will need to be adjusted for each patient experiencing symptoms[45,52].

Controlling for problems

In order to attribute symptoms occurring only to the ingestion of the challenge food, it is important to ensure avoidance of any other influencing factors. Urticaria, itching, redness and eczema are all symptoms that may be triggered by food allergy. However, they can also be caused by a range of other factors such as temperature changes, stress or contact sensitivity. It may therefore be useful to avoid water/sand/dough play during the challenge[52].

Ingestion of other foods during a food challenge can cause practical problems. Ideally, no food other than the challenge foods or food used for blinding should be

Table 3.2 Common problems which occur during challenges.

Problem	Solution
Patient/parent anxiety	Full discussion at time of agreed challenge Reassurance on the day Promote benefits of challenge
Food refusal	Identify fussy patient prior to challenge and mask/hide allergen Use of play leaders for children Rewards (children), e.g. chocolate buttons
Non-visual symptoms, e.g. nausea, stomach ache	Lengthen observation time and then proceed with same size (not double) dose Rearrange challenge and do blind
No symptoms on day but self-reported symptoms at home later	Encourage patients to return to ward if symptoms occur so they can be documented Allow continued ingestions of food but in smaller quantities than on day of challenge Repeat challenge with overnight observation
Patient does not attend challenge	Acceptable dates, e.g. school holidays Written information

ingested. This can cause a problem for patients who have travelled a long distance, or when challenges continue for a few hours. Young children can be particularly difficult to handle when feeling hungry. For this reason, patients are allowed a light breakfast prior to challenge. If they should get hungry or thirsty during the challenge, only food that they have previously tolerated and that is not contaminated with any of the challenge food should be allowed. Other problems which can occur during a food challenge are summarised in Table 3.2.

3.6.3 Performing the challenge

See Appendices 2–6 for details of challenge protocols, documentation and symptom scoring.

Challenge food

In any challenge, the food used should mimic the history as closely as possible. In open challenges, dried, cooked or raw food as indicated by the history should be used. Cooking, canning and roasting can have different effects on the allergenicity of different foods, and any form of processing used for the challenge food could potentially influence the challenge outcome. This highlights the importance of replicating the history when doing food challenges with regards to using cooked, processed or raw food. In order to eliminate many of the issues raised about cooking, digestion etc., a negative challenge, either open or DBPCFC, should always be followed up by consumption of a normal portion of the food.

Capsules can be used as the challenge vehicle when using dried food to perform a challenge, but this is not the preferred option, especially for patients suffering from oral allergy syndrome (OAS), as contact with the oral mucosa and oesophagus is prevented. In addition, capsules are not suitable for young children, who are likely to be unable or unwilling to swallow them[37]. They are also not suitable for home challenges, as capsules can be opened.

Challenge dose

There is no recommended 'starting dose' that should be used for all patients/challenges, but it should be at least half of the dose the patient reacted to in the past[45]. Some clinicians prefer to start the challenge with a labial rub (applying the challenge food to the inside of the lip). The development of symptoms is considered a positive test, and a negative labial rub can be followed by the oral challenge doses[53]. For immediate symptoms it has been suggested that the dose may be doubled at each interval or increased logarithmically, as guided by the patient's history. A time span of 15 but preferably 30 minutes can be allowed between each dose. The timing between doses should be sufficient to allow symptoms to develop, and based on the reported history of the reactions. For prolonged challenges, usually just one dose of food per day is recommended, although some studies have continued to use a gradual increase of the dosages after day one of the challenge. Apart from taking account of the amount reported by the history, there are no specific recommendations regarding the dose used when performing food challenges in order to diagnose delayed symptoms such as eczema or constipation[16].

It is recommended that the final dose for all challenges should be 'the normal daily intake in a serving of the food in question, adjusted for the age of the patient'[45]. However, for DBPCFC, these high total doses are very difficult to disguise. If the patient, particularly a child, refuses the food at the time, the parents should be asked to give a normal portion of the food at home, on the same day[54]. However, if severe reactions cannot be ruled out, the final dose should be administered in an open fashion, on a separate occasion, after breaking the code. In principle, the food challenge should provide a sufficient amount of the allergenic food to rule out food allergy. In some cases, however, subsequent reactions may still be experienced at home, even after consumption of a normal portion of food on the challenge day[55]. Sometimes, these reactions experienced at home after a negative DBPCFC may be false positives.

Challenge duration

It has been suggested that when dealing with immediate-type symptoms, a positive reaction should be obtained within 2 hours. A longer challenge period (1–4 weeks) is recommended when looking for delayed reactions and in case of repeated consumption. The timing between two challenges should allow for symptoms to develop and/or subside as well as taking the disease pattern into account. A waiting time of 3–4 hours is recommended when dealing with immediate symptoms, and at least 1 week when dealing with delayed symptoms.

Specific issues relating to DBPCFC

The active and placebo challenges are preferably conducted on separate days and in random order. The active food is disguised in a test food matrix with similar sensory properties to the placebo test food. The active and placebo challenges should be identical regarding taste, appearance, smell, viscosity, texture, structure and volume[45,48]. It is therefore important that the blinding capacities of the recipes are validated. For reliable results, this should be done by a professional panel of food tasters in a food laboratory[48], by standard procedures using for example the duo-test/paired comparison test and triangle test, but to date this method has been used in only a limited number of studies. Although this seems to be a reasonable standard in adults and older children, it will most probably not be possible for most of the allergy services in the UK, and for very young children such stringent standards may not be necessary, although it remains true for the observers[37]. However, if blinding is inadequate or incomplete, one should be aware that the double-blind nature of the test may be compromised, resulting in false-positive test results.

Unequivocal tolerance to the food matrix has to be ascertained by dietary history. When challenging children, special care needs to be taken to ensure acceptable taste and volume of the test food, so that even choosy eaters will actually eat the test food and the challenge test can be completed.

In a blind challenge, any vehicle used for masking the food must enable the clinician to perform a truly blind challenge, masking the smell, flavour and texture of the food. The blinding procedure should be well planned, e.g. to ensure that the fat content of the vehicle does not influence the challenge outcome[56]. The vehicle must also allow for enough challenge food to be used. A variety of foods can be used for blinding (Table 3.3). Many commercial products such as egg-free, milk-free, wheat-free cakes, biscuits or pastas can be used as placebo. It can be very difficult to find a suitable placebo and/or vehicle when dealing with children with multiple food allergies, i.e. finding a food that is well tolerated and accepted by the child[37]. For

Table 3.3 Ways in which foods may be disguised for blind food challenge.

Test food	Suitable base materials for disguise
Cow's milk	Soya formula, mashed potato, pureed lentils, soups, casseroles
Soya formula	Cow's milk, pureed lentils
Egg	Mashed potato, pureed lentils
Wheat	Pureed lentils, oatcakes, flapjacks, gluten-free foods
Corn	Oatcakes, flapjacks, soups, casseroles
Rye, oats and barley	Gluten-free bread, soups, casseroles
Orange juice	Carrot juice
Sugar	Carrot juice, 'diet' drinks
Food colours	Carrot juice, orange juice
Preservatives	Orange juice
Strong taste	Peppermint oil
Dark colour	Beetroot juice, blackcurrant juice

cow's milk challenges in young infants, cow's milk hydrolysates the child usually drinks can be used as a food matrix for disguising the milk, whereas in older children solid recipes, such as pancakes, meat recipes or cookies are suitable[48,57].

There is no international agreement on the incremental scales to be used. Several incremental scales have been published over the years, some of which start with only a few milligrams of allergenic food, while others have higher initial doses[23,46,50,58]. For optimal safety of the patient, it is advisable to start with low initial doses (a few milligrams) and to use sufficiently long time intervals. Time intervals of 30 minutes between the doses seem appropriate to avoid severe reactions[50]. It is agreed that the maximum dose should reflect one normal portion of the challenge foods, but these high amounts are hard to disguise, and no studies have been performed on the desirable top discrete or cumulative dose.

To check for false-negative challenges, a negative DBPCFC should be followed by an open food challenge with the challenge food, or by introduction of the food into the diet until the food is consumed in a meal-size portion or in amounts in which it is normally eaten. In the case of a positive DBPCFC, the patient is advised to continue the elimination of the offending food, whereas in the case of (less frequent) dubious results the test has to be repeated.

3.6.4   Interpretation of food challenge results

This is not always easy, as there are some confounding effects. Diseases such as eczema and chronic urticaria go into remission from time to time. It is possible that the results of a food challenge could be falsely negative when the disease is in remission or falsely positive when the disease is active. Allergic reactions to inhalant allergens can also affect the challenge outcome.

Symptoms experienced during food challenges should be recorded on a symptom score chart in hospital or in symptom diaries at home. There are no clear guidelines regarding at what point a challenge should be considered positive, and whether the food challenge should be terminated in case of repeated subjective symptoms or in case of objective symptoms[50]. The clinician should therefore make the final decision based on clinical discretion and the safety of the patient. Challenges are considered positive when the patient experiences symptoms in line with the history during the food challenge, or when allergic symptoms related to FHS are experienced during the challenge and verified by the supervising clinician.

The assessment of the outcome of a DBPCFC should occur in a blinded fashion. Subsequently, the code is broken, and the final outcome is assessed. Recently, a proposal for a standardised assessment of challenge sessions and DBPCFC was published, for optimal consistency in the evaluation of the test results[50]. This guidance suggests that in exceptional cases a challenge session or total DBPCFC may be assessed as questionable, when it remains inconclusive whether or not the observed, usually mild symptoms after the last challenge dose were caused by the food challenge. A questionable DBPCFC should be repeated (Figure 3.3, Table 3.4).

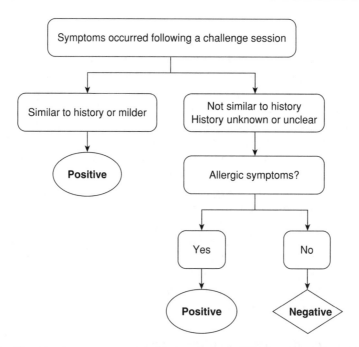

Figure 3.3 Algorithm for assessment of allergic symptoms following a challenge session in DBPCFC (with the exception of non-IgE-mediated allergic disorders).

Table 3.4 Assessment protocol for the outcome of DBPCFC.

Active food challenge	Placebo challenge	Assessment of DBPCFC
Positive	negative	positive
Positive (clearly more positive than placebo)	positive	positive
Negative	negative	negative
Negative (or positive, but clearly less positive than placebo)	positive	negative

There are a number of factors that could lead to false-negative or false-positive challenges, which should be taken into account[59]:

- the symptoms experienced: some objective symptoms, such as vomiting, may be of psychological origin;
- difficulty in distinguishing contact urticaria from urticaria caused by oral intake;
- insufficient consumption of the challenge food;
- insufficient challenge duration;
- how to interpret subjective symptoms such as palpitations, tongue burning or abdominal discomfort, itching in the mouth or on the skin without other visible symptoms;

- use of medication during the food challenge, or insufficient withdrawal of medication;
- the possibility, suggested by some authors, that a food challenge may lead to a temporary effect similar to oral immunotherapy;
- mistakes made with food preparation and provision during the food challenge;
- interference by other staff or patients during the food challenge;
- confounding factors after the last challenge dose, such as viral infections or contact with inhalant allergens once at home.

3.6.5   Management strategies after the challenge

Most food challenges will give a clear answer as to whether the patient is able to eat the food or not. If no reaction has occurred the patient must feel confident to eat the food again, and should be encouraged to do so. This may be difficult where strict avoidance measures have been adhered to for some time. The outcome of a challenge will either be that the food can be reintroduced, or that the food needs to continue to be partially or fully excluded, with a plan for whether a further challenge will take place in the future.

3.7   Conclusion

The diagnosis of FHS is a difficult area, as the mechanisms involved are often not understood and multiple symptoms (immediate and/or delayed onset) and triggers can be involved. Furthermore, there is no perfect diagnostic test, and health professionals often have different opinions regarding the use of tests and food challenges. The situation may be further complicated by the involvement of non-professionals performing non-validated tests.

References

1. Venter C, Pereira B, Grundy J et al. Incidence of parentally reported and clinically diagnosed food hypersensitivity in the first year of life. *J Allergy Clin Immunol* 2006; **117**: 1118–24.
2. Venter C, Pereira B, Grundy J et al. Prevalence of sensitization reported and objectively assessed food hypersensitivity amongst six-year-old children: a population-based study. *Pediatr Allergy Immunol* 2006; **17**: 356–63.
3. Pereira B, Venter C, Grundy J et al. Prevalence of sensitization to food allergens, reported adverse reaction to foods, food avoidance, and food hypersensitivity among teenagers. *J Allergy Clin Immunol* 2005; **116**: 884–92.
4. Christie L, Hine RJ, Parker JG, Burks W. Food allergies in children affect nutrient intake and growth. *J Am Diet Assoc* 2002; **102**: 1648–51.
5. Eggesbo M, Botten G, Stigum H. Restricted diets in children with reactions to milk and egg perceived by their parents. *J Pediatr* 2001; **139**: 583–7.
6. Sicherer SH, Noone SA, Munoz-Furlong A. The impact of childhood food allergy on quality of life. *Ann Allergy Asthma Immunol* 2001; **87**: 461–4.
7. Bernstein IL. Proceedings of the Task Force on Guidelines for Standardizing Old and New Technologies Used for the Diagnosis and Treatment of Allergic Diseases. *J Allergy Clin Immunol* 1988; **82**: 487–526.

8. Ortolani C, Ispano M, Pastorello EA, Ansaloni R, Magri GC. Comparison of results of skin prick tests (with fresh foods and commercial food extracts) and RAST in 100 patients with oral allergy syndrome. *J Allergy Clin Immunol* 1989; **83**: 683–90.

9. Rosen JP, Selcow JE, Mendelson LM *et al*. Skin testing with natural foods in patients suspected of having food allergies: is it a necessity? *J Allergy Clin Immunol* 1994; **93**: 1068–70.

10. Zuberbier T, Edenharter G, Worm M *et al*. Prevalence of adverse reactions to food in Germany: a population study. *Allergy* 2004; **59**: 338–45.

11. Bock SA, Buckley J, Holst A, May CD. Proper use of skin tests with food extracts in diagnosis of hypersensitivity to food in children. *Clin Allergy* 1977; **7**: 375–83.

12. Bock SA, Atkins FM. Patterns of food hypersensitivity during sixteen years of double-blind, placebo-controlled food challenges. *J Pediatr* 1990; **117**: 561–7.

13. Eigenmann PA, Sampson HA. Interpreting skin prick tests in the evaluation of food allergy in children. *Pediatr Allergy Immunol* 1998; **9**: 186–91.

14. Menardo JL, Bousquet J, Rodiere M, Astruc J, Michel FB. Skin test reactivity in infancy. *J Allergy Clin Immunol* 1985; **75**: 646–51.

15. Sampson HA. Food allergy. Part 2: diagnosis and management. *J Allergy Clin Immunol* 1999; **103**: 981–9.

16. Bock SA, Sampson HA. Evaluation of food allergy. In: Leung DYM, Sampson HA, Geha R, Szefler SJ, eds. *Pediatric Allergy: Principles and Practice*. St Louis, MO: Mosby, 2003: 478–87.

17. Sporik R, Hill DJ, Hosking CS. Specificity of allergen skin testing in predicting positive open food challenges to milk, egg and peanut in children. *Clin Exp Allergy* 2000; **30**: 1540–6.

18. Sampson HA. Utility of food-specific IgE concentrations in predicting symptomatic food allergy. *J Allergy Clin Immunol* 2001; **107**: 891–6.

19. Boyano-Martinez T, Garcia-Ara C, Diaz-Pena JM, Martin-Esteban M. Prediction of tolerance on the basis of quantification of egg white-specific IgE antibodies in children with egg allergy. *J Allergy Clin Immunol* 2002; **110**: 304–9.

20. Garcia-Ara C, Boyano-Martinez T, Diaz-Pena JM *et al*. Specific IgE levels in the diagnosis of immediate hypersensitivity to cows' milk protein in the infant. *J Allergy Clin Immunol* 2001; **107**: 185–90.

21. Verstege A, Mehl A, Rolinck-Werninghaus C *et al*. The predictive value of the skin prick test weal size for the outcome of oral food challenges. *Clin Exp Allergy* 2005; **35**: 1220–6.

22. Wainstein BK, Yee A, Jelley D, Ziegler M, Ziegler JB. Combining skin prick, immediate skin application and specific-IgE testing in the diagnosis of peanut allergy in children. *Pediatr Allergy Immunol* 2007; **18**: 231–9.

23. Perry TT, Matsui EC, Conover-Walker KM, Wood RA. The relationship of allergen-specific IgE levels and oral food challenge outcome. *J Allergy Clin Immunol* 2004; **114**: 144–9.

24. Roberts G, Lack G. Diagnosing peanut allergy with skin prick and specific IgE testing. *J Allergy Clin Immunol* 2005; **115**: 1291–6.

25. Mauro C, Claudia A, Tullio F *et al*. Correlation between skin prick test using commercial extract of cow's milk protein and fresh milk and food challenges. *Pediatr Allergy Immunol* 2007; **15**: 583–8.

26. Roehr CC, Reibel S, Ziegert M *et al*. Atopy patch tests, together with determination of specific IgE levels, reduce the need for oral food challenges in children with atopic dermatitis. *J Allergy Clin Immunol* 2001; **107**: 548–53; as discussed in Mauro *et al*.[25].

27. Niggemann B, Reibel S, Wahn U. The atopy patch test (APT): a useful tool for the diagnosis of food allergy in children with atopic dermatitis. *Allergy* 2000; **55**: 281–5.

28. Spergel JM, Beausoleil JL, Mascarenhas M, Liacouras CA. The use of skin prick tests and patch tests to identify causative foods in eosinophilic esophagitis. *J Allergy Clin Immunol* 2002; **109**: 363–8.

29. Michaelis LJ, Woods P, Fox A, Cox H. The use of complementary medicine among children. *Arch Dis Child* 2006; **91**: A68.

30. Ko J, Lee JI, Munoz-Furlong A, Li XM, Sicherer SH. Use of complementary and alternative medicine by food-allergic patients. *Ann Allergy Asthma Immunol* 2006; **97**: 365–9.

31. Krop J, Lewith GT, Gziut W, Radulescu C. A double blind, randomized, controlled investigation of electrodermal testing in the diagnosis of allergies. *J Altern Complement Med* 1997; **3**: 241–8.

32. Pothmann R, von Frankenberg S, Hoicke C, Weingarten H, Ludtke R. [Evaluation of applied kinesiology in nutritional intolerance of childhood]. *Forsch Komplementarmed Klass Naturheilkd* 2001; 8: 336–44.

33. Zuo XL, Li YQ, Li WJ *et al.* Alterations of food antigen-specific serum immunoglobulins G and E antibodies in patients with irritable bowel syndrome and functional dyspepsia. *Clin Exp Allergy* 2007; 37: 823–30.

34. Atkinson W, Sheldon TA, Shaath N, Whorwell PJ. Food elimination based on IgG antibodies in irritable bowel syndrome: a randomised controlled trial. *Gut* 2004; 53: 1459–64.

35. Teuber SS, Porch-Curren C. Unproved diagnostic and therapeutic approaches to food allergy and intolerance. *Curr Opin Allergy Clin Immunol* 2003; 3: 217–21.

36. Isolauri E, Turjanmaa K. Combined skin prick and patch testing enhances identification of food allergy in infants with atopic dermatitis. *J Allergy Clin Immunol* 1996; 97: 9–15.

37. Carter C. Double-blind food challenges in children: a dietitian's perspective. *Current Medical Literature (Allergy)* 1995; 4: 95–9.

38. Werfel T, Breuer K. Role of food allergy in atopic dermatitis. *Curr Opin Allergy Clin Immunol* 2004; 4: 379–85.

39. Sampson HA. Update on food allergy. *J Allergy Clin Immunol* 2004; 113: 805–19.

40. Crevel RW, Briggs D, Hefle SL, Knulst AC, Taylor SL. Hazard characterisation in food allergen risk assessment: the application of statistical approach and the use of clinical data. *Food Chem Toxicol* 2007; 45: 691–701.

41. Hourihane JO, Knulst AC. Thresholds of allergenic proteins in foods. *Toxicol Appl Pharmacol* 2005; 207: 152–6.

42. Vierk K, Falci K, Wolyniak C, Klontz KC. Recalls of foods containing undeclared allergens reported to the US Food and Drug Administration, fiscal year 1999. *J Allergy Clin Immunol* 2002; 109: 1022–6.

43. Venter C, Pereira B, Voigt K *et al.* Comparison of open and double-blind placebo-controlled food challenges in diagnosis of food hypersensitivity amongst children. *J Hum Nutr Diet* 2007; 20: 565–79.

44. Bock SA, Sampson HA, Atkins FM *et al.* Double-blind, placebo-controlled food challenge (DBPCFC) as an office procedure: a manual. *J Allergy Clin Immunol* 1988; 82: 986–97.

45. Bindslev-Jensen C, Ballmer-Weber BK, Bengtsson U *et al.* Standardization of food challenges in patients with immediate reactions to foods: position paper from the European Academy of Allergology and Clinical Immunology. *Allergy* 2004; 59: 690–7.

46. Mofidi S, Bock SA. *A Health Professional's Guide to Food Challenges.* Fairfax, VA: Food Allergy & Anaphylaxis Network, 2005.

47. Taylor SL, Hefle SL, Bindslev-Jensen C *et al.* A consensus protocol for the determination of the threshold doses for allergenic foods: how much is too much? *Clin Exp Allergy* 2004; 34: 689–95.

48. Vlieg-Boerstra BJ, Bijleveld CM, van der Heide S *et al.* Development and validation of challenge materials for double-blind, placebo-controlled food challenges in children. *J Allergy Clin Immunol* 2004; 113: 341–6.

49. Bindslev-Jensen C. Standardization of double-blind, placebo-controlled food challenges. *Allergy* 2001; 56: 75–7.

50. Vlieg-Boerstra BJ, van der Heide S, Bijleveld CMA *et al.* Placebo reactions in double-blind, placebo-controlled food challenges in children. *Allergy* 2007; 62: 905–12.

51. Brouwer ML, Wolt-Plompen SAA, Dubois AEJ *et al.* No effects of probiotics on atopic dermatitis in infancy: a randomized placebo-controlled trial. *Clin Exp Allergy* 2006; 36: 899–906.

52. Ball H, Food Challenges for Children, a Practical Guide; Leicestershire Nutrition and Dietetic Service 11/12 Warren Parkway, Enderby, Leic, 2005.

53. Rancé F, Dutau G. Peanut hypersensitivity in children. *Pediatr Pulmonol Suppl* 1999; 18: 165–7.

54. Sampson HA. Adverse reactions to food. In: Middleton E, Reed CE, Ellis EF *et al.*, eds. *Allergy: Principles and Practice.* St Louis, MO: Mosby, 1998: 1162–82.

55. Caffarelli C, Petroccione T. False-negative food challenges in children with suspected food allergy. *Lancet* 2001; 358: 1871–2.

56. Grimshaw KE, King RM, Nordlee JA *et al.* Presentation of allergen in different food preparations affects the nature of the allergic reaction: a case series. *Clin Exp Allergy* 2003; 33: 1581–5.
57. Asero R, Ballmer-Weber BK, Beyer K *et al.* IgE-mediated food allergy diagnosis: current status and new perspectives. *Mol Nutr Food Res* 2007; 51: 135–47.
58. Perry TT, Conover-Walker MK, Pomes A *et al.* Dose-response in double-blind placebo-controlled oral food challenges in children with atopic dermatitis. *J Allergy Clin Immunol* 2000; 105: 582–6.
59. Niggemann B, Beyer K. Pitfalls in double-blind, placebo-controlled oral food challenges. *Allergy* 2007; 62: 729–32.

4 Triggers of Food Hypersensitivity

Isabel Skypala

4.1 Introduction

There are a multitude of triggers which could be involved in food hypersensitivity (FHS). For immune-mediated conditions, food allergens (proteins) are the key trigger for the reactions, and food allergens are the main focus of this chapter. Food allergens can precipitate both IgE-mediated and non-IgE-mediated food allergy, although the mechanism of inducing a response will be different and may involve different constituent parts of the food. For example, IgE-mediated wheat allergy involves the insoluble wheat gliadins (see Chapter 9), whereas it is the alcohol-soluble gluten fragments that precipitate coeliac disease (see Chapter 9). Non-allergic FHS can be provoked by a much greater variety of triggers; milk can provoke lactose intolerance due to the carbohydrate fraction (lactose) rather than the casein or whey proteins (see Chapter 5). Other foods contain naturally occurring substances such as vasoactive amines or salicylates, which are also known to trigger FHS in sensitive individuals. Finally, food additives can elicit a response, but the mechanisms of action are not well understood. Some may act in combination with a food allergen to provoke an IgE-mediated response or mast cell degranulation, whereas others may induce a mechanistic response, such as the inhalation of sulphur dioxide causing bronchospasm. This chapter will concentrate on the structure and function of food allergens; food additives, salicylates and vasoactive amines are described in Chapter 10.

4.2 Allergens and the immune system

The main cells of the adaptive immune system, the T and B lymphocytes, recognise substances produced by microbes and non-infectious molecules. These substances are known as antigens[1]. In some people, antigens from pollens, animal dander or food proteins can elicit immune responses known as hypersensitivity reactions; when this happens, the antigens are known as allergens[2]. Although foods are composed of proteins, carbohydrates and lipids, the allergens involved in food allergy are usually proteins or haptenated proteins, where a small organic molecule or hapten becomes covalently attached to proteins in the tissues.

Only a small proportion of those exposed to a protein allergen will become sensitised. Lack[3] suggests that differences in population genetics, host immune responses, patterns of breast-feeding, age of weaning, consumption of novel foods and processing of novel foods may all interact to determine whether the introduction of a particular food into a population will lead to sensitisation. Bischoff and Crowe[4] conjecture that, given the large number of food proteins in the human diet, it is surprising that so small a number of foods account for most food allergic reactions, although they suggest that reactions are generally dependent on age and local eating habits. Analysis of animal proteins shows that if sequence identity to a homologous human protein is above 62%, the protein is rarely allergenic[5].

4.3   Food allergen classes and nomenclature

Sensitisation to food and food particles occurs through the ingested, inhaled or cutaneous routes. Food allergens are graded as either class 1 or class 2 allergens[6]. Class 1 allergens are water-soluble glycoproteins 10–70 kD in size, stable to heat, acids and proteases, and they include caseins (milk), vicilins (legumes and nuts), ovomucoid (eggs) and non-specific lipid transfer proteins (many different plant foods). Their robust nature allows them to sensitise during ingestion, breaching the normal immune tolerance to foods, although for some class 1 allergens sensitisation can also occur through the skin[7,8]. Allergies provoked by class 2 allergens usually occur due to pollen-sensitisation in the respiratory tract leading to symptoms in the oral mucosa, caused by cross-reactivity to plant foods due to homologous epitopes. Class 2 allergens are usually heat-labile, difficult to isolate and susceptible to enzymatic degradation, which means they cannot sensitise upon ingestion[6]. They are thought to be highly soluble, with some able to be absorbed in the oral mucosa, allowing immediate symptoms to occur in sensitised individuals.

Allergen nomenclature is standard for all allergens that cause IgE-mediated allergy in humans. A designation is composed of the first three letters of the genus, a space, the first letter of the species name, a space and an Arabic number. In the event that two species names have identical designations, they are discriminated from one another by adding one or more letters (as necessary) to each species designation[9]. For example, *Arachis hypogaea* is the scientific name for peanut; nine allergens have been identified in peanut, and they are labelled Ara h 1, Ara h 2 etc.

4.4   How does a food allergen induce allergy?

It is still unknown what structural and biochemical properties are needed for a given protein to induce allergy, and it is unclear whether a detailed knowledge of the protein structure–function relationships for individual allergens predict allergenicity of novel foods. However, it is known that there are several different structural proteins that are important in food allergy. These include:

1 alpha-helical proteins such as 2S-albumins from seeds and non-specific lipid transfer proteins (nsLTPs);
2 beta-sheet proteins with a prominent helix in close contact, such as lipocalins, profilins and Bet v 1-related proteins;

3 alpha + beta structures in which the alpha and beta structural elements are not intimately associated, such as lactalbumin;

4 serine protease inhibitors.

In addition to the 3D structure of intact proteins, the sugar side-chain may also be responsible for cross-reactions amongst foods from vegetables and invertebrates[10].

Food allergens contain one or more sequences of amino acids, which are recognised by the antibody; these binding sites on the allergen are known as epitopes. There are two types of epitopes, sequential (linear) epitopes and conformational epitopes. Sequential epitopes are antigenic determinants composed of single segments of sequential amino acids along the polypeptide chain. Conformational epitopes are antigenic determinants composed of amino acids from different parts of the protein sequence, brought together by folding. Conformational epitopes can be destroyed when the protein is altered, whereas sequential epitopes are not affected. Class 1 allergens are more likely to contain sequential epitopes, while class 2 allergens will probably contain conformational epitopes. The mapping of epitopes has shown that both sequential and conformational epitopes cause allergic reactions[6]. More than 1,000 epitopes have now been mapped, some of which have been cloned and sequenced using recombinant DNA and monoclonal antibody technologies[4,11].

Although the match of an antibody to an antigen is specific, because only the epitope is involved in the reaction, another allergen with a very similar or homologous epitope can also bind to that antibody. This phenomenon is known as cross-reactivity, and it is very common in food allergy. Cross-reactivity is manifest when an individual already sensitised to one food allergen experiences symptoms after exposure to a different food allergen, due to binding between the antibody against the first food and the epitope of the second. However, cross-reactivity needs to be distinguished from co-sensitisation, where an individual is sensitised to more than one allergen.

4.5 Classification of food allergens

Allergens from both plant and animal sources have been analysed to ascertain the relationships between them, including their protein structure, sequence and allergenic properties. Work by Breiteneder, Radauer, Mills and Jenkins has shown that both animal and plant food allergens can be classified into groups according to the protein structures, and that some proteins are more allergenic than others[5,12–16].

4.5.1 Animal food allergens

These can be classified into three major families – tropomyosins, EF-hand proteins and caseins – and 14 minor families containing 1–3 allergens[5]. Tropomyosins are muscle proteins; those found in mammals, birds and fish are very similar to human tropomyosin and are not reported to be allergenic. However, invertebrate tropomyosin, in molluscs and arthropods such as crustaceans and insects, is allergenic and also accounts for the cross-reactivity seen in these groups[17]. There is no cross-reactivity between shellfish and fish, largely because the main fish allergens come from a different family; the EF-hand allergens include the parvalbumins, and it is the beta parvalbumins which are the main allergens in cod, salmon and mackerel[18]. The other main animal family is the caseins, which are found in mammalian milks and account for the very high degree of cross-reactivity between milks, due to over 90% sequence identity between alpha and beta caseins from cow, goat and sheep[19,20]. It is the percentage of sequence identity here that dictates which milks will cross-react. For example, mare's milk has a very low sequence identity to cow's milk, and children with a cow's milk allergy can generally tolerate mare's milk[21], and only a small percentage of children who have a cow's milk allergy will have specific IgE antibodies to beta casein, which has the highest sequence identity with human casein[22].

4.5.2   Plant food allergens

Plant food allergens are classified as belonging to one of several superfamilies[14]. Some, such as peanut, have major and minor allergens in all of these superfamilies. The cupin superfamily includes vicilins and legumins and contains some of the major allergens in legumes, tree nuts and seeds. The prolamin superfamily includes cereal prolamins, seed storage proteins and nsLTPs. Both of these groups of allergens are generally resistant to proteolysis, pH change and thermal treatments, making them class 1 allergens and so likely to cause food allergy through primary sensitisation in the gastrointestinal tract. The other two families are the plant defence system and profilin families. The plant defence system contains the pathogenesis-related (PR) proteins, defined as plant proteins induced in response to infections by pathogens such as fungi, bacteria and viruses, or due to adverse environmental conditions[14]. PR proteins are divided into groups, several of which, PR2, PR3, PR5 and PR10, are involved in IgE-mediated food allergy reactions, and some groups of allergens are highly homologous and cross-reactive to allergens from latex and pollens, especially the main birch tree pollen allergen Bet v 1 (see Chapter 7). The final plant superfamily, the profilins, are highly conserved in plant cells with 70–85% identical residues in sequences of different species, with profilins found not only in plant foods but also trees, grasses, weeds and latex (see Chapter 7).

4.6   Advances in food allergen technology

Increased knowledge and understanding of food allergens can in turn lead to improved diagnostic tests. This will enable clinicians to be more robust in their diagnosis and to give better advice on food avoidance and the likelihood of resolution of an allergy. Many allergens have been characterised, and recombinant DNA technology has been used to produce allergen extracts containing individual allergens[4,11]. Purified recombinant allergen extracts are highly effective in the diagnosis of allergy to some foods, especially where this involves labile allergens[23,24]. Such allergens are now becoming commercially available and in the future will be especially important in the diagnosis of plant food allergies. The development of individual allergens for testing will also help to improve their specificity and sensitivity. The egg allergen, Gal d 1 (ovomucoid) is resistant to heat and contains linear epitopes; one study[25] showed that the presence of serum-specific IgE antibodies to Gal d 1 could be used as a marker of persistent egg allergy.

The epitope-binding capacity of some allergens has been shown to be predictive in terms of the longevity of the allergy. It is known that children who do not outgrow egg allergy have IgE antibodies to sequential epitopes, whereas those who do make IgE antibodies to conformational epitopes[26]; a similar picture has emerged with regard to milk allergy[27]. The epitope-binding domains of the wheat gliadins may also differ depending on the type of symptoms elicited by wheat. Those with WDEIA, anaphylaxis and urticarial reactions to wheat recognise sequential epitopes on gliadins, whereas those suffering from atopic dermatitis related to wheat recognise conformational epitopes[28]. Epitopes on different allergens can have a degree of amino acid sequence similarity or homology that allows an antibody specific to one allergen to bind with another structurally similar allergen epitope. Homologous epitopes are common in food allergy, accounting for the frequent cross-reactivity between different foods and also between food allergens and allergens from pollens or insects.

4.7 Peanut allergens

In the clinical setting, the peanut allergens are probably the best characterised and most extensively studied of the allergens, and provide a useful illustration of the diversity and characteristics of allergens. Up to nine peanut allergens have been sequenced, with the main allergen, Ara h 1, first identified in 1991[29]. Ara h 1 is highly resistant to thermal processing, and is protected from protease digestion and denaturation by another peanut allergen, Ara h 2, allowing it to pass across the small intestine[14,30].

All peanut allergens respond to heat in a different way. For example, Ara h 1 levels increase when the peanut is roasted, with levels over 20 times greater in roasted than in raw peanuts. The increase in Ara h 1 in roasted peanuts is accompanied by a decrease in total protein, indicating that other proteins in peanuts are not heat-stable[31]. Two allergens which may be affected by heat are Ara h 5 and Ara h 8. Ara h 5 is a profilin, and one study has shown that 13% of a group of peanut-allergic patients were sensitised to this profilin, with those who had monosensitivity to Ara h 5 exhibiting only mild OAS-type symptoms[32]. Ara h 8 has a 45.9% identity with the Bet v 1 amino acid sequence, and studies suggest that Ara h 8 has a very low stability to roasting but is not fully inactivated by heat application[29]. These differences in peanut allergens may help to explain why, although the per capita consumption of peanuts in the USA is the same as in China, there is no peanut allergy in China. The Chinese eat boiled or fried peanuts, whereas those eaten most frequently in the USA are dry roasted peanuts, which are thought to be more allergenic due to the higher heat, maturation and curing used in their production[6].

Sensitisation rates to allergens can also vary, and it is often useful to look at individual allergen responses. All peanut-allergic individuals appear to be sensitised to Ara h 2, compared to less than 10% of those tolerant of peanuts[23,33,34]. Peeters and colleagues[33] showed that those with severe symptoms had a greater response to Ara h 2 and Ara h 6 at lower concentrations, recognised a greater number of peanut allergens, and showed a greater cumulative response than those with mild symptoms. A study by Beyer *et al.*[34] showed that regardless of their specific IgE level, most symptomatic patients showed IgE binding to the three immunodominant epitopes on Ara h 2, as compared to less than 10% of those patients who were tolerant of peanuts. In another study[23], all patients with peanut allergy showed positive SPT to Ara h 2; 53% of them were monosensitised, with significantly lower severity scores than polysensitised subjects.

4.8   Food labelling

Although a wide range of food allergens, additives and naturally occurring substances are implicated in the spectrum of adverse food reactions, most reactions are triggered by 8–9 foods, although the EU identified 14 major allergens or food groups; peanuts and tree nuts are the most common cause of anaphylaxis, and, together with cow's milk, eggs, fish and shellfish, soya, wheat and seeds, account for 90% of IgE-mediated food reactions[35]. The recognition that these foods are all significant provokers of food allergic responses was acknowledged by their listing in a European ingredient rule (Directive 2003/89/EC)[36], which became law in November 2005, stating that specified allergens must be declared on pre-packaged foods if they have been added deliberately, however small the amount. The foods covered include cereals containing gluten, crustaceans, egg, fish, peanut, soya, milk, nuts, celery, mustard, sesame seed, and sulphur dioxide and sulphites at more than 10 mg/litre or 10 mg/kg. The directive was updated to include lupin and molluscs in 2007 (Directive 2006/142/EC; Table 4.1)[37]. Although only a small number of foods

Table 4.1   Ingredients that must be labelled if added to a food (European Commission Directive 2006/142/EC).

- Milk and milk products including lactose
- Eggs
- Fish
- Crustaceans, e.g. prawns, crab, lobster
- Molluscs, e.g. mussels, oysters, scallops
- Cereals containing gluten, including wheat, rye, barley, oats and spelt
- Peanuts
- Tree nuts, i.e. almond, hazelnut, walnut, cashew, pecan, brazil, pistachio, macadamia
- Soybeans and products containing soya
- Lupin flour
- Sesame seeds
- Mustard
- Celery
- Sulphur dioxide and sulphites at concentrations of more than 10 mg/kg

are thought to be implicated in food hypersensitivity, it seems that almost any food can cause symptoms, with case reports of allergic reactions to a diverse range of foods including seal meat[38].

References

1. Abbas AK, Lichtman AH. *Basic Immunology: Functions and Disorders of the Immune System*. Philadelphia, PA: Saunders, 2001.
2. Chaplin DD. Overview of the human immune response. *J Allergy Clin Immunol* 2006; **117**: S430–5.
3. Lack G. New developments in food allergy – old questions remain. *J Allergy Clin Immunol* 2004; **114**: 127–30.
4. Bischoff S, Crowe SE. Food allergy and the gastrointestinal tract. *Curr Opin Gastroenterol* 2004; **20**: 156–67.
5. Jenkins JA, Breiteneder H, Mills ENC. Evolutionary distance from human homologs reflects allergenicity of animal food proteins *J Allergy Clin Immunol* 2007; **120**: 1399–405.
6. Sampson HA. Update on food allergy. *J Allergy Clin Immunol* 2004; **113**: 805–19.
7. Sicherer SH, Sampson HA. Food allergy. *J Allergy Clin Immunol* 2006; **117**: S470–5.
8. Lack G, Fox D, Northstone K, Golding J. Factors associated with the development of peanut allergy in childhood. *N Eng J Med* 2003; **348**: 977–85.
9. International Union of Immunological Societies Allergen Nomenclature Sub-Committee. *Allergen Nomenclature*. www.allergen.org.
10. Aalberse RC, Stapel SO. Structure of food allergens in relation to allergenicity *Pediatr Allergy Immunol* 2001; **12** (Suppl 14): 10–14.
11. Thompson PJ, Stewart GA, Samet JM. Allergies and pollutants. In: Holgate ST, Church MK, Lichtenstein LM, eds. *Allergy*. Edinburgh: Elsevier, 2002: 3–16.
12. Breiteneder H, Ebner C. Molecular and biochemical classifications of plant-derived food allergens. *J Allergy Clin Immunol* 2000; **106**: 27–36.
13. Breiteneder H, Mills ENC. Molecular properties of food allergens. *J Allergy Clin Immunol* 2005; **115**: 14–23.
14. Breiteneder H, Radauer C. A classification of plant food allergens *J Allergy Clin Immunol* 2004; **113**: 821–30.
15. Mills ENC, Jenkins JA, Shewry PR. The role of common properties in determining plant food protein allergenicity. In: Mills ENC, Shrewy PR, eds. *Plant Food Allergens*. Oxford: Blackwell, 2004: 158–70.
16. Radauer C, Breiteneder H. Evolutionary biology of plant food allergens. *J Allergy Clin Immunol* 2007; **120**: 518–25.
17. Reese G, Ayuso R, Lehrer SB. Tropomyosin: an invertebrate pan-allergen. *Int Arch Allergy Immunol* 1999; **119**: 247–58.
18. Hansen TK, Bindslev-Jensen C, Skov PS, Poulsen LK. Codfish allergy in adults: IgE cross-reactivity among fish species. *Ann Allergy Asthma Immunol* 1997; **78**: 187–94.
19. Restani P, Gaiaschi A, Plebani A *et al*. Cross-reactivity between milk proteins from different animal species. *Clin Exp Allergy* 1999; **29**: 997–1004.
20. Bellioni-Businco B, Paganelli R, Lucenti P *et al*. Allergenicity of goat's milk in children with cow's milk allergy. *J Allergy Clin Immunol* 1999; **103**: 1191–4.
21. Businco L, Giampietro PG, Lucenti P *et al*. Allergenicity of mare's milk in children with cow's milk allergy. *J Allergy Clin Immunol* 2000; **105**: 1031–4.
22. Natale M, Bisson C, Monti G *et al*. Cow's milk allergens identification by two-dimensional immunoblotting and mass spectrometry. *Mol Nutr Food Res* 2004; **48**: 363–9.
23. Astier C, Morisset M, Roitel O *et al*. Predictive value of skin prick tests using recombinant allergens for diagnosis of peanut allergy. *J Allergy Clin Immunol* 2006; **118**: 250–6.
24. Mari A, Ballmer-Weber BK, Veiths S. The oral allergy syndrome: improved diagnostic and treatment methods. *Curr Opin Allergy Clin Immunol* 2005; **5**: 267–73.
25. Järvinen KM, Beyer K, Vila L *et al*. Specificity of IgE antibodies to sequential epitopes of hen's egg ovomucoid as a marker for persistence of egg allergy. *Allergy* 2007: **62**: 758–65.

26. Cooke SK, Sampson HA. Allergenic properties of ovomucoid in man. *J Immunol* 1997; **159**: 2026–32.
27. Vila L, Beyer K, Järvinen KM *et al*. Role of conformational and linear epitopes in the achievement of tolerance in cow's milk allergy. *Clin Exp Allergy* 2001; **31**: 1599–606.
28. Battais F, Mothes T, Moneret-Vautrin DA *et al*. Identification of IgE-binding epitopes on gliadins for patients with food allergy to wheat. *Allergy* 2005; **60**: 815–21.
29. Mittag D, Akkerdass J, Ballmer-Weber B *et al*. Ara h 8, a Bet v 1-homologous allergen from peanut, is a major allergen in patients with combined birch pollen and peanut allergy. *J Allergy Clin Immunol* 2004; **114**: 1410–17.
30. Maleki SJ, Viquez O, Jacks T *et al*. The major peanut allergen, Ara H 2, functions as a trypsin inhibitor, and roasting enhances this function. *J Allergy Clin Immunol* 2003; **112**: 190–5.
31. Pomés A, Butts CL, Chapman MD. Quantification of Ara h 1 in peanuts: why roasting makes a difference. *Clin Exp Allergy* 2006; **36**: 824–30.
32. Kleber-Janke T, Crameri R, Scheurer S, Veiths S, Becker WM. Patient-tailored cloning of allergens by phage display: peanut (*Arachis hypogaea*) profilin, a food allergen derived from a rare mRNA. *J Chromatogr B Biomed Sci Appl* 2001; **756**: 295–305.
33. Peeters KABM, Kopplemann SJ, van Hoffen E *et al*. Does skin prick test reactivity to purified allergens correlate with clinical severity of peanut allergy? *Clin Exp Allergy* 2007; **37**: 108–15.
34. Beyer KB, Ellman-Grunther L, Järvinen KM *et al*. Measurement of peptide-specific IgE as an additional tool in identifying patients with clinical reactivity to peanuts. *J Allergy Clin Immunol* 2003; **112**: 202–7.
35. Bock SA, Sampson HA, Atkins FM *et al*. Double-blind, placebo-controlled food challenge (DBPCFC) as an office procedure: a manual. *J Allergy Clin Immunol* 1988; **82**: 986–97.
36. European Union. Directive 2003/89/EC of the European Parliament and of the Council of 10 November 2003 amending Directive 2000/13/EC as regards indication of the ingredients present in foodstuffs. *Official Journal of the European Union* 2003; L308: 15–18.
37. European Union. Commission Directive 2006/142/EC of 22 December 2006 amending Annex IIIa of Directive 2000/13/EC of the European Parliament and of the Council listing the ingredients which must under all circumstances appear on the labelling of foodstuffs. *Official Journal of the European Union* 2006; L368: 110–11.
38. Moore LM, Rathkopf MM, Sanner CJ, Whisman BA, Demain JG. Seal and whale meat: two newly recognized food allergies. *Ann Allergy Asthma Immunol* 2007; **98**: 92–6.

Part 2
Dietary Management

5 Milk and Eggs

Tanya Wright and Rosan Meyer

Hypersensitivity reactions to cow's milk and hen's egg are seen both in children and in adults. These reactions can be IgE- and/or non-IgE-mediated in the case of both cow's-milk protein (CMP) and egg allergies. Additionally, symptoms to cow's milk can also occur as a result of lactase deficiency (i.e. lactose intolerance), which is a non-allergic food hypersensitivity reaction[1,2]. Cow's-milk protein allergy (CMPA) and egg allergy are the most common allergies seen in childhood, with a documented prevalence of 2–3% and 1.6% respectively in the first three years of life[3].

In adults, however, IgE-mediated allergy to CMP is rare. A population study by Woods *et al.* found that only 0.7% of atopic adults have a positive skin prick test (SPT) to CMP, and none of those patients reported symptoms associated with the consumption of cow's milk[4]. The most common reactions in adulthood are non-immune-mediated, with about 4.8% of adults reporting non-specific 'illness', ranging from abdominal bloating (see irritable bowel syndrome, Chapter 2) to diarrhoea (see lactose intolerance, below). Egg allergy follows a similar trend, with 1.6% of an adult atopic population with a positive SPT, but only 0.2% of those individuals reporting associated symptoms[4,5].

This chapter is aimed at providing guidelines on the diagnosis and management of immune-mediated CMP and hen's egg allergy, in addition to presenting information on the most commonly seen non-immune responses to both these foods in children and adults.

5.2 Cow's milk

5.2.1 Cow's-milk protein allergy

CMPA usually develops in the first year of life[6]. A review by Høst *et al.* on 229 peer-reviewed articles on CMPA from 1967 to 2001 found that most infants with CMPA develop symptoms before 1 month of age, and the incidence of CMPA at 1 year of age was 2–2.5%[7]. This concurs with most clinical experience that CMP-allergic infants typically present after their first or second known exposure to CMP, which is usually taken as an infant formula, yoghurt, or commercial or home-cooked baby foods. It is common practice for maternity units to offer a CMP-based formula to newborns as their first ever feed if breast-feeding is delayed post partum. This early feed may represent the sensitising event which leads to the development of 'immune memory', i.e. specific-IgE formation[1,8]. Additional routes of CMP exposure (or sensitisation) include skin contact reactions (e.g. kiss-induced reactions) and inhalation of CMP via cooking vapours (a cause of allergic asthmatic reactions)[9].

Numerous milk proteins have been implicated in allergic responses (Table 5.1). Casein accounts for about 80% of the total protein content in cow's milk, and whey for the rest. Casein consists of five protein fractions, α_{s1}-, α_{s2}-, β-, κ- and γ-casein, and whey fractions contain globular proteins, α-lactalbumin and β-lactoglobulin[10]. The allergenicity of each of these proteins remains unclear, with casein being a major milk allergen. However, significant reactivity to both α-lactalbumin and β-lactoglobulin from whey protein has also been documented[11]. β-Lactoglobulin is acid-stable and is likely to remain intact after passage through the stomach, which may explain its role as an allergen in CMPA[6]. New research on the different milk proteins, specifically on IgE- and IgG-binding epitopes, have provided some useful information regarding persistent CMPA[11]. Some of the IgE-binding regions on α_{s1}-, β- and κ-casein were recognised only by older children with CMPA but not by patients under 3 years of age[6]. Some epitopes of β-lactoglobulin, but none from α-lactalbumin, were associated with the persistence of CMPA. These are potential useful markers for identifying patients that will continue to have CMPA in future.

It is important to note that research performed on other mammalian species has shown that animals that are phylogenetically related, like sheep, goat, water buffalo, horse and donkey, have quite similar milk proteins to cow's milk. β-Lactoglobulin, a major allergen in cow's milk, is present in all studied mammalian milks[12]. These milks harbour an allergic potential, and are for this reason not suitable as an alternative in patients with CMPA.

Clinical presentation of CMP-induced disease

CMP can induce both acute IgE-mediated reactions (within 2 hours) and delayed reactions that may be either non-IgE-mediated or mixed (> 2 hours). Current data

Table 5.1 Proteins in cow's milk[11].

Protein	Cow's milk (mg/mL)
α_{s1}-casein	11.6
α_{s2}-casein	3.0
β-casein	9.6
κ-casein	3.6
γ-casein	1.6
α-lactalbumin	1.2
β-lactoglobulin	3.0
immunoglobulins	0.6
lactoferrin	0.3
lysozyme	trace
serum albumin	0.4

suggest that 58% of CMPA individuals displayed an early reaction and the remaining 42% had a delayed, non-IgE-mediated reaction[13-16]. A broad range of clinical symptoms and syndromes have been reported with CMPA[6]. The clinical spectrum ranges from acute anaphylactic manifestations to atopic dermatitis, food-associated wheeze, infantile colic, gastro-oesophageal reflux (GOR) related to eosinophilic oesophagitis, cow's-milk enterocolitis, food-associated proctocolitis and constipation[17]. Table 5.2 provides a summary of reactions and their immune classification. CMPA usually affects at least two systems: 50–60% of CMPA individuals have cutaneous symptoms, 50–60% have gastrointestinal symptoms, and approximately 20–30% respiratory symptoms[7].

Typically breast-fed infants with CMPA present very soon after birth with eczema and/or proctocolitis, or they present after exposure to a CMP-based infant formula or weaning foods that contain this protein[18]. It is estimated that about 15% of infants with CMPA retain their sensitivity to CMP into adult life[10]. Although adult onset of IgE-mediated CMPA has been reported in the medical literature, this occurrence remains rare[21]. Immediate IgE reactions are usually easy to identify and verify, and have received more attention in diagnosis and management from healthcare professionals. In contrast, non-IgE-mediated reactions, such as GOR, Heiner's syndrome and constipation, are often not well recognised and remain a source of debate amongst clinicians, as the underlying pathophysiology is often not as well defined as IgE-mediated reactions[22,23]. Current research indicates that CMPA is present in 16–42% of infants with GOR[24]. Chronic constipation is seen in 3–16% of children and is related to CMPA in 30–55% of these patients[25]. CMP as a cause

Table 5.2 Classification of cow's milk protein-induced immune reactions[1,6,18-20].

IgE-mediated	
Gastrointestinal	Gastrointestinal anaphylaxis: symptoms include vomiting, pain and/or diarrhoea
Cutaneous	Urticaria, angio-oedema, pruritus, morbilliform rashes and flushing
Respiratory	Acute rhinoconjunctivitis, wheezing, coughing and stridor
Generalized	Anaphylaxis
Mixed IgE- and non-IgE-mediated	
Gastrointestinal	Eosinophilic oesophagitis, colitis and/or proctocolitis
Cutaneous	Atopic eczema
Respiratory	Asthma
Non-IgE-mediated	
Gastrointestinal	Food-protein-induced enterocolitis, food-protein-induced proctocolitis and food-protein-induced enteropathy syndrome – which may present with a clinical picture of 'sepsis'
Cutaneous	CMP-induced contact dermatitis.
Respiratory	Food-induced pulmonary haemosiderosis (Heiner's syndrome) (rare) – pulmonary haemosiderosis or bleeding in the lower respiratory tract.
Mechanism uncertain	
	Excess mucous production – the 'snuffly child' (association remains controversial, but commonly suspected by parents); constipation (association remains controversial); intestinal colic; Heiner's syndrome

of chronic constipation in adults has been documented by Carroccio *et al.*, but it is reported only in a very small number of patients, and other causes for constipation need to be ruled out first[26]. Heiner's syndrome is a food hypersensitivity pulmonary disease that primarily affects infants, and is mostly caused by CMP (see also Chapter 2). However, its occurrence is extremely rare and it should only be suspected in young children with chronic pulmonary disease of obscure cause[19].

Diagnosis of CMPA

To prevent needless suffering, an early and accurate diagnosis of CMPA is essential. The diagnosis of CMPA relies on a detailed clinical history (Table 5.3), physical examination and, depending on the type of reaction, SPT and/or specific IgE testing can be performed[1]. The physical examination is helpful to assess the growth of the child[27], to exclude signs suggestive of nutritional deficiency such as iron deficiency and rickets related to vitamin D deficiency[28,29], and lastly to determine whether the patient has any other clinical signs of atopy (e.g. Dennie–Morgan folds). The respiratory and dermatological examination should also seek to document the presence or absence of concomitant allergic conditions such as asthma and/or eczema, which may impact on the management of the patient with CMPA.

Allergy tests (SPT and specific IgE testing) are particularly useful in making the diagnosis of IgE-mediated CMPA[1]. Guidelines have been published to assist clinicians

Table 5.3   Taking an effective clinical history[6,30,31].

Questions should aim to establish the following	Significance
What is the suspected food allergen causing the reported reaction?	Is the allergen typical for age? Allergies to CMP are common in young children but rare in adulthood.
What is the timing of the reaction post exposure?	IgE-mediated CMPA reactions usually occur within 2 hours. Enterocolitis syndromes and eczema exacerbations are typically more delayed in onset.
What are the allergic symptoms?	If symptoms are not typical of an immediate-onset IgE-mediated reaction, then a differential diagnosis must be considered.
What is the route of allergen exposure?	Does the patient react on ingestion of CMP and/or after skin contact?
Is there a prior history of CMP tolerance?	It is rare to have a history of ongoing tolerance to CMP prior to developing an allergy. Most CMPA presents during infancy.
Concomitant allergic disease?	At least 25% of CMPA will go on to develop additional food allergies. Food-allergic infants, particularly egg-allergic infants, are at risk of the development of asthma (which is a risk factor for future severe food-induced allergic reactions).

in making the diagnosis[32–35] (see Chapter 2 and Table 3.1). However, results frequently fall below these published predictive cut-off values in spite of reported symptomatology. Because of these limitations, elimination diets and double-blind randomised controlled food challenges remain the gold standard[1]. An elimination diet should ideally be followed under the supervision of a dietitian, and care should be taken to ensure nutritional adequacy[36]. Food challenges should only be performed in a controlled environment with emergency treatment at hand[37] (see Chapter 3).

Non-IgE-mediated reactions commonly yield negative allergy tests and require empirical CMP avoidance to confirm diagnosis[23]. It is generally recommended that an elimination diet should be followed for at least 4 weeks before a decision is made on symptom improvement and reintroduction is considered[23]. There is a suggestion that allergy patch testing could aid the diagnosis of these types of reactions. However, this is not yet part of routine practice, as the patch test method has not yet been standardised[1].

Managing CMPA

The mainstay of treatment for CMPA is the avoidance of CMP in addition to other mammalian milks (e.g. goat, sheep, donkey and buffalo products)[12]. Cow's milk contributes protein, calcium, phosphorous, thiamine, riboflavin, niacin, vitamin A (in full-cream milk) and D (in full-cream milk) to the diet[38]. Avoidance therefore should always aim to maintain nutritional adequacy by introducing suitable alternatives or supplementing nutrients (e.g. calcium)[28,29,39]. Dietary exclusion must be complete, including traces of milk, and measures to reduce accidental exposure from cross-contamination should also be implemented. Avoidance of CMP requires the ingredients of all foods to be known. This means reading and knowing all the different terms used to label CMP (Table 5.4). It is also important to be aware that product recipes change, so these labels need to be checked with every new food opened. The labelling law in the European Union (EU) requires milk products to be labelled in the ingredients panel of pre-packed foods if they are intentionally present

Table 5.4 Foods that list any of these ingredients on their label need to be avoided in CMPA patients.

Cow's milk (fresh, UHT, evaporated, condensed, dried)
Butter, butter oil, butter milk
Cream
Cheese
Yogurt, fromage frais
Casein, caseinates, hydrolysed casein, sodium caseinate
Curd
Ghee
Lactoglobulin
Lactose (this is milk sugar; you need only avoid if extremely allergic to milk)
Milk solids, non-fat milk solids
Whey, hydrolysed whey, whey powder, whey syrup sweetener
Unspecified 'flavourings' (if very allergic)

in the product, however tiny the amount. This legislation does not include any traces of milk during manufacturing, but manufacturers are increasingly labelling this voluntarily. Such labels should be heeded by the severely milk-allergic population. Patients may also wish to contact the manufacturers directly to ascertain the level of milk protein contamination.

There are also increasing numbers of foods made specifically for special diets on the supermarket shelves (Table 5.5). Other outlets, including health-food shops and special diet food suppliers also have a variety of 'free from' foods. Kosher foods are often dairy-free and manufactured under strict regulations, and may be consumed by patients with a CMPA. It is important to note that many of the replacement products have an inferior nutritional content (e.g. rice milk, pea milk, oat milk) when compared to full-cream milk. These replacements are not only lacking in energy and protein density, but also have low or absent fat-soluble vitamins and minerals. Nutrient supplementation might therefore be required, and patients should be advised to purchase the calcium-enriched variety of the milk replacements.

Managing a CMP-free diet in infants is significantly more complicated than in adults, as the avoidance diet impacts on the breast-feeding mother, the choice of formula and weaning foods. Breast milk remains the ideal choice for the CMPA infant[40]. Although CMP β-lactoglobulin can be detected in the breast milk of 95% of lactating women (0.9–150 µg/l) it remains well tolerated in most CMPA infants. The infant will, however, be exposed to CMP not only in the mother's breast milk but also through skin contact. Therefore, if CMPA symptoms persist in the breast-fed infant, a strict maternal CMP exclusion diet is indicated, avoiding all products in Table 5.4[1,41]. Studies, particularly in infants with severe atopic eczema and enterocolitis related to CMPA, have indicated improvements on this diet[1,41]. It is important to consider the adequacy of the lactating mother's calcium intake when this strategy is adopted, as the recommended requirement for breast-feeding mothers exceeds 1,000 mg/day (Table 5.6), which may be difficult to achieve on an un-supplemented diet. The inclusion of non-dairy foods high in calcium may also help in increasing calcium intake naturally (Table 5.7).

Table 5.5 Products specifically manufactured for the dairy-free market.

To replace	Suitable replacement product
Milk	Oat milk, pea milk, rice milk, soya milk, quinoa milk, nut milks (only if nuts are already being tolerated), coconut milks (note that organic milk-free products do not have calcium added)
Spreading fats	Dairy-free and vegan spreads
Cheese	Hard, soft, melting, spreading and Parmesan varieties of soya cheese*
Yogurts	Soya
Ice creams	Soya, oat, rice, hemp
Cream	Soya, oat, coconut

* Rice cheese usually contains casein, which is a milk protein and therefore unsuitable for those avoiding milk protein, but it will be suitable for someone with a lactose intolerance.

Table 5.6   Daily calcium requirements[42].

Age	Calcium required (mg)
0–12 months	525 mg
1–3 years	350 mg
4–6 years	450 mg
7–10 years	550 mg
Males 11–18 years	1000 mg
Males 19+ years	700 mg
Females 11–18 years	800 mg
Females 19+ years	700 mg
Breast-feeding	Female requirements + 550 mg

Table 5.7   Calcium-rich CMP-free foods.

Food	Calcium (mg)
1 glass/200 ml calcium-enriched soya milk	250
1 glass/200 ml rice milk	26
1 glass/200 ml calcium-enriched rice milk	240
1 glass/200 ml calcium-enriched oat milk	240
1 glass/200 ml pea milk	84
1 glass/200 ml almond milk	32
30 g soya cheese hard (melting variety)	90
30 g soya cheese hard (non-melting variety)	30–60
125 g soya yogurt	125
1 glass/200 ml calcium-fortified orange juice	245
1 glass/200 ml calcium-enriched soya fruit drink	240
1 glass/200 ml calcium-fortified water	60
100 g sardines (tinned – where bones eaten)	500
40 g instant porridge (dry – before milk added)	480
50 g tofu (soya bean curd)	255
100 g (1 large bowl) muesli	200
3 dried figs	170
100 g spinach	160
2 heaped tablespoons red kidney beans	100
100 g (3 slices) white bread	100
30 g breakfast cereals	100
25 g Brazil nuts (7 whole nuts)	90
60 g shelled prawns	90
14 g (1 tablespoon) sunflower/sesame seeds	85
1 medium orange	75
150 g (small tin) baked beans	75
25 g almonds (12 whole nuts)	65
3 slices whole meal bread	50
25 g watercress	55
100 g dark green vegetables	50

In addition to adequate calcium intake, adequate consumption of foods rich in vitamin D (e.g. oily fish, egg yolk, fortified dairy-free margarine) and sunlight exposure will assist in maintaining the calcium homeostasis. If the infant's symptoms do not improve after approximately 2 weeks of maternal avoidance, CMP should be reintroduced[1]. Healthcare professionals must be aware, however, of the very small but significant number of infants who may continue to react, in spite of maternal exclusion (especially patients with enterocolitis and severe atopic dermatitis) and these may require an amino acid formula[43,44]. However, this decision should be taken together with a paediatric allergist, as breast-feeding should never be stopped unless to do so is of benefit to the child.

For CMPA infants who are unable to receive breast milk (which remains the ideal infant feed), an appropriate and safe hypoallergenic infant formula needs to be selected. There are strict criteria which distinguish between hypoallergenic and non-hypoallergenic formulas. The European Society of Paediatric Gastroenterology, Hepatology and Nutrition (ESPGHAN) and the European Society of Paediatric Allergy and Clinical Immunology (ESPACI) stipulate that hypoallergenic formulas for the treatment of CMPA should be tolerated by 90% of infants with CMPA, with a 95% confidence interval[40]. Only amino acid (AA) and extensively hydrolysed formulas (eHF) (Table 5.8) are suitable to treat CMPA. Within the category of eHF, both casein- and whey-based formulas are commercially available and have become the mainstay formulas for treating infants with CMPA[45]. It is important to note that although partially hydrolysed formulas are available in the UK they are *not* hypoallergenic and should not be used for an infant with diagnosed CMPA[40].

It is estimated that up to 10% of infants will continue to react to eHF[46,47]. This is as a consequence of the residual allergenicity in eHF, related to residual CMP peptides and/or aggregation of smaller peptides due incomplete hydrolysis[40]. A recent systematic review by Hill *et al.* found AA-based formula especially useful in patients with non-IgE-mediated food enterocolitis/proctitis syndromes with faltering growth, severe atopic dermatitis and symptoms during exclusive breast-feeding[44]. A major hurdle in the use of hypoallergenic formulas is their poor taste[48]; this is however less of an issue for younger infants (< 6 months of age) with a relatively 'naive' taste repertoire. Older infants, and infants who were previously enjoying the pleasant taste of breast milk, commonly reject the introduction of hypoallergenic formula. Therefore:

1   introduce the hypoallergenic formula as soon as possible, or if breast-feeding is to continue, transition the introduction with incremental mixing of the milks;
2   offer the hypoallergenic formula as the only fluid source;
3   if the infant is above 6 months, introduce the formula in a feeder beaker that has good flow (avoid beakers with valves);
4   mask the smell with a good-quality vanilla essence (a few drops only);
5   commercial chocolate, banana or strawberry milkshake powders should only be used as a last option, as they are very high in sugar and create a habit of 'sweet preference'. When this method is used to introduce the hypoallergenic formulas, gradually reduce the amount of milkshake powder until the formula is tolerated neat.

Milk and Eggs 125

Table 5.8 Hypoallergenic formulas available in the UK.

Type of formula	Indications/comments	Examples
Extensively hydrolysed whey	Whey empties the stomach faster and may therefore be of benefit to patients with gastrointestinal symptoms. Contains a higher percentage of peptides above 1.5 kD. The addition of lactose into whey hydrolysate improves taste.	Pepti (Cow & Gate) – contains lactose Pepti junior (Cow & Gate) – contains medium chain triglycerides (MCT) as fat source
Extensively hydrolysed casein	Most protein < 1.5 kD. Well tolerated by children with IgE mediated allergy. Has a distinct taste. Lactose-free.	Nutramigen 1 (Mead Johnson) (up to 6 months) Nutramigen 2 (Mead Johnson) (over 6 months) Pregestimil (Mead Johnson) (54% MCT)
Soya formulas (non-hydrolysed protein)	Not recommended for infants under 6 months. Not recommended as the first choice of formula for 6–12 months. May be given to those refusing extensively hydrolysed formulas. Lactose-free. Suitable for vegans.	Infasoy (Cow & Gate) Farley's soya formula (Heinz) Isomil (Abbott) Prosobee (Mead Johnson) Wysoy (SMA)
Non-milk-based extensively hydrolysed formulas	Not suitable for some cultures, religions or vegetarians (because contains meat derivatives). Seldom used for treating CMPA, due to poor taste. Suitable for malabsorption disorders.	Prejomin (Milupa) Pepdite (SHS) (under 1 year) Pepdite 1+ (SHS) (over 1 year) MCT Pepdite (SHS) (75% MCT)
Elemental amino-acid-based formula	Suitable for multiple, severe food allergies and when other formulas are unsuitable: enterocolitis, proctitis, persistent severe atopic eczema and faltering growth. For children with persistent symptoms in on eHF.	Neocate (SHS) (up to 1 year) Neocate Active (SHS) (1–10 years) – better taste, more calcium and iron Neocate Advance (SHS) (1–10 years)

It is important also to mention the role of soya formulas in patients with CMPA, as this has been a source of great controversy over the last few years. Prior to the availability of hypoallergenic formulas, the only alternative to CMP-based formula for infants with CMPA were formulas derived from soya. Soya-based infant formulas remain popular, with clear advantages and disadvantages. Soya is lactose-free, making it ideal for vegan families, and soya formulas have a favourable taste. However, soya protein is a relatively common food allergen, with some 3–14% of young children with IgE-mediated and up to 40% of those with non-IgE-mediated CMPA having concomitant soya allergy[49,50]. Initial concerns that soya may induce peanut allergy (both are pulses) have not been substantiated[51,52]. Recent concerns, based on animal studies, relate to the possible effects on young infants of soya-containing phyto-oestrogens[49]. As a precaution, the Committee on Toxicity of

Chemicals in Food recommended that soya formula should only be consumed after the age of 6 months. In the light of other hypoallergenic formulas being available for these patients, both the British Dietetic Association Paediatric Group and ESPGHAN recommend that alternative hypoallergenic formulas should be used as first-line treatment in younger infants (< 6 months)[49,53]. The cross-reactivity between CMP and soya is significant in non IgE-mediated food allergy, and the use of soya-based formula is therefore totally contraindicated in these conditions[52].

Resolution of CMPA

The prognosis of CMPA is good, with a remission rate of approximately 45–50% at 1 year, 60–75% at 2 years, and 85–90% at 3 years, 92% at 5 and 10 years and 97% at 15 years of age[54,55]. Individuals with delayed reactions have been shown to develop tolerance sooner than those with immediate reactions: 64%, 92% and 96% versus 31%, 53% and 63%, respectively[56]. Monitoring the development of tolerance is an essential part of managing food allergy[34]. CMPA allergy is commonly outgrown, so retesting and reassessment is required annually. Several studies have investigated the value of SPT and specific IgE tests in predicting tolerance to CMPA. Vanto *et al.* found that a wheal size of < 5 mm in SPT correctly identified 83% of infants who developed tolerance to CMP by the age of 4 years, and a wheal size of ≥ 5 mm in SPT correctly identified 71% of infants with persistent CMPA. CMP-specific IgE < 2 kU_A/L correctly identified 82% of infants who developed tolerance to CMP, while conversely a CMP-specific IgE ≥ 2 kU_A/L correctly identified 71% of infants with persistent CMPA[56]. Vassilopoulou *et al.* found that SPT ≤ 4 mm (specific IgE ≤ 3.94 kU_A/L) could correctly predict a negative challenge whereas SPT ≥ 7.5 mm and specific IgE ≥ 25.4 kU_A/L were predictive of a positive milk challenge[57]. The decision to expose a child to a food challenge should not only rely on the reduction of SPT and specific IgE towards CMP, but also on the length of CMP exclusion and the outcome of any accidental ingestion of CMP-containing foods (e.g. cakes, croissants)[34]. A discussion with the parents may also influence the decision on whether to proceed with the food challenge. Cut-offs may also need to be adjusted to your local clinic population.

Once tolerance has been established, it is important that CMP is reintroduced into the patient's diet. In practice this is often done with processed dairy products (e.g. cheese, cakes) first before introducing fresh milk.

5.2.2 Lactose intolerance

Lactose intolerance is often confused with CMPA. It is distinctly different, however, in that it is not immune-mediated and is due to an intolerance to the carbohydrate lactose in cow's milk[31]. The cause is the absence or deficiency, to a varying degree, of the enzyme lactase in the gastrointestinal tract. Three major types of lactose intolerance exist: congenital, primary and secondary. Congenital lactose intolerance has the least lactase activity and is a lifelong disorder characterised by poor growth and infantile diarrhoea from the first exposure to breast milk, which contains lactose[58].

This form of lactase deficiency is extremely rare. Conversely, primary lactose intolerance occurs in 70% of humans and usually occurs, over a period of years, never before 2–5 years of age and often not until young adulthood. Patients suffering from primary lactose intolerance have low (not absent) levels of lactase and usually tolerate foods that have lower lactose content. Secondary lactose intolerance refers to those patients that lose lactase activity as a result of gastrointestinal illness that damages the brush border of the small intestine, e.g. viral gastroenteritis, giardiasis or coeliac disease. This is usually reversible, and lactose can often be reintroduced after following a lactose-free diet for a few weeks.

Symptoms experienced with lactose intolerance include diarrhoea, bloating and cramping[31]. This is due to the deficiency of intestinal lactase, which prevents hydrolysis of ingested lactose. The osmotic load of the unabsorbed lactose causes secretion of fluid and electrolytes, which induces an acceleration of small intestinal transit. In the large intestine, the lactose is fermented by colonic bacteria to yield short-chain fatty acids and hydrogen gas – thus leading to intestinal bloating[59]. Symptoms experienced with lactose intolerance are very similar to those seen in patients with irritable bowel syndrome (IBS). Although lactose intolerance does not lead to IBS, research has shown that 24–27% of patients with IBS have lactose intolerance[60]. It is important to note, however, that only 52% of these patients experienced symptom relief on a lactose-free diet[61]. For more information on IBS see Chapter 2.

Lactose intolerance is usually diagnosed using one of three methods: the lactose intolerance test, which is performed after an 8–12 hour fast followed by the ingestion of a solution containing lactose, with blood sugar levels measured before and after; the hydrogen breath test, which detects hydrogen from undigested lactose; and testing for reducing substances in stools, which indicates the presence of undigested lactose in the stool[61]. A diagnosis of lactose intolerance if often also made on the basis of a clinical history (e.g. severe gastroenteritis) and is confirmed by the exclusion of lactose-containing foods and subsequent improvement of symptoms. In practice it is not always considered necessary to have one of these tests if it is known that a low-lactose diet resolves symptoms. Instead, an incremental exclusion and reintroduction diet alongside a detailed diary can identify the lactose tolerance level, and specific dietary advice given accordingly.

Lactose intolerance is treated with a lactose-free diet or lactose-reduced diet. The type of lactose intolerance predicts the level of lactose avoidance. In patients with congenital lactose intolerance, all lactose as well as traces of lactose should be avoided[61]. The principles are the same as managing a patient on a CMP-free diet (see above). The only difference is that infants with this condition require a lactose-free formula, and adults may tolerate commercial lactose-free milk. Patients with secondary lactose intolerance also require total lactose avoidance, but this condition is transient and lactose should be reintroduced after an avoidance diet of 4–8 weeks[58]. Individuals with primary lactose intolerance usually tolerate some lactose in their diet; however, the level of tolerance is very individual and should be treated as such. It is not uncommon for some of them to tolerate a small amount of cow's milk on cereal, Cheddar cheese and live yoghurts, whilst others cannot even tolerate minuscule amounts of low-lactose milk[61]. Thus, for individuals with

Table 5.9 Low-lactose foods.

Food type	Low-lactose example
Milk	Soya, rice, oat, nut, coconut, potato and pea milks Lactose-reduced and lactose-free milks
Fat	Pure butter, dairy-free spreads, soya spread, vegetable oils
Cheese	Edam, Gouda, Roquefort, Brie, Cheddar, blue cheese, soya cheese, rice cheese
Yoghurt	Cow's milk yoghurt (low lactose), soya yoghurt (no lactose)
Cream	Soya cream, oat cream

primary lactose intolerance, low-lactose cow's milk and low-lactose dairy products such as Cheddar cheese and fermented yoghurts (Table 5.9) can often be tolerated, but tolerance levels need to be established for effective management of this diet. It is also important to limit overzealous restriction of lactose.

5.3   Egg allergy

Egg allergy is one of the most prevalent food allergies in children. The estimated prevalence varies between 1.6% and 3.2% depending on the classification and nomenclature of food hypersensitivity reactions used[62]. Egg allergy is much less common in older children and the adult population[63]. Pereira *et al.* reported that 1% of their adolescents (*n* = 649) were sensitised to egg[63], whereas Woods *et al.* found that 1.6% of their adult population had a positive SPT to egg, although only 0.2% had had illness associated with the ingestion of egg[4].

5.3.1   Clinical presentation of egg-induced disease

Atopic dermatitis represents the main clinical manifestation[3] of egg allergy in infancy, although several authors have reported urticaria, angio-oedema, acute vomiting, violent diarrhoea or even anaphylaxis (all IgE-mediated reactions) on first known exposure to egg in infants' weaning diets[62,64,65]. These findings indicate that children may be sensitised to eggs, even though they have never eaten them. It has in fact been shown that egg proteins can cross the placenta to induce a specific immune response in the fetus, in addition to being transferred through breast milk in breast-fed infants[66].

The impact of egg protein on gastrointestinal reactions is much less well defined, and the evidence base is limited to case reports[67]. Anecdotally, parents often report exacerbation of gastrointestinal symptoms in children with allergic colitis when egg is introduced as part of a weaning diet, and resolution of symptoms when egg is removed[23]. It is therefore important not to dismiss these symptoms, if they are reported by parents.

Eggs are composed of 56–61% egg white and 27–32% egg yolk. Clinically relevant allergens are found in both egg yolk and egg white, but egg-white allergy is more commonly seen[68]. The allergenic components of egg white include ovoalbumin

(Gal d 2: 54% of egg white), ovotransferrin (12%), ovomucoid (Gal d 1: 11%), ovomucin (3.5%) and lysozyme (Gal d 4: 3.4%)[3]. Egg yolk also contains a variety of components that are allergenic: ovoflavoprotein, apovitellenins I and IV, phosvitin and α-livetin[5]. Research has identified four distinct sets of proteins that egg-allergic children commonly react to[69]:

1 lysosyme and ovalbumin;
2 ovomucoid;
3 ovomucin;
4 all egg-white proteins and the egg-yolk proteins apovitellenins I and IV, phosvitin.

Adults most commonly react to ovotransferrin (53%), then ovomucoid (38%), followed by ovalbumin (32%) and lysozyme (15%)[3]. Research has also found a difference in the allergenicity between cooked and raw egg. It is therefore not uncommon for egg-allergic individuals to tolerate cooked egg in small amounts (e.g. cake, biscuits), but not raw egg (e.g. fresh sorbet, mayonnaise, royal icing)[70].

5.3.2 Diagnosis

The diagnosis of egg allergy relies on a thorough patient history, including the type of egg-containing food (raw, partially cooked or cooked egg) the individual reacts to, the symptoms experienced and the time it takes for the reaction to occur. A detailed dietary assessment is most probably the most useful tool and will often identify suspected culprit foods that are inadvertently being ingested. A dietary history also helps identify those patients whose egg hypersensitivity allows foods to be tolerated in small amounts.

In addition to the clinical history, diagnostic testing procedures (SPT and/or specific IgE testing) are useful, especially in patients with IgE-mediated egg allergy. Although these tests have been shown to be sensitive indicators for when a child has a reaction to egg, they are not necessarily predictive of the likelihood or severity of clinical reactions[3]. A wheal of > 7 mm to egg has been shown to be a strong predictor of the development of an adverse reaction on egg consumption, whilst a wheal < 3 mm has been shown to be useful in excluding egg allergy[71]. Patients with a wheal size of 3–7 mm are in the diagnostic 'grey zone', and in these cases the clinical history should guide diagnosis or a food challenge should be considered. Additionally, egg-specific antibody levels ≥ 7 kU_A/L indicate $\geq 95\%$ likelihood for the individual to react to egg on challenge[62] (see also Chapter 3).

In patients with non-IgE-mediated reactions to egg, a period of egg exclusion (for at least four weeks) followed by reintroduction should be considered. The reintroduction should commence slowly and gradually over three days, with cooked egg products first, whilst keeping a symptom diary. The diary will reveal whether a tolerance level exists or whether total egg exclusion should be recommended. Atopy patch testing has also been suggested as an alternative test in patients with non-IgE-mediated egg allergy. However, this form of testing has not been standardised, and whilst having a high degree of specificity (95%) it has a low sensitivity (more or less 10%)[5].

Table 5.10 Foods that list any of these ingredients on their labels need to be avoided in patients with egg allergy.

Egg/fresh egg (including those from all birds)
Egg powder, dried egg, frozen egg, pasteurised egg
Egg proteins (albumin, ovalbumin, globulin, ovoglobulin, livetin, ovomucin, vitellin, ovovitellin)
Egg white, egg yolk

Table 5.11 Classification of egg-containing foods.

Well-cooked egg	Loosely cooked egg	Raw egg
Cakes	Meringues	Fresh mousse
Biscuits	Lemon curd	Fresh mayonnaise
Dried egg pasta	Quiche	Fresh ice cream
Egg in sausages and prepared meat dishes	Scrambled egg	Fresh sorbet
Well-cooked fresh egg pasta	Boiled egg	Royal icing (both homemade royal icing and commercial powdered icing-sugar mix)
Egg glaze on pastry	Fried egg	Horseradish sauce
Sponge fingers	Omelette	Tartar sauce
Quorn	Poached egg	Raw egg in cake mix and other dishes awaiting cooking (children of all ages love to taste!)
Nougat, Milky Way, Mars bar, Chewits	Egg in batter	'Frico' Edam cheese or other cheeses containing egg-white lysozyme
Egg in some gravy granules	Egg in breadcrumbs	
Dried egg noodles	Hollandaise sauce Egg custard Pancakes and Yorkshire pudding – some patients who can eat well-cooked egg can tolerate these, but it depends on how well cooked they are and if they contain any 'sticky' batter inside	

5.3.3   Management of egg allergy

The mainstay of managing individuals with egg allergy (egg-white or yolk allergy) is the avoidance of all egg and egg-containing products. Eggs are an important source of high-biological-value protein, fat, vitamin E, riboflavin, thiamine and folic acid. Dietary avoidance should therefore aim to ensure replacement of these nutrients,

Table 5.12 Examples of egg-free products.

Egg-free mayonnaise	
Egg-free cakes and muffins	
Egg-free puddings	
Egg-free omelette mix	
Egg replacers	
Whole-egg replacers	Whole egg replacer (Allergycare)
	Ener-G egg replacer (General Dietary)
	Loprofin egg replacer (SHS International)
	No-egg replacer (Orgran)
Egg-white replacer	Loprofin egg white replacer (SHS International)

especially in vegetarian patients. In the European Union (EU) manufacturers are legally bound to declare egg on the ingredients list of pre-packaged foods, however much or little egg the food contains (Table 5.10). The word *egg* must be used rather than names of the individual proteins, which may not be recognised by some consumers. Outside the EU different food labelling laws are in place, and egg can legally be omitted from the ingredients list altogether or disguised as flavourings. The degree of care and element of risk when eating these foods will depend on the severity of the reaction. This is another reason why older children and adults following egg-free diets who have not reacted for many years should have their allergy reassessed. Following unwarranted restricted diets for longer than necessary can impact on nutritional status.

Some patients tolerate cooked egg and even small amounts of raw egg in their diet. Table 5.11 provides a list of foods that can be consumed, depending on the level of tolerance. The resolution of an egg allergy often starts with tolerance to well-cooked egg. This may progress to all forms of egg, but this is not always the case[71].

A variety of egg-free products are available from health-food shops and supermarkets to make this exclusion diet more user-friendly (Table 5.12).

Manufacturers and supermarkets often also produce a list of own-brand products that are free from egg and other allergens (CMP, nuts, soya etc). These are available free of charge. They help to identify which foods are safe to eat, and including them in the diet can make the diet more interesting and nutritious. Patients should be advised to read ingredient labels every time they buy a particular product, as recipes can change.

5.3.4 Other considerations in patients with egg allergy

Some of the vaccines, including MMR, yellow fever and influenza, may contain traces of egg derivatives. It is therefore important to take this into account when egg-allergic patients require these vaccines[72,73]. The British Society for Allergy and Clinical Immunology has published the following recommendations for MMR vaccination in egg-allergic children[74]:

Table 5.13 Probability of developing egg tolerance, based on decrease in specific IgE over 12 months.

Decrease in IgE (%)	Probability of developing tolerance
50	0.52
75	0.65
90	0.78
99	0.95

1   The administration of the MMR vaccine to egg-allergic children has an excellent safety record and may be administered to all egg-allergic children as a routine procedure in primary care.
2   The MMR vaccine is grown on cultured-embryo-chick fibroblasts and is therefore generally free of hen's egg protein. When traces of hen's egg protein are found, the protein is highly processed and the concentrations are too low to represent a risk.
3   As with the administration of other vaccines, MMR administration should be postponed if children are unwell. Adrenaline should be readily available at the clinical site in all cases because anaphylaxis – although rare and unpredictable – can occur.
4   If previous vaccination (MMR or other) resulted in a severe allergic reaction (any breathing problems or collapse) then a specialist allergy assessment is required prior to repeat – hospital-based – MMR administration, in order to exclude allergy to specific vaccine components such as neomycin or gelatine.

Non-food items (cosmetics, toiletries, perfumes and medications) containing egg should only be avoided if they cause irritation. They are required to be labelled, but the labelling may be in Latin, with the words *ovum* or *ovo* represent egg.

5.3.5   Resolution of egg allergy

The prognosis for children with egg allergy is good. Approximately half of egg-allergic children will be tolerant by the age of 3 years, and 66% by 5 years of age[71].

Annual follow-up of patients with egg allergy is required to monitor tolerance. In general, a combination of the outcome of accidental ingestion, a reduction in SPT (based on serial measurement) and specific IgE to egg will predict whether a food challenge should be performed (Table 5.13). A discussion with the parents may also influence the decision on whether to proceed with the food challenge. As a guide to when egg allergy might have resolved, cut-off levels for SPT and specific IgE for egg have been published (see Chapter 3, Table 3.1), but it is important to note that these may require adjusting for your specific clinic population[34].

References

1. Vandenplas Y, Brueton M, Dupont C *et al.* Guidelines for the diagnosis and management of cow's milk protein allergy in infants. *Arch Dis Child* 2007; **92**: 902–8.

2. Johansson SG, Bieber T, Dahl R *et al*. Revised nomenclature for allergy for global use. Report of the Nomenclature Review Committee of the World Allergy Organization, October 2003. *J Allergy Clin Immunol* 2004; **113**: 832–6.
3. Allen CW, Campbell DE, Kemp AS. Egg allergy: are all childhood food allergies the same? *J Paediatr Child Health* 2007; **43**: 214–18.
4. Woods RK, Stoney RM, Raven J *et al*. Reported adverse food reactions overestimate true food allergy in the community. *Eur J Clin Nutr* 2002; **56**: 31–6.
5. Hu W, Katelaris CH, Kemp AS. Recurrent egg allergy in adulthood. *Allergy* 2007; **62**: 709.
6. Heine RG, Elsayed S, Hosking CS, Hill DJ. Cow's milk allergy in infancy. *Curr Opin Allergy Clin Immunol* 2002; **2**: 217–25.
7. Høst A. Frequency of cow's milk allergy in childhood. *Ann Allergy Asthma Immunol* 2002; **89** (6 Suppl 1): 33–7.
8. Høst A. Primary and secondary dietary prevention. *Pediatr Allergy Immunol* 2001; **12** (Suppl 14): 78–84.
9. Virtanen T, Zeiler T, Rautiainen J *et al*. Immune reactivity of cow-asthmatic dairy farmers to the major allergen of cow (BDA20) and to other cow-derived proteins: the use of purified BDA20 increases the performance of diagnostic tests in respiratory cow allergy. *Clin Exp Allergy* 1996; **26**: 188–96.
10. Jarvinen KM, Beyer K, Vila L *et al*. B-cell epitopes as a screening instrument for persistent cow's milk allergy. *J Allergy Clin Immunol* 2002; **110**: 293–7.
11. Busse PJ, Jarvinen KM, Vila L, Beyer K, Sampson HA. Identification of sequential IgE-binding epitopes on bovine alpha(s2)-casein in cow's milk allergic patients. *Int Arch Allergy Immunol* 2002; **129**: 93–6.
12. Restani P, Beretta B, Fiocchi A, Ballabio C, Galli CL. Cross-reactivity between mammalian proteins. *Ann Allergy Asthma Immunol* 2002; **89** (6 Suppl 1): 11–15.
13. Breuer K, Heratizadeh A, Wulf A *et al*. Late eczematous reactions to food in children with atopic dermatitis. *Clin Exp Allergy* 2004; **34**: 817–24.
14. Sampson HA. Immediate hypersensitivity reactions to foods: blinded food challenges in children with atopic dermatitis. *Ann Allergy* 1986; **57**: 209–12.
15. Zuberbier T, Edenharter G, Worm M *et al*. Prevalence of adverse reactions to food in Germany: a population study. *Allergy* 2004; **59**: 338–45.
16. Bishop JM, Hill DJ, Hosking CS. Natural history of cow milk allergy: clinical outcome. *J Pediatr* 1990; **116**: 862–7.
17. Hill DJ, Hosking CS. Cow milk allergy in infancy and early childhood. *Clin Exp Allergy* 1996; **26**: 243–6.
18. Lee LA, Burks AW. Food allergies: prevalence, molecular characterization, and treatment/prevention strategies. *Annu Rev Nutr* 2006; **26**: 539–65.
19. Moissidis I, Chaidaroon D, Vichyanond P, Bahna SL. Milk-induced pulmonary disease in infants (Heiner syndrome). *Pediatr Allergy Immunol* 2005; **16**: 545–52.
20. Hill DJ, Hosking CS. The cow milk allergy complex: overlapping disease profiles in infancy. *Eur J Clin Nutr* 1995; **49** (Suppl 1): S1–12.
21. Levy FS, Bircher AJ, Gebbers JO. Adult onset of cow's milk protein allergy with small-intestinal mucosal IgE mast cells. *Allergy* 1996; **51**: 417–20.
22. Sicherer SH. Food allergy. *Lancet* 2002; **360**: 701–10.
23. Ferreira CT, Seidman E. Food allergy: a practical update from the gastroenterological viewpoint. *J Pediatr (Rio J)* 2007; **83**: 7–20.
24. Salvatore S, Vandenplas Y. Gastroesophageal reflux and cow milk allergy: is there a link? *Pediatrics* 2002; **110**: 972–84.
25. Iacono G, Carroccio A, Cavataio F *et al*. Chronic constipation as a symptom of cow milk allergy. *J Pediatr* 1995; **126**: 34–9.
26. Carroccio A, Iacono G. Review article: chronic constipation and food hypersensitivity: an intriguing relationship. *Aliment Pharmacol Ther* 2006; **24**: 1295–304.
27. D'Auria E. A follow-up study of nutrient intake, nutritional status, and growth in infants with cow milk allergy fed either a soy formula or an extensively hydrolysed whey formula. *J Pediatr Gastroenterol Nutr* 2006; **42**: 594–5.

28. Levy Y, Davidovits M. Nutritional rickets in children with cow's milk allergy: calcium deficiency or vitamin D deficiency. *Pediatr Allergy Immunol* 2005; **16**: 553.

29. Fox AT, Du TG, Lang A, Lack G. Food allergy as a risk factor for nutritional rickets. *Pediatr Allergy Immunol* 2004; **15**: 566–9.

30. Bakirtas A, Turktas I, Dalgic B. Cow milk allergy presenting as colitis. *Eur J Pediatr* 2003; **162**: 653.

31. Bahna SL. Cow's milk allergy versus cow milk intolerance. *Ann Allergy Asthma Immunol* 2002; **89** (6 Suppl 1): 56–60.

32. Thong BY, Hourihane JO. Monitoring of IgE-mediated food allergy in childhood. *Acta Paediatr* 2004; **93**: 759–64.

33. Sporik R, Hill DJ, Hosking CS. Specificity of allergen skin testing in predicting positive open food challenges to milk, egg and peanut in children. *Clin Exp Allergy* 2000; **30**: 1540–6.

34. Hill DJ, Heine RG, Hosking CS. The diagnostic value of skin prick testing in children with food allergy. *Pediatr Allergy Immunol* 2004; **15**: 435–41.

35. Garcia-Ara MC, Boyano-Martinez MT, Az-Pena JM, Martin-Munoz MF, Martin-Esteban M. Cow's milk-specific immunoglobulin E levels as predictors of clinical reactivity in the follow-up of the cow's milk allergy infants. *Clin Exp Allergy* 2004; **34**: 866–70.

36. Businco L, Cantani A. Management of infants with cow milk allergy. *Adv Exp Med Biol* 1991; **310**: 437–43.

37. Niggemann B, Beyer K. Diagnosis of food allergy in children: toward a standardization of food challenge. *J Pediatr Gastroenterol Nutr* 2007; **45**: 399–404.

38. Michaelsen KF. Cows' milk in complementary feeding. *Pediatrics* 2000; **106**: 1302–3.

39. Noimark L, Cox HE. Nutritional problems related to food allergy in childhood. *Pediatr Allergy Immunol* 2008; **19**: 188–95.

40. Høst A, Halken S. Hypoallergenic formulas: when, to whom and how long. After more than 15 years we know the right indication! *Allergy* 2004; **59** (Suppl 78): 45–52.

41. Kramer MS, Kakuma R. Maternal dietary antigen avoidance during pregnancy or lactation, or both, for preventing or treating atopic disease in the child. *Cochrane Database Syst Rev* 2006; (3): CD000133.

42. Department of Health. Nutrition and bone health with particular reference to calcium and vitamin D: report of the Subgroup on Bone Health (Working Group on the Nutritional Status of the Population) of the Committee on Medical Aspects of Food and Nutrition Policy. London: Stationery Office, 1998.

43. Restani P, Gaiaschi A, Plebani A *et al.* Evaluation of the presence of bovine proteins in human milk as a possible cause of allergic symptoms in breast-fed children. *Ann Allergy Asthma Immunol* 2000; **84**: 353–60.

44. Hill DJ, Murch SH, Rafferty K, Wallis P, Green CJ. The efficacy of amino acid-based formulas in relieving the symptoms of cow's milk allergy: a systematic review. *Clin Exp Allergy* 2007; **37**: 808–22.

45. Klemola T, Vanto T, Juntunen-Backman K *et al.* Allergy to soy formula and to extensively hydrolyzed whey formula in infants with cow's milk allergy: a prospective, randomized study with a follow-up to the age of 2 years. *J Pediatr* 2002; **140**: 219–24.

46. de Boissieu D, Matarazzo P, Dupont C. Allergy to extensively hydrolyzed cow milk proteins in infants: identification and treatment with an amino acid-based formula. *J Pediatr* 1997; **131**: 744–47.

47. Iacono G, Carroccio A, Cavataio F *et al.* Gastroesophageal reflux and cow's milk allergy in infants: a prospective study. *J Allergy Clin Immunol* 1996; **97**: 822–7.

48. Pedrosa M, Pascual CY, Larco JI, Martin Esteban M. Cow's milk allergic children: a comparative study of taste, smell, and texture evaluated by healthy volunteers. *J Investig Allergol Clin Immunol* 2006; **16**: 351–6.

49. Agostoni C, Axelsson I, Goulet O *et al.* Soy protein infant formulae and follow-on formulae: a commentary by the ESPGHAN Committee on Nutrition. *J Pediatr Gastroenterol Nutr* 2006; **42**: 352–61.

50. Zeiger RS, Sampson HA, Bock SA *et al.* Soy allergy in infants and children with IgE-associated cow's milk allergy. *J Pediatr* 1999; **134**: 614–22.

51. Lack G, Fox D, Northstone K, Golding J. Factors associated with the development of peanut allergy in childhood. *N Engl J Med* 2003; **348**: 977–85.
52. Klemola T, Kalimo K, Poussa T *et al*. Feeding a soy formula to children with cow's milk allergy: the development of immunoglobulin E-mediated allergy to soy and peanuts. *Pediatr Allergy Immunol* 2005; **16**: 641–6.
53. British Dietetic Association. Paediatric group position statement on the use of soya protein for infants. *J Fam Health Care* 2003; **13**: 93.
54. James JM, Sampson HA. Immunologic changes associated with the development of tolerance in children with cow milk allergy. *J Pediatr* 1992; **121**: 371–7.
55. Isolauri E, Suomalainen H, Kaila M *et al*. Local immune response in patients with cow milk allergy: follow-up of patients retaining allergy or becoming tolerant. *J Pediatr* 1992; **120**: 9–15.
56. Vanto T, Helppila S, Juntunen-Backman K *et al*. Prediction of the development of tolerance to milk in children with cow's milk hypersensitivity. *J Pediatr* 2004; **144**: 218–22.
57. Vassilopoulou E, Konstantinou G, Kassimos D *et al*. Reintroduction of cow's milk in milk-allergic children: safety and risk factors. *Int Arch Allergy Immunol* 2008; **146**: 156–61.
58. Buller HA, Rings EH, Montgomery RK, Grand RJ. Clinical aspects of lactose intolerance in children and adults. *Scand J Gastroenterol Suppl* 1991; **188**: 73–80.
59. Bianchi PG, Parente F, Sangaletti O. Lactose intolerance in adults with chronic unspecific abdominal complaints. *Hepatogastroenterology* 1983; **30**: 254–57.
60. Parker TJ, Woolner JT, Prevost AT *et al*. Irritable bowel syndrome: is the search for lactose intolerance justified? *Eur J Gastroenterol Hepatol* 2001; **13**: 219–25.
61. Lomer MC, Parkes GC, Sanderson JD. Review article: lactose intolerance in clinical practice: myths and realities. *Aliment Pharmacol Ther* 2007; **27**: 93–103.
62. Heine RG, Laske N, Hill DJ. The diagnosis and management of egg allergy. *Curr Allergy Asthma Rep* 2006; **6**: 145–52.
63. Pereira B, Venter C, Grundy J *et al*. Prevalence of sensitization to food allergens, reported adverse reaction to foods, food avoidance, and food hypersensitivity among teenagers. *J Allergy Clin Immunol* 2005; **116**: 884–92.
64. de Boissieu D, Dupont C. Natural course of sensitization to hen's egg in children not previously exposed to egg ingestion. *Eur Ann Allergy Clin Immunol* 2006; **38**: 113–17.
65. Cant A, Marsden RA, Kilshaw PJ. Egg and cows' milk hypersensitivity in exclusively breast fed infants with eczema, and detection of egg protein in breast milk. *Br Med J* 1985; **291**: 932–5.
66. Monti G, Muratore MC, Peltran A *et al*. High incidence of adverse reactions to egg challenge on first known exposure in young atopic dermatitis children: predictive value of skin prick test and radioallergosorbent test to egg proteins. *Clin Exp Allergy* 2002; **32**: 1515–19.
67. Kondo M, Fukao T, Omoya K *et al*. Protein-losing enteropathy associated with egg allergy in a 5-month-old boy. *J Investig Allergol Clin Immunol* 2008; **18**: 63–6.
68. Anet J, Back JF, Baker RS *et al*. Allergens in the white and yolk of hen's egg: a study of IgE binding by egg proteins. *Int Arch Allergy Appl Immunol* 1985; **77**: 364–71.
69. Aabin B, Poulsen LK, Ebbehoj K *et al*. Identification of IgE-binding egg white proteins: comparison of results obtained by different methods. *Int Arch Allergy Immunol* 1996; **109**: 50–7.
70. Potamianou-Taprantzi P, Zanikou S, Psarros P *et al*. Relationship between egg-specific serum IgE concentration and the outcome of specific provocation to egg allergic children. *Allergy* 2002; **57** (Suppl 73): 79.
71. Boyano-Martinez T, García-Ara C, Díaz-Pena JM, Martin-Esteban M. Prediction of tolerance on the basis of quantification of egg white-specific IgE antibodies in children with egg allergy. *J Allergy Clin Immunol* 2002; **110**: 304–9.
72. Mosimann B, Stoll B, Francillon C, Pecoud A. Yellow fever vaccine and egg allergy. *J Allergy Clin Immunol* 1995; **95**: 1064.
73. James JM, Zeiger RS, Lester MR *et al*. Safe administration of influenza vaccine to patients with egg allergy. *J Pediatr* 1998; **133**: 624–8.
74. British Society for Allergy and Clinical Immunology. Recommendations for combined measles, mumps and rubella (MMR) vaccination in egg-allergic children. London: BSACI, 2007. www.bsaci.org.

6 Seafood

Isabel Skypala

6.1 Introduction

Fish allergy affects both children and adults, whereas allergy to crustaceans tends to occur in older children and adults but less commonly in young children, probably due to exposure being much lower in this age group in the UK. The prevalence varies around the world and is linked to the consumption of particular types of seafood. Seafood allergy is usually only associated with immediate symptoms related to an IgE-mediated food hypersensitivity response, and is not normally implicated in delayed reactions. Seafood allergy is also more likely to occur in people who are atopic and sensitised to other aeroallergens, or have rhinitis or asthma. Reactions to both fish and shellfish are potentially severe and cross-reactivity is common, often meaning that those diagnosed with a single-species allergy have to avoid all fish or all shellfish. Although they are all now required by European Union (EU) legislation to be labelled, fish, crustaceans and molluscs can appear in some unusual foods, and because of the longevity of shrimp allergens contamination can be a major problem, especially when eating out. There are some differential diagnoses which are important to take into consideration when diagnosing allergy to seafood, and therefore it is important to check specific IgE levels, as these are a good indicator of the presence or absence of a seafood allergy. Unlike other food allergies, allergy to seafood tends to be lifelong.

6.2 Prevalence and natural history

The prevalence of fish and seafood allergy varies depending on the age of the cohort and the consumption patterns of the population. Allergic reactions to fish are common where fish constitutes a major source of food protein in the diet[1]. Fish and crustacean allergy is more common than that reported to molluscs, and seafood allergy tends to be more common in adults than in children. The prevalence of reported allergy to seafood in UK children aged 11 or 15 years was 1.3% for fish and 0.5% for shellfish, with fish accounting for 11.4% of reported reactions, whereas shellfish only accounted for 3.8% of reactions[2]. A Danish study on a cohort of 3-year-old children and their older siblings reported they were unable to confirm any reported reactions to cod or shrimp in these children, although the actual prevalence of the same foods in their parents was reported to be 0.2% to cod and 0.3% to shrimp[3].

A study of adults in Germany[4] showed the prevalence of positive reactions to crab was 1.2%, herring and mackerel 0.45%, and mussels 0.1%, whereas a study of adults in Portugal suggested that reported prevalence to fish was 11.5% and molluscs 5.8%[5]. Results from a US telephone survey indicate a prevalence of 0.4% for fish allergy, and 2% for allergy to shellfish[6], although a more recent study reports that the prevalence of shellfish allergy is lower, at 0.6% for self-reported and 0.3% for doctor-diagnosed[7]. In Singapore, where a great deal of fish and shellfish is consumed, shellfish was the second most common sensitising allergen after egg, affecting 27% of a cohort of 227 children referred for reported food allergy[1], and was the most common allergen reported to cause immediate hypersensitivity in adults, affecting 33% of a cohort of 74 adults[8]. A study of Thai children reported that fish and seafood, especially shrimp, were the commonest reported allergens in older children[9].

In a study looking at self-reported food allergy in both adults and children in Russia, Estonia, Lithuania, Norway and Sweden, 19% of the cohorts reported an allergy to fish, ranging from 39% in Russia to 11% in Denmark, whereas the rate for shrimp was much higher in Denmark (20%) compared to the Russian reported rate of 8.7%[10].

Seafood allergy is thought to be usually lifelong in both children and adults, but some studies and case reports suggest remission may be possible. Solensky reported a case of resolution of fish allergy in an adult with a history of fish anaphylaxis[11], and in another study of 32 children with fish allergy, five seemed to lose their allergy[12]. In contrast, this has yet to be reported for those who are allergic to shellfish, with no change in specific IgE antibody levels to shrimp reported in 11 shrimp-allergic subjects over a 2-year period[13].

6.3   Foods involved

Wide ranges of seafood have been implicated in food-allergic responses, but generally the foods causing symptoms reflect local or national availability and consumption patterns. Species tested in European studies tend to be similar to those foods consumed in the UK, such as cod, tuna, salmon, trout, plaice, although other species such as pollack and wolf-fish are less well known in the UK. However, studies and case reports from around the world include reported reactions to sea urchin roe, boiled razor-shell and krill[14–16]. Other studies, looking at the allergenicity of fish commonly consumed in both Japan and India, examined fish varieties not familiar to Europeans such as bonito, yellowtail, saurel, skipper, pomfret, hilsa and bhetki[17,18].

6.3.1   Fish

Studies suggest that there is strong cross-reactivity between fish species, both fresh- and salt-water varieties. Parvalbumin is the dominant allergen in finned fish, and cod, mackerel, herring and plaice have all been shown to share a common parvalbumin antigenic determinant[19]. Van Do and colleagues studied nine parvalbumins and

Table 6.1   Cross-reactivity of fish and shellfish species.

Seafood	Cross-reacting species
Cod	Tuna, mackerel, herring, plaice, sole, bass, eel
Tuna	Cod, trout, salmon
Salmon	Sardine, mackerel, tuna
Mackerel	Anchovy, cod, salmon, herring, sardine, plaice
Prawns	Lobster, crab, crayfish
Mussels	Octopus, squid
Shellfish	Cockroach, house dust mite, snails

showed that the cod allergen Gad c 1 had the highest Ig-E binding affinity, making it the most allergenic fish, together with salmon, pollack, herring and wolf-fish[20]. *In vitro* studies have suggested a strong cross-reactivity between cod, mackerel, herring and plaice, and also between pollack, salmon, trout and tuna, and finally between mackerel and anchovy[21].

Half of all cod-allergic children in a classic study into fish allergy reported reactions to other fish[22], although others reported eating other species without difficulty. Helbling and colleagues challenged subjects known to be fish-allergic with several different species and demonstrated that some subjects reacted to two or three different fish species[21]. Tanaka *et al.* suggest that there are several different clusters of cross-reactivity, such as cod and tuna, and salmon, sardine and mackerel[23]. Helbling *et al.* found that adult patients reacted to several fish species challenged[24], but other groups have found that actual symptoms to cross-reacting fish species are far less common[25]. There are other members of the parvalbumin family which can be implicated in food allergy outside the fish species, with one case report[26] of anaphylaxis to frog's legs, which contain α-parvalbumin. Table 6.1 shows the clusters of fish and shellfish reported to cross-react with each other.

6.3.2   Crustaceans and molluscs

Crustaceans are a subphylum of Arthropoda (arthropods), a phylum which also includes spiders, scorpions, cockroaches, mites, centipedes and insects. Crayfish, crab, lobster and shrimp are all classified in the order Decapoda. Molluscs are all in the phylum Mollusca, in which the classes Bivalvia (clams, mussels and oysters), Cephalopoda (octopus and squid) and Gastropoda (snails) are the most relevant for mollusc allergy. Crustaceans and molluscs share a common allergenic protein called invertebrate tropomyosin.

The main allergen in shrimp was identified many years ago as Pen a 1, and studies have shown it to be similar to other allergens in crab, lobster and crayfish – but also show IgE-binding to house-dust mite and cockroaches[27]. This high degree of cross-reactivity is also more prevalent in patients who are atopic. Tanaka and colleagues showed that octopus and squid, and crab and shrimp, were the two main cross-reacting clusters of shellfish[23] (Table 6.1). Although most patients will be sensitised to the pan-allergen tropomyosin, some patients may be monosensitised to a specific shrimp allergen[28]. Allergy to a crustacean species can be severe, with a high risk of reactions between different crustaceans as well as between crustaceans and molluscs. Allergy to molluscs is less common than to crustaceans, and cross-reactivity between molluscs is not well established. Allergy to barnacles has also been reported, although the allergen appears to be specific only for barnacles[29].

Invertebrate tropomyosin is also found in airborne insect allergens such as those of cockroach and house-dust mite, and in the fish muscle parasite *Anisakis*, although mammalian tropomyosins are non-allergenic[27]. Allergy to both molluscs and crustaceans has been linked to reactions to house-dust mite and cockroaches, with one study showing that five limpet-allergic individuals with asthma were sensitised to house-dust mite, and another showing that 28 individuals who developed asthmatic symptoms after the consumption of snails were all sensitised to house-dust mite[30].

The allergens involved in both fish and shellfish allergy are similar in that they are highly cross-reactive, involve pan-allergens and can cause sensitisation or symptoms through aerosolisation and inhalation[31]. These allergens can also cause occupational allergies such as asthma and dermatitis in workers exposed to crustaceans, molluscs and bony fish[32]. However, fish and shellfish allergens differ when exposed to heat. Fish allergens can be degraded on exposure to heat, meaning that some patients reacting to salmon and tuna may safely consume canned varieties[33]. In contrast, allergens from crustaceans and molluscs remain potent allergens after cooking. Shrimp allergenic activity has been detected in oil used to cook shrimp[34], and there have been reports of adults experiencing symptoms after the inhalation of vapours from cooking squid[35]. Although there is strong inter-species cross-reactivity in both fish and crustacean allergy, there is no cross-reactivity between crustaceans and vertebrate fish[36].

6.4 Diagnosis

6.4.1 History

In common with other suspected food allergies, history is a crucial part of the diagnostic pathway for seafood allergy. Fish and shellfish are usually quite obvious ingredients in a meal or snack, and therefore patients often present with symptoms they already suspect are due to fish or shellfish, which they are often avoiding.

Seafood allergy usually manifests itself as immediate symptoms of an IgE-mediated allergic nature. It is therefore helpful to go through the reaction in detail, establishing the precise nature of symptoms, presence or absence of allergic symptoms such as itching, flushing, hives or urticarial rash, angio-oedema and whether any more severe symptoms such as tracheal obstruction, vomiting, wheeze or asthma, tachycardia or hypotension were noted. A study by Helbling and colleagues showed that the commonest observed sign of a positive reaction to a fish challenge was vomiting, and the most prevalent symptom itching of the mouth and throat[24]. Seafood is often involved in the most severe food allergic reactions; crustaceans are reported to cause 10% of all cases of anaphylaxis to foods in France[37] and seafood 8% of fatal anaphylaxis in the UK[38].

Information on the type of fish or seafood eaten is important, as is knowledge of whether anyone else also experienced symptoms. Given the globalisation of food markets and possibilities of sensitisation to foods during trips abroad, it will be important to consider other fish species, and it may be difficult to confirm suspicions about an unfamiliar seafood item as skin prick or serum IgE-specific tests may not be available. Furthermore, the food may not always be obvious. Some people who may not routinely eat seafood may have occupational exposure to seafood in a kitchen or processing plant, or may be exposed to cross-reacting allergens found in fish gelatine. Others may be able to consume cooked fish, but react to sushi (Japanese raw fish dishes); oral allergy syndrome has been reported in a sushi bar worker who probably became sensitised through handling raw fish[39].

6.4.2   Differential diagnoses

A differential diagnosis is a very important consideration in suspected seafood allergy. There may be components in the seafood that can cause true IgE-mediated reactions. Some people may have reactions to fish but are actually sensitised to nematode worms such as *Anisakis* which are present in the fish, and may affect workers in a fish processing plant[40] or sushi bar[41]. Exposure to live fish bait has been reported to cause allergies in some people, and symptoms after eating chickens fed with fishmeal have also been reported, although these were thought to be symptoms to the *Anisakis simplex* nematode worm contaminating the fishmeal, rather than to the fishmeal itself[42,43]. It has also been reported that some people may develop an allergy to fish roe without concomitant fish allergy[44].

However, the commonest differential diagnosis is seafood poisoning, including reactions to natural toxins; the gastroenteritis and systemic symptoms caused by bacterial toxins can easily be confused with food allergy[45]. Fish poisoning can be generally divided into two categories: scombroid poisoning, where the toxin is not present in the live fish but produced in the flesh of caught fish, and ciguatera poisoning, where the toxin is present in the live fish[46]. Five types of shellfish toxins have been identified, although paralytic shellfish poisoning is the best known and causes the most severe symptoms.

Scombroid poisoning is possibly the most easily confused with fish allergy, due to the typical symptoms it causes of flushing, sweating, urticaria, gastrointestinal symptoms, palpitations and in severe cases bronchospasm[47]. Marine bacteria decarboxylate the histidine which is present in certain species of fish, both scombroid (tuna, mackerel, skipjack and bonito) and non-scombroid (herring, sardines, marlin and anchovies), and this increases the histamine content of these fish[48]. The fish may look and smell normal, and histamine is resistant to heat, so cooking or canning such fish will not remove the histamine[49]. Symptoms usually begin within one hour of eating the fish and can be mistaken at their most severe for anaphylaxis. Proper handling and refrigeration of fish can prevent the build-up of histamine.

6.4.3   Estimation of specific IgE using skin prick tests and serum analysis

In addition to taking a history it is very important, given the likelihood of a differential diagnosis, to undertake some specific IgE estimation to ascertain the presence or absence of IgE antibodies to suspected seafood allergens.

There is a wide range of seafood allergens available in both skin prick test solutions and CAP-RAST FEIA tests. However, in contrast with other common allergens such as milk, egg and peanut, very little work has been carried out on the validation of specific IgE estimation for fish or crustaceans. For skin prick tests, several studies have suggested that the predictive accuracy of a positive skin prick test to fish was 84%, and 78% for specific IgE[21,33]. Sampson suggests that a specific IgE level for fish of 20 kU$_A$/L has a 95% positive predictive value (PPV) for the presence of fish allergy in someone reporting symptoms to fish, with 100% specificity[50]. He also showed that even a low level of 3 kU$_A$/L specific IgE antibody to fish was sufficient to have a 90% specificity, although the PPV in this case was only 56%.

This work suggests that skin prick and serum estimations of specific IgE for fish are very useful in making a diagnosis of fish allergy. For shellfish, despite the absence of any studies, it can be surmised that since the tropomyosin allergens are very robust the allergens are likely not to have been affected by heat treatments. As with fruits and vegetables, it is possible to use fresh seafood for skin prick testing, although there have been no studies examining the potential consequences of increased histamine levels in fish affecting the results. However, one study has looked at the effectiveness of raw and boiled extracts of shrimp, showing that the boiled extracts were more effective than the raw extracts[51]. Therefore reagents are likely to be the best choice for skin prick testing, although, given the known specificity of some shrimp allergens, negative test results for prawn, in the face of a good clinical history of reactions to prawns, need to be interpreted with caution and possibly confirmed with cooked fresh prawns and/or oral food challenge.

It may also be useful to establish whether the patient has any other allergies. A study in 2002 showed that in young adults there was a relationship between nasal allergy and shrimp allergy which may be a reflection of the cross-reaction between house-dust mite and crustaceans[52]. Skin prick test or specific IgE estimation of house-dust mite might therefore be very useful in the diagnostic process. One study looking at shellfish allergy found that 90% of subjects with suspected shellfish allergy had a positive skin test to house-dust mites[53].

6.4.4   Oral food challenge (see also Chapter 3)

The presence of specific IgE antibodies to seafood, as evidenced by positive SPT or positive CAP-RAST FEIA test, are usually sufficient to make a diagnosis. However, due to the often very severe reported symptoms, and the possibility of a differential diagnosis, a negative specific IgE screen needs confirmation by an oral food challenge, prior to advising the patient to reintroduce seafood into his or her diet.

European guidelines recommend that all oral food challenges be carried out by qualified personnel and with access to equipment for resuscitation[54]. This is especially important for seafood allergy, due to the often severe symptoms elicited. However, the symptom type usually means that it is only necessary to perform an open challenge with fish or shellfish, as it is suggested this is sufficient when dealing with suspected IgE-mediated acute reactions manifesting with objective signs and the expectation of a negative outcome.

Seafood allergens are generally very stable, which means that whether given in open form or processed in order to blind the allergen, the resulting challenge will be a reliable test of the patient's tolerance to seafood. The European guidelines propose starting doses for oral challenge to seafood of 5 mg for both cod and shrimp, although another consensus protocol for low-dose oral food challenge recommends starting at 10 µg of the allergenic food[55]. Challenge guidelines[56] recommend that up to the equivalent of a normal portion should be consumed without a reaction before the challenge can be said to be negative; for seafood a normal portion is suggested to be 60–80 g (2–3 oz). Should it be necessary to undertake a blinded challenge, the same dosages of seafood are recommended. For blinding, some recommend that the test fish is added to a fish patty or burger contain a fish known to be tolerated, and others recommend adding fish or seafood to a meat burger[56,57].

6.5 Avoidance

Once the diagnosis has been made, then advice will need to be given on avoidance. On the face of it this may appear to be relatively simple, but there are a number of food products that may contain seafood or seafood derivatives which may need to be taken into account. Fish, crustaceans and molluscs are all required by EU labelling laws to be declared on all products to which they have been deliberately added, however small the amount. This makes them much easier to spot, especially in products which are not an obvious source; for example, both Worcestershire sauce and Patum Peperium (Gentleman's Relish) may contain anchovies. However, some sources of fish in foods are not required to be labelled as they are considered to be a very low risk for allergic reactions. These exemptions include fish gelatine used as a carrier for vitamins/flavours, or in alcohol production, where it is added to fine the wine or beer and may be called isinglass.

6.5.1 Fish

A confirmed allergy to one fish species may not mean that the sufferer will react to other fish species. However, the evidence suggests that it would be unsafe to advise consumption of fish not known to cause a reaction, without first undertaking further tests of specific IgE estimation and possibly oral food challenges. Many patients may have already evaluated other fish species and found that they can be consumed with safety, and given the labile nature of some fish allergens, it may be possible for canned tuna and salmon to be eaten. But raw wet fish are liable to cross-

Table 6.2 Foods containing fish and seafood.

Fish	All white and oily fish, surimi (processed seafood product that may be found in pizza toppings), Caesar salad, Worcestershire sauce, Gentleman's Relish, kedgeree, Caponata (a traditional sweet and sour Sicilian relish), fish sauce, paella, bouillabaisse, gumbo
Crustaceans	Prawns, crab, crayfish, langoustine, lobster
Molluscs	Bivalves – mussels, oysters, scallops, clams Gastropods – limpets, periwinkles, snails Cephalopods – squid, cuttlefish, octopus

contamination, and therefore people with a fish allergy should avoid purchasing fresh fish from a mixed fish stall, even though they may be safe eating some varieties. Should they be allergic only to fish, given the lack of cross-reactivity between fish and crustaceans, such patients could be advised to eat crustaceans, but again they will need to be careful of cross-contamination, either from a wet fish stall or in a restaurant kitchen. Fish-oil capsules may not be advisable for some who are highly sensitive to small amounts of fish, as some fish protein could be present, and they should be advised to find other sources of omega-3 fat supplementation such as linseed (flax seed) or algae oil[58].

6.5.2   Crustaceans and molluscs

Due to the high likelihood of inter-species cross-reactivity, an allergy to one crustacean usually requires avoidance of all crustaceans. There may be no need to avoid molluscs, but again cross-contamination is an issue. Should someone with a known allergy to crustaceans wish to consume molluscs, it is advisable that the individual specific IgE level of the desired molluscs be undertaken first to just ensure no cross-reactivity exists, and then consumption advised with extreme caution. Due to the robust nature of crustacean allergens and the fact that they may be present in cooking vapours, it is extremely important that someone with a prawn allergy does not eat in a restaurant where prawns may be cooked in the same pan as other dishes, or in a restaurant where food is cooked on display in communal woks.

For both fish and shellfish allergy, it is very important that the allergy has been confirmed as being due to fish or shellfish. If this has not been done, there is the potential for continued exposure to the actual food causing the problem. For a list of foods likely to contain seafood see Table 6.2.

References

1. Chiang WC, Kidon MI, Liew WK *et al*. The changing face of food hypersensitivity in an Asian community. *Clin Exp Allergy* 2007; **37**: 1055–61.
2. Pereira B, Venter C, Grundy J *et al*. Prevalence of sensitization to food allergens, reported adverse reaction to foods, food avoidance, and food hypersensitivity among teenagers. *J Allergy Clin Immunol* 2005; **116**: 884–92.

3. Osterballe M, Hansen TK, Mortz CG, Høst A, Bindslev-Jensen C. The prevalence of food hypersensitivity in an unselected population of children and adults. *Pediatr Allergy Immunol* 2005; **16**: 567–73.
4. Zuberbier T, Edenharter G, Worm M *et al*. Prevalence of adverse reactions to food in Germany: a population study. *Allergy* 2004; **59**: 338–45.
5. Falcão H, Lunet N, Lopes C, Barros H. Food hypersensitivity in Portuguese adults. *Eur J Clin Nutr* 2004; **58**: 1621–5.
6. Sicherer SH, Muñoz-Furlong A, Sampson HA. Prevalence of seafood allergy in the United States determined by a random telephone survey. *J Allergy Clin Immunol* 2004; **114**: 159–65.
7. Vierk KA, Koehler KM, Fein SB, Street DA. Prevalence of self-reported food allergy in American adults and use of food labels. *J Allergy Clin Immunol* 2007; **119**: 1504–10.
8. Thong BYH, Cheng YK, Leong KP, Tang CY, Chng HH. Immediate food hypersensitivity among adults attending a clinical immunology/allergy centre in Singapore. *Singapore Med J* 2007; **48**: 236–40.
9. Santadusit S, Atthapaisalsarudee S, Vichyanond P. Prevalence of adverse food reactions and food allergy among Thai children. *J Med Assoc Thai* 2005; **88**: S27–32.
10. Eriksson NE, Möller C, Werner S *et al*. Self-reported food hypersensitivity in Sweden, Denmark, Estonia, Lithuania and Russia. *J Investig Allergol Clin Immunol* 2004; **14**: 70–9.
11. Solensky R. Resolution of fish allergy: a case report. *Ann Allergy Asthma Immunol* 2003; **91**: 411–12.
12. Dannaeus A, Inganäs M. A follow-up study of children with food allergy. Clinical course in relation to serum IgE- and IgG-antibody levels to milk, egg and fish. *Clin Exp Allergy* 1981; **11**: 533–9.
13. Daul CB, Morgan JE, Lehrer SB. The natural history of shrimp-specific immunity. *J Allergy Clin Immunol* 1990; **86**: 88–93.
14. Rodriguez V, Bartolomé B, Armisén M, Vidal C. Food allergy to *Paracentrotus lividus* (sea urchin roe). *Ann Allergy Asthma Immunol* 2007; **98**: 393–6.
15. Martin-Garcia C, Carnés J, Blanco R *et al*. Selective hypersensitivity to boiled razor shell. *J Investig Allergol Clin Immunol* 2007; **17**: 271–3.
16. Nakano S, Yoshinuma T, Yamada T. Reactivity of shrimp allergy-related IgE antibodies to krill tropomyosin. *Int Arch Allergy Immunol* 2007; **145**: 175–81.
17. Koyama H, Kakami M, Kawamura M *et al*. Grades of 43 fish species in Japan based on IgE–binding activity. *Allergol Int* 2006; **55**: 311–16.
18. Chatterjee U, Mondal G, Chakraborti P, Patra HK, Chatterjee BP. Changes in the allergenicity during different preparations of pomfret, hilsa, bhetki and mackerel fish as illustrated by enzyme-linked immunosorbent assay and immunoblotting. *Int Arch Allergy Immunol* 2006; **141**: 1–10.
19. Hansen TK, Bindslev-Jensen C, Skov PS, Poulsen LK. Codfish allergy in adults: IgE cross-reactivity among fish species. *Ann Allergy Asthma Immunol* 1997; **78**: 187–94.
20. Van Do T, Elsayed S, Florvaag E, Hordvik I, Endresen C. Allergy to fish parvalbumins: studies on the cross-reactivity of allergens from 9 commonly consumed fish. *J Allergy Clin Immunol* 2005; **116**: 1314–20.
21. Helbling A, McCants ML, Musmand JJ, Schwartz HJ, Lehrer SB. Immunopathogenesis of fish allergy: identification of fish-allergic adults by skin test and radioallergosorbent test. *Ann Allergy Asthma Immunol* 1996: **77**: 48–54.
22. Aas K. Studies of hypersensitivity to fish: a clinical study. *Int Arch Allergy Appl Immunol* 1966; **29**: 346–63.
23. Tanaka R, Ichikawa K, Hamano K. Clinical characteristics of seafood allergy and classification of 10 seafood allergens by cluster analysis. *Arerugi* 2000; **49**: 479–86.
24. Helbling A, Haydel R, McCants ML *et al*. Fish allergy: is cross-reactivity among fish species relevant? Double-blind placebo-controlled food challenge studies of fish allergic adults. *Ann Allergy Asthma Immunol* 1999; **83**: 517–23.
25. De Martino M, Novembre E, Galli L *et al*. Allergy to different fish species in cod allergic children: in vivo and in vitro studies. *J Allergy Clin Immunol* 1990; **86**: 909–14.
26. Hilger C, Grigioni F, Thill L, Mertens L, Hentges F. Severe IgE-mediated anaphylaxis following consumption of fried frog legs. *Allergy* 2002; **57**: 1053–8.

27. Reese G, Ayuso R, Lehrer SB. Tropomyosin: an invertebrate pan-allergen. *Int Arch Allergy Immunol* 1999; **119**: 247–58.
28. Morgan JE, O'Neil CE, Daul CB, Lehrer SB. Species-specific shrimp allergens: RAST and RAST-inhibition studies. *J Allergy Clin Immunol* 1989; **83**: 1112–17.
29. Moreno EMC, Alonso LE, Sánchez AA *et al*. Barnacle hypersensitivity. *Allergol Immunopathol Madr* 2002; **30**: 100–3.
30. van Ree R, Antonicelli L, Akkerdaas JH *et al*. Asthma after consumption of snails in house-dust-mite-allergic patients: a case of IgE cross-reactivity. *Allergy* 1996; **51**: 387–93.
31. James JM, Crespo JF. Allergic reactions to foods by inhalation. *Curr Allergy Asthma Rep* 2007; **7**: 167–74.
32. Jeebhay MF, Robins TG, Lehrer SB, Lopata AL. Occupational seafood allergy: a review. *Occup Environ Med* 2001; **58**: 553–62.
33. Bernhisel-Broadbent J, Scanlon SM, Sampson HA. Fish hypersensitivity. I. In vitro and oral challenge results in fish-allergic patients. *J Allergy Clin Immunol* 1992; **89**: 730–7.
34. Lehrer SB, Kim L, Rice T *et al*. Transfer of shrimp allergens to other foods through cooking oil. *J Allergy Clin Immunol* 2007; **119**: S112.
35. Carrillo T, Rodriguez de Castro F, Blanco C *et al*. Anaphylaxis due to limpet ingestion. *Ann Allergy* 1994; **73**: 504–8.
36. Chapman JA, Bernstein IL, Lee RE *et al*. Food allergy: a practice parameter. *Ann Allergy Asthma Immunol* 2006; **96**: S1–68.
37. Moneret-Vautrin DA, Morisset M. Adult food allergy. *Curr Allergy Asthma Rep* 2005; **5**: 80–5.
38. Pumphrey RSH. Lessons for management of anaphylaxis from a study of fatal reactions. *Clin Exp Allergy* 2000; **30**: 1144–50.
39. Sugita K, Kabashima K, Nakashima D, Tokura Y. Oral allergy syndrome caused by raw fish in a Japanese sushi bar worker. *Contact Dermatitis* 2007; **56**: 369–70.
40. Nieuwenhuizen N, Lopata AL, Jeebhay MF *et al*. Exposure to the fish parasite *Anisakis* causes allergic airway hyper reactivity and dermatitis. *J Allergy Clin Immunol* 2006; **117**: 1098–105.
41. Weir E. Sushi, nematodes and allergies. *CMAJ* 2005; **172**: 329.
42. Siracusa A, Marcucci F, Spinozzi F *et al*. Prevalence of occupational allergy due to live fish bait. *Clin Exp Allergy* 2003; **33**: 507–10.
43. Armentia A, Martin-Gil FJ, Pascual C *et al*. *Anisakis simplex* allergy after eating chicken meat. *J Investig Allergol Clinn Immunol* 2006; **16**: 258–63.
44. Mäkinen-Kiljunen S, Kiistala R, Varjonen E. Severe reactions from roe without concomitant fish allergy. *Ann Allergy Asthma Immunol* 2003; **91**: 413–16.
45. Chegini S, Metcalfe DD. Seafood toxins. In: Metcalfe DD, Sampson HJ, Simon RA, eds. *Food Allergy: Adverse Reactions to Foods and Food Additives*. Oxford: Blackwell, 2003: 487–510.
46. Chegini S, Metcalfe DD. Contemporary issues in food allergy: seafood toxin-induced disease in the differential diagnosis of allergic reactions. *Allergy Asthma Proc* 2005; **26**: 183–90.
47. Attaran RR, Probst F. Histamine fish poisoning: a common but frequently misdiagnosed condition. *Emerg Med J* 2000; **19**: 474–5.
48. Fritz SB, Baldwin JL. Pharmacologic food reactions. In: Metcalfe DD, Sampson HJ, Simon RA, eds. *Food Allergy: Adverse Reactions to Foods and Food Additives*. Oxford: Blackwell, 2003: 395–407.
49. Lehane L. Update on histamine fish poisoning. *Med J Aust* 2000; **173**: 149–52.
50. Sampson H. Utility of food-specific IgE concentrations in predicting symptomatic food allergy. *J Allergy Clin Immunol* 2001; **107**: 891–6.
51. Carnés J, Ferrer A, Huertas AJ *et al*. The use of raw or boiled crustacean extracts for the diagnosis of seafood allergic individuals. *Ann Allergy Asthma Immunol* 2007; **98**: 349–54.
52. Woods RKA, Thien F, Raven J, Walters EH, Abramson M. Prevalence of food allergies in young adults and their relationship to asthma, nasal allergies and eczema. *Ann Allergy Asthma Immunol* 2002; **88**: 183–9.
53. Wu AY, Williams GA. Clinical characteristics and pattern of skin test reactivities in shellfish allergy patients in Hong Kong. *Allergy Asthma Proc* 2004; **25**: 237–42.
54. Bindslev-Jensen C, Ballmer-Webber BK, Bengtsson U *et al*. Standardisation of food challenges in patients with immediate reactions to foods: position paper from the European Academy of Allergology and Clinical Immunology. *Allergy* 2004; **59**: 690–7.

55. Taylor SL, Hefle SL, Bindeslev-Jensen C *et al.* A consensus protocol for the determination of the threshold doses for allergenic foods: how much is too much? *Clin Exp Allergy* 2004; **34**: 689–95.
56. Mofidi S, Bock SA. *A Health Professional's Guide to Food Challenges.* Fairfax, VA: Food Allergy & Anaphylaxis Network, 2005.
57. Noè D, Bartemucci L, Mariani N, Cantari D. Practical aspects of preparation of foods for double-blind, placebo-controlled food challenge. *Allergy* 1998: **53** (46 Suppl); 75–7.
58. Food Standards Agency. Can someone with a fish allergy take fish-oil supplements? www.eatwell.gov.uk/asksam/healthissues/foodintolerance/fishoilsupp. Accessed September 2008.

7 Fruits and Vegetables

Isabel Skypala

7.1 Introduction

Allergy to fruits and vegetables either involves a primary sensitisation to an allergen in the plant food, usually one which is stable to heat and digestion, or it is a secondary reaction caused by a cross-reaction between a plant food allergen and an antibody to pollen or latex. The first type of allergy may be mediated by a group of allergens known collectively as non-specific lipid transfer proteins (nsLTPs), which have been sequenced in a wide range of plant foods, although it can also involve other allergens. The sensitisation will occur in the gastrointestinal tract and the symptoms can be as severe as those involved in other primary food allergies[1]. This type of plant food allergy is much less common, however, than the second type, caused by cross-reacting allergen epitopes. This type of reaction falls into a group of conditions known collectively as oral allergy syndrome (OAS).

OAS is an IgE-mediated food hypersensitivity which has been defined as 'a complex of symptoms induced by exposure of the oral and pharyngeal mucosa to food allergens'[2]. Although any reaction triggered by mucosal exposure to food of either plant or animal origin can be classified as OAS, the term is most closely associated with symptoms caused by cross-reactions between pollens and plant foods[3]. The pollens involved are most commonly tree pollens, especially birch trees, but grass and weed pollens including mugwort and ragweed also cross-react with foods to cause OAS. Other plant-derived allergens such as latex also cross-react with plant food allergens and the latex–food cross-reaction is the other main cause of OAS. Most of the research information on fruit and vegetable allergy and OAS comes from continental Europe rather than the UK, where the prevalence of these allergies and the main foods involved are not well characterised.

7.2 Prevalence and natural history

Fruit and vegetables have become an increasingly common cause of both primary and cross-reactive food allergic symptoms in all ages. In early prevalence studies, common food allergens cited would rarely include fruits or vegetables. Eriksson's classic study in 1982, however, showed that they were a common cause of food allergic reactions, particularly in those who were also sensitised and/or symptomatic to birch pollen[4]. A large pan-European study showed that, of those foods reported to cause symptoms, fruit and vegetables were in the top four (together with milk and egg), with 29.5% of reported reactions being to fruits and 13.5% to vegetables[5].

The type of foods reported to cause reactions may vary considerably from country to country. A study of food allergy prevalence in Germany showed, through skin prick test confirmation of reported symptoms in 800 people, that 21% had a confirmed allergy to apple, 19.3% to raw potato, 13.9% to carrot and 13.6% to celery[6]. In a five-country study[7] (Russia, Estonia, Lithuania, Sweden and Denmark), self-reported food hypersensitivity to apple was the second most common cause of reported food hypersensitivity, but that varied from 56% of the cohort in Sweden to 25% of the cohort in Lithuania. Similarly, strawberry hypersensitivity was reported in 43% of Russians, but only 21% of Lithuanians.

The specificity of fruits and vegetables to different countries is well illustrated by the example of peach allergy being the most common form of allergy to fresh fruits in Spain[8], carrot allergy affecting up to 25% of food-allergic subjects in central Europe[9], and Swiss and French subjects being commonly sensitised to celery[10], which can lead to severe reactions on exposure including anaphylaxis. Some fruits and vegetables are becoming increasingly reported as causing reactions, due to rising consumption: for example, kiwi fruit allergy appears to be growing in frequency[11,12].

The rates of allergic reactions to fruits and vegetables varies according to age, with children being overall less likely to react, possibly because the reactions are often associated with pollen sensitisation. Although it is suggested that adults are more likely to have allergies to shellfish, peanuts, tree nuts and fish, allergy to fruits and vegetables is also thought to be highly prevalent at 5%[13]. A study of Portuguese adults showed fruits to be the most common food to cause reported symptoms[14].

A study by Osterballe and colleagues showed the prevalence of allergy to fruit and vegetables was 3.2% of the adult cohort of an unselected population, compared to 1.0% in children older than 3 years[15]. This prevalence rate is similar to that reported by Vierk and colleagues, who found that 2.8% of their adult cohort reported reactions to fruits and vegetables, although the prevalence rate fell to 1.6% for those who had a doctor-diagnosed allergy to those foods[16].

The dominance of fruit and vegetable allergies in adults is supported by two studies from the Isle of Wight. The first, on a birth cohort, showed that at the age of 3 years the main foods reported to cause reactions did include some fruits and vegetables such as potatoes and tomatoes, but mainly involved milk, egg, peanut and cereals such as wheat and corn[17]. A second study on school-aged children showed the commonest foods reported to cause reactions to be milk, additives, eggs, peanuts, tree nuts, wheat, fish and shellfish, although banana, kiwi, tomatoes and green beans were also reported to cause reactions[18].

Nuts, fruit and milk were the commonest foods cited to cause adverse effects in adults in another study by Schäfer and colleagues[19], frequently with concomitant sensitisation to aeroallergens, which supports the assertion that food allergy in adults is associated with other atopic conditions. The commonest manifestation of OAS involves cross-reacting homologues to allergens from the silver birch tree (*Betula pendula*, also known by the synonym *Betula verrucosa*). It has been suggested that more than 50% of birch-pollen-allergic patients could have OAS, with one estimate placing the figure as high as 93%[20–22]. A UK survey found the prevalence of confirmed allergic rhinitis or hay fever to be of the order of 26%[23], and it is thought that approximately 20–25% of those with allergic rhinitis are affected by birch pollen[24,25], giving a theoretical prevalence of 5–7% of UK subjects with birch pollen allergy. Veiths *et al.* have suggested that the estimated prevalence of pollen–food syndrome (PFS) is 1% of the population[22]; however, if 5–7% of the UK population have birch-pollen allergy, and upwards of 50% of these have PFS, then a PFS prevalence of 3–5% may be more likely.

In terms of the natural history, it is unknown whether fruit or vegetable allergies resolve over time. Those associated with pollen sensitivity and OAS have anecdotally been reported to resolve, which may be linked to the changing sensitisations to aeroallergens.

7.3 Foods involved

For both primary sensitisation and OAS, it is the actual structure of the plant food allergens that plays the most important part in determining which foods are more likely to cause problems. Unlike some other food allergies, it is quite common for people to report an allergy to more than one fruit or vegetable, which again is due to the epitope structure and the highly cross-reactive nature of fruit and vegetable allergens. So, although botanical relationships are still relevant, it is the allergen type that will determine, for example, whether apple will cause mild OAS symptoms or more severe systemic symptoms associated with a primary fruit allergy.

The botanical classification of plant foods is shown in Table 7.1; however, many plant foods from unrelated botanical families have very similar homologous allergens. Breiteneder and Radauder[26,27] showed that plant food allergens could be classified as belonging to one of several superfamilies (Tables 7.2 and 7.3). Some foods, such as peanut, have major and minor allergens in all of these superfamilies. The cupin superfamily contains some of the major allergens in legumes, tree nuts and seeds, often involved in primary food allergy but not in pollen–food cross-reactivity such as OAS. The prolamin superfamily includes cereal prolamins, seed storage proteins and nsLTPs, the last of which are resistant to proteolysis, pH change and thermal treatments.

The main allergens involved in OAS are found in the plant defence system and profilin families. The plant defence system contains the pathogenesis-related (PR) proteins, defined as plant proteins induced in response to infections by pathogens such as fungi, bacteria and viruses, or due to adverse environmental conditions[26]. PR proteins are divided into groups, several of which, PR2, PR3, PR5 and PR10, are involved in IgE-mediated food allergy reactions. PR5 proteins or thaumatin-like proteins (TLPs) are heat-stable and present in many pollens and plant foods. They may be major allergens in some cases of primary food hypersensitivity to fruits and vegetables. In OAS, however, the most significant group is the PR10 proteins or Bet v 1 homologues[20]. Profilins are the other plant food family of allergens to be involved in OAS. Profilins are small proteins found in all eukaryotic cells, and there is 70–85% similarity between different species[29].

Table 7.1 Botanical classification of fruits and vegetables (adapted from Vaughan and Geissler[28]).

Family	Fruits, vegetables and nuts
Actinidiaceae	Kiwi
Adoxaceae	Elderberry
Alliaceae (lily)	Onions, chives, shallots, leeks, garlic
Anacardiaceae	Mango, cashew nut, pistachio nut
Apiaceae	Carrot, celery, dill, parsley, coriander, fennel, aniseed, caraway, coriander, cumin, dill, angelica, celeriac, parsnip, chervil
Arecaceae	Betal nut, dates, coconut, palm hearts, sago
Asparagaceae	Asparagus
Asteraceae (Compositae)	Lettuce, endive, chicory, artichoke, guava, tarragon, sunflower, chamomile, Jerusalem artichoke
Brassicaceae (Cruciferae)	Cabbage, turnip, black and white mustard seed, rape seed, horse-radish, watercress, mustard cress, rocket, pak choi, kale, Brussels sprout, cauliflower, broccoli, kohlrabi, radish, swede
Bromeliaceae	Pineapple
Capparaceae	Capers
Chenopodiaceae (goosefoot)	Spinach, seakale or chard, beetroot
Convolvulaceae	Sweet potato, yam
Corylaceae (Betulaceae)	Hazel nuts (filbert nuts, cob nuts)
Cucurbitaceae	Melon, cucumber, pumpkin, watermelon, courgette, marrow, squash
Cyperaceae	Chinese water chestnut
Ericaceae	Bilberry, blueberry, cranberry
Fabaceae (Leguminosae)	Peanut, soya, pigeon pea, Goa bean, runner bean, French bean, haricot bean, butter bean, lima bean, chickpea, mung bean, fava bean, pea, lentil, tamarind, guar gum, fenugreek, liquorice, gum arabic
Fagaceae	Chestnut
Grossulariaceae	Blackcurrants, redcurrants, gooseberries
Iridaceae	Saffron
Junglandaceae	Walnut, pecan nut
Lamiaceae (Labiatae)	Peppermint, spearmint, sage, oregano, marjoram, thyme, rosemary, basil, lemon balm
Lauraceae	Avocado, bay leaves, cinnamon
Lecythidaceae	Brazil nut
Malvaceae	Okra
Moraceae	Fig, mulberry, breadfruit
Musaceae	Banana, plantain

Table 7.1   *(cont'd)*

Family	Fruits, vegetables and nuts
Myrtaceae	Cloves
Oleaceae	Olive
Orchidaceae	Vanilla
Pedaliaceae	Sesame
Pinaceae	Pine nut
Piperaceae	White and black peppercorns
Polygonaceae	Rhubarb, buckwheat
Proteaceae	Macadamia nut
Punicaceae	Pomegranate
Rosaceae	Apple, pear, strawberry, cherry, apricot, peach, plum, nectarine, almond, quince, sloe, damson, greengage, loquat, raspberry, blackberry, loganberry, boysenberry, dewberry, cloudberry
Rutaceae	Orange, lemon, grapefruit, tangerine, kumquat, clementine, ugil
Sapindaceae	Ackee, lychee
Solanaceae	Tomato, aubergine, potato, sweet pepper, chilli pepper, cayenne pepper
Vitaceae	Grape
Zingiberaceae	Ginger, cardamom, turmeric

7.3.1   Primary food allergy

Primary food allergy involving fruits and vegetables is caused by sensitisation to an allergen that is not affected by proteolysis, such as nsLTP or TLP. Although the clinical relevance of TLP has yet to be well established, several allergenic TLPs from fruits have been described, including cherry, pepper, kiwi, grape and apples, with Mal d 2, the TLP found in apples, reported to induce symptoms in apple-allergic individuals[30]. There have been considerably more nsLTP allergens identified as being causative of food-allergic reactions to a variety of plant foods including apples, peaches, pears, apricots, cherries, grapes, strawberries, oranges, tomatoes and lettuce. Sensitisation to nsLTPs is much more common in southern Europe, where there is little birch-pollen sensitisation; Salcedo and colleagues showed that only 3% of German patients but 100% of Italian patients are sensitised to nsLTPs[31], making them the most likely cause of an allergy to fruits and vegetables in the absence of pollen sensitisation. It has been shown that those people sensitised to peach nsLTP are more likely to have clinical cross-reactivity to other foods containing nsLTP[32].

Apples are one of the commonest fruits eaten in Europe and the commonest reported cause of fruit allergy in Europe, except Spain, where peach allergy is more prevalent. A large pan-European study of apple allergy[33] showed that in Spain apple

Table 7.2 Plant food superfamilies: cupins and 2S-albumins. Main allergens in nuts and seeds (adapted from references[22,26,27], and from www.allergen.org and and www.allergome.com).

Food	Cupins		Prolamins
	Vicilins	Legumins	2S-albumins
Peanut	Ara h 1	Ara h 3, Ara h 4	Ara h 2, Ara h 6, Ara h 7
Soya	Gly m BD	Glycinin G1	
Hazelnut	Cor a 11	Cor a 9	
Almond			Pru du 2S-albumin
Walnut	Jug r 2		Jug r 1
Brazil nut		Ber e 2	Ber e 1
Cashew nut	Ana o 1	Ana o 2	Ana o 3
Pistachio nut	Pis v 2		Pis v 1
Sesame seed	Ses i 3	Ses i 6, Ses i 7	Ses i 1, Ses i 2
Oriental mustard			Bra j 1
Yellow mustard			Sin a 1

Table 7.3 Plant food superfamilies: prolamins, plant defence system and profilins. Main allergens in nuts and seeds (adapted from references[22,26,27], and from www.allergen.org and and www.allergome.com).

Food	Prolamins	Plant defence system		Profilins
	nsLTP	Other PR proteins	PR10/Bet v 1 homologues	
Peanut	Ara h 9		Ara h 8	Ara h 5
Soya			Gly m 4	Gly m 3
Hazelnut	Cor a 8		Cor a 1	Cor a 2
Almond	Pru du 8			Pru du 4
Walnut	Jug r 3			
Chestnut	Cas s 8	Cas s 5		
Avocado		Pers a 1		
Apple	Mal d 3	Mal d 2	Mal d 1	Mal d 4
Pear	Pyr c 3		Pyr c 1	Pyr c 4
Peach	Pru p 3		Pru p 1	Pru p 4
Plum	Pru d 3			Pru d 4
Apricot	Pru ar 3		Pru ar 1	
Cherry	Pru av 3	Pru av 2	Pru av 1	Pru av 4
Strawberry	Fra a 3		Fra a 1	Fra a 4
Orange	Cit s 3			Cit s 2
Kiwi		Act d 1, Act d 2	Act d 8	
Melon		Cuc m 3, Cuc m 1		Cuc m 2
Pineapple				Ana c 1
Lychee				Lit c 1
Banana		Ba 1, Ba 2		Mus x p 1
Grape	Vit v 1			
Tomato	Lyc e 3			Lyc e 1
Celery			Api g 1	Api g 4
Carrot	Carrot LTP		Dau c 1	Dau c 4
Pepper		Cap a 1		Cap a 2
Lettuce	Lac s 1			
Barley	Barley nsLTP 1 & 2			Hor v 12
Wheat	Wheat nsLTP 1 & 2			
Maize	Zea m 14			Zea m 12

allergy is associated with severe systemic reactions, with sufferers sensitised to the nsLTP in apples, Mal d 3. The authors suggest that apple allergy in Spain is a result of primary sensitisation to the peach nsLTP allergen Pru p 3, and is more likely to be systemic as Mal d 3 and Pru p 3 behave as class 1 food allergens, being resistant to proteolytic attack in the digestive tract (see Chapter 4).

Apart from apples and peaches, other fruits associated with primary fruit allergy include grapes and kiwi fruit. Grapes contain an nsLTP and have been reported[34] as being causative of reactions not only to grapes but also to raisins, grape juice, wine vinegar and wine. However, although it is known that sensitisation and clinical reactions to nsLTPs are more likely in Mediterranean countries, anaphylaxis to grapes has also been reported in Germany[35]. Kiwi is also an increasing cause of primary food allergy, and although it is reported to cause mild symptoms in adult patients with OAS, studies suggest it is capable of causing severe reactions, especially in young children and in adults who are not pollen-sensitised[11,12]. The allergen in kiwi thought to cause most of the reactions (Act d 1) is apparently not so important in UK subjects with kiwi allergy, illustrating once again that allergen sensitisation may vary between population groups[36]. With regard to other fruits, there have been case reports of severe reactions including anaphylaxis to banana, lychee, logan fruit, mandarin, blueberry and mango.

Vegetable allergy is well recognised in some parts of Europe; celery and carrots are reported to be common causes of food hypersensitivity reactions in Europe, often in association with pollen sensitisation and OAS[9,10]. However, celery can cause severe systemic reactions; in France, 30% of a cohort of 580 subjects thought their severe anaphylactic reactions were due to celery consumption[37]. The reason for this may be that celery root still retains its allergenicity even after extended heat treatment, and celery spice is allergenic for patients with an allergy to raw celery[38]. Clinical allergy to other vegetables is less well reported, although allergy to lettuce[39] and cabbage[40] have been reported to involve lipid transfer proteins. Allergy to cooked potato has been reported only in children and can cause severe reactions, with anaphylaxis in some cases[41]. Other vegetables which have been reported to cause anaphylaxis in isolated cases include courgette, coriander, garlic and aubergine.

7.3.2 Oral allergy syndrome (OAS)

In sensitised individuals, cross-reactions between pollens and foods, latex and foods, mites and foods or food and food can result in an instant allergic reaction taking place in the oral mucosa. These reactions are all manifestations of oral allergy syndrome (OAS), and they most commonly involve fruits, vegetables and nuts. OAS involving pollens cross-reacting to foods is very common, and several authors have suggested that the term pollen–food syndrome (PFS) should be used to describe OAS symptoms related to pollen cross-reactivity[42,43].

Pollen–food syndrome (PFS)

PFS is the type of food allergy often referred to as a class 2 food allergy, and it is the predominant food allergy of adulthood[42,44,45]. Those who suffer from PFS have a primary sensitisation to a pollen allergen due to exposure via the lungs, and their symptoms on eating plant foods are due to a wide variety of plant food allergens having very similar (homologous) epitopes to those of pollen allergens. These food allergens are usually from the PR or profilin families of plant food allergens, being generally heat-sensitive and susceptible to digestion by proteases, making them unlikely to elicit primary food allergy[46]. However, although they cannot stimulate the formation of food-specific IgE antibodies, these food allergens have sufficiently similar epitopes to allow them to bind to pollen-specific IgE antibodies on mast cells, triggering the release of histamine and causing the classic symptoms of PFS[47].

The commonest manifestation of PFS involves foods which cross-react to birch-pollen allergens. It has been suggested that more than 50% of birch-pollen-allergic patients could have PFS, with one estimate placing the figure as high as 93%[3,21,22,28]. Other pollens, such as ragweed, mugwort and grass, also cross-react with food[48] (Table 7.4). Generally grass and weed pollens are less common causes of PFS than birch, although food-allergic patients are often sensitised to these pollens; Mortz *et al.* showed that 96% of peanut-sensitised individuals had concomitant reactions to grass pollen[49]. There are no reports of the prevalence of PFS in people sensitised to tree pollens other than birch, although associations between plane tree pollenosis and food allergy, and cypress allergy and peach, have been reported[22,50–52]. The prevalence of PFS is influenced by the different pollens and dietary habits which predominate in a given geographical area, and it can change over time[42,53].

Whatever pollen is involved, the cross-reacting allergens in PFS are all found in fruits, vegetables and nuts. The main allergens involved in PFS are PR proteins and profilins (Table 7.3). For PFS, the most significant group is the PR10 proteins, as many of these are homologous to the main birch pollen allergen Bet v 1. About 90%

Table 7.4 Foods which can cross-react to different types of pollen and latex[22,51,54].

Birch pollen	Apple, pear, cherry, peach, nectarine, apricot, plum, kiwi, hazelnut, other nuts, almond, celery, carrot, potato
Birch/mugwort	Celery, carrot, spices, sunflower seed, honey
Grass	Melon, watermelon, orange, tomato, potato, peanut, Swiss chard
Ragweed	Watermelon and other melon, banana, courgette, cucumber
Plane	Hazelnut, peach, apple, melon, kiwi, peanuts, maize, chickpea, lettuce, green beans
Latex	Avocado, chestnut, banana, passion fruit, kiwi fruit, papaya, mango, tomato, pepper, potato, celery

of birch-pollen-allergic subjects have specific IgE antibodies against Bet v 1, and this allergen shares 35–60% amino acid sequence identity with PR10 proteins[26,55,56]. Bet v 1 homologues mainly cause reactions in the oral mucosa, and heat-treated foods do not cause symptoms in Bet-v-1-allergic patients due to the cross-reacting allergen's susceptibility to heat and proteolysis. Studies suggest that between 59% and 96% of allergy to apple, stone fruits, kiwi, celery, carrot, pear, cherry and hazelnut in birch-sensitised subjects is due to cross-reactivity between Bet v 1 and its homologues[22,28].

Profilins are the other plant food family of allergens to be involved in PFS. Although 70% or more of the symptoms in PFS can be attributed to Bet v 1 homologues, profilin cross-reactivity plays a role in about 20% of sufferers, with profilin-specific IgE detected in 10–30% of those with pollen-related food allergy[26,29]. The other main birch-pollen allergen, Bet v 2, is a profilin, and profilins are also found in other trees, grasses, weeds, latex and foods. Bet v 2 cross-reacts with the profilin in celery, the major allergen in melon is a profilin, and it has been suggested that profilins could be responsible for allergies to tomatoes, melon, citrus fruits and bananas[42,57,58]. PFS affecting mugwort- and/or grass-pollen-sensitised individuals may be mediated by profilins. This has been confirmed in Spanish patients with peach and apple sensitivity, and in ragweed-free areas melon and watermelon are associated with patients who have grass-pollen allergy[59,60].

Several prevalence studies have indicated that the commonest foods to elicit symptoms in PFS are apple, peach, tree nuts, peanut and carrot (Table 7.5)[4,61,62]. The Rosaceae family (apples, pears, stone fruits, strawberries), kiwi fruit and tree nuts are probably the commonest foods to elicit PFS, but the Apiaceae (carrots, celery, herbs and spices), the Fabaceae (peanuts, soya, bean sprouts) and the

Table 7.5 Foods which most commonly cause OAS.

Sweden (questionnaire to 600 subjects, 380 with birch-pollen allergy[4])	Italy (100 subjects with history of OAS[60])	Switzerland (383 case histories[61])
Hazelnut	Apple	Hazelnut
Apple	Hazelnut	Celery
Peach	Peanut	Apple
Cherry	Walnut	Carrot
Almond	Peach	Peanut
Walnut	Fennel	Almond
Pear	Orange	Peach
Carrot	Tomato	Soybean
Plum	Pear	
Potato peel	Cherry	
Brazil nut	Carrot	
Peanut	Pea	
Almond	Potato	
Apricot	Melon	
Coconut	Banana	

Solanaceae (potatoes, peppers and tomatoes) families can all be involved (Table 7.4). Homologues of Bet v 1 and Bet v 2 are found in spices of the Apiaceae family[63]. There are both Bet v 1 homologues and profilin in carrots, which can affect pollen-sensitised individuals; carrot allergy is associated with sensitisation to celery, spices, mugwort and birch pollen[9]. Data from France showed that food allergy to spices was not common; the spices reported included coriander, caraway, fennel, garlic and onion[64]. The authors suggest that patients at risk of spice allergy are young adults sensitised to mugwort and birch allergens, There have also been case reports of severe reactions to dill and coriander[65,66] (see also Chapter 10).

Peanut allergy is traditionally associated with the main allergens Ara h 1, Ara h 2 and Ara h 3, but there is also a profilin (Ara h 5) which has been shown to be the cause of mild OAS symptoms in monosensitised peanut-allergic individuals, and a Bet v 1 homologue which could also be responsible for OAS symptoms[67,68]. It has been suggested that hazelnut allergy is usually associated with birch or hazel pollen allergy, probably due to one of the main hazelnut allergens, Cor a 1, being a PR10 protein homologous to Bet v 1[69]. The potato allergen Sol t 1 is heat-labile but can cause contact urticaria in sensitised individuals, with a pollen allergy, when peeling potatoes.

The work on apple allergy in Europe sums up the differences between primary food allergy and PFS very nicely[33]. This published work suggests that people in the Netherlands, Austria and most of Italy have mild reactions to apple, responding to Mal d 1, a Bet v 1 homologue, whereas subjects from Spain showed severe systemic symptoms to apple, correlated with a response to Mal d 3, an nsLTP, but also to Pru p3, an nsLTP in peach. The conclusion is that apple allergy in Spain is a result of primary sensitisation to peach and is more likely to be systemic, whereas apple allergy in northern Europe is predominately mild, probably due to the presence of large numbers of birch trees sensitising the population to Bet v 1 via the inhaled route.

Latex–food syndrome (LFS)

Allergy to natural latex rubber (*Hevea brasiliensis*) is widespread, and high in certain risk groups such as healthcare workers. There are 13 main latex allergens but only five are considered to be the major allergens: Hev b 1 (rubber elongation factor), Hev b 2 (β1,3-glucanase), Hev b 5, Hev b 6.01 and 6.02 (hevein precursor and hevein) and Hev b 13 (early nodule-specific protein)[70]. These allergens cover the spectrum of allergens and include profilins, nsLTPs and PR allergens. This means they have potential cross-reactivity with a wide range of foods. It is thought that about 30–50% of those allergic to natural latex rubber will have associated hypersensitivity reactions to plant foods, and Wagner *et al.* suggest that a pre-existing fruit allergy could represent an additional risk factor for the development of a latex allergy[54]. Hev b 6.02 shows sequence identity with several class 1 chitinases (PR3 proteins) such as Pers a 1 (avocado), Ba1 and Ba2 (bananas) and Cas s 5 (chestnut). Hev b 7 (patatin-like protein) has 50% similarity to the potato allergen patatin (Sola t 1), and may also cross-react to an allergen in tomatoes[71]. Hev b 8 (profilin) has been linked to cross-reactivity with celery, banana, pineapple and pepper, and most recently to chestnut. Hev b 11 (class 1 chitinase) is associated with cross-reactivity to avocado[71]. Cassava, turnip and courgette have also been linked to cross-reactivity to latex[72,73] (Table 7.4).

Moulds, yeast and mushrooms

There are some case reports of anaphylaxis to white button mushrooms[74] and other mushrooms, especially shitake mushrooms, inducing allergic asthma[75], contact dermatitis[76], eosinophilia and gastrointestinal symptoms[77]. However, it has also been reported that reactions to mushrooms appear as a type of oral allergy syndrome[78,79], symptoms being related to concomitant mould allergy. A review in 1988 concluded that the prevalence of mushroom allergy was probably about 1% but could be much more common, due to large numbers of spores in August and September[80]. Helbling et al. showed that 48 of a cohort of 1,207 people with respiratory conditions had positive skin prick tests to mushroom[81]. Patients with oral allergy syndrome to mushrooms have been sensitised to various moulds including *Alternaria*, *Cladosporium* and *Aspergillus*; one patient had a clustered sensitisation to fungi, including mushrooms, moulds and yeast extracts[82]. Ingested yeast allergy is very rare.

7.4   Presenting symptoms and diagnosis

Patients reacting to fruits and vegetables can have varying degrees of clinical reactivity to foods. Primary food allergy to fruits and vegetables can manifest itself in symptoms of varying degrees, ranging from mild urticaria to anaphylaxis, the onset being occasionally rapid and usually within 15 minutes of eating, although it may occur up to one hour after eating. The main difference between this and symptoms in PFS is that the latter occur almost immediately, either on contact or up to five minutes after eating, and usually resolve rapidly and spontaneously, although some sufferers do report subsequent gastric or systemic symptoms[3,83]. A second highly characteristic feature of PFS symptoms is that the symptoms are localised to the oro-pharynx and usually involve labial, pharyngeal, gingival and palatal pruritis, often intense and sometimes accompanied by local angio-oedema, papulae, blisters and most severely glottal oedema[3,4,21]. Latex–food cross-reactions may fall into both categories.

The foods involved in both primary food allergy to fruits and vegetables and PFS may also be similar, and so it is important to ask additional questions about whether the foods elicit symptoms in both their raw and cooked state. Most foods causing PFS do not cause reactions when cooked, although there is evidence that they could provoke atopic dermatitis reactions in sensitised individuals even when cooked or digested[84,85]. However, asking whether cooked apples provoke symptoms could be the key question in deciding whether someone has an apple allergy or PFS involving apples. Since most of the nsLTP in apple (and probably other fruits) is known to be in the skin of the fruit, asking whether people tolerate peeled apples is also helpful.

One of the difficulties in diagnosing PFS is that the measurement of specific IgE by using CAP-RAST FEIA and/or SPT using commercial reagents often does not detect PFS involving fruits or vegetables, due to the labile nature of the class 2 allergens involved. Asero and colleagues showed that those who were likely to have reactivity to non-Rosaceae plants and to be sensitised to nsLTP were those who had a high level of specific IgE to peach[32]. Therefore cross-reactivity to botanically unrelated plants is more likely in those with a high level of specific IgE to peach. It is for this reason that he proposes that if skin prick tests are performed using the prick-to-prick test (PPT) method with fresh foods, they should be followed by SPT to commercial peach reagent to determine whether nsLTPs are involved[58]. Reagents are much more useful for diagnosing primary food allergy, as the allergens involved are heat-stable. But, given the variation in sensitisation to individual allergens, and the possibility that the reagent may not contain all of the relevant allergens, it is important to confirm a negative reagent test with a PPT using the fresh food. Similarly, *in vitro* tests for specific IgE estimation will also be useful for primary allergy to fruits and vegetables, but variable in their accuracy in PFS diagnosis.

Apart from taking a good clinical history, the best diagnostic test currently available for PFS is to undertake PPT using fresh fruits and vegetables in place of reagents[86]. Like SPT, PPTs have a high sensitivity but low specificity, with overall only a 50% positive predictive value, although the negative predictive value is more than 90%[87]. However, this varies with different foods, and sensitivities of 97%, 92% and 89% to hazelnut, apple and melon respectively have been reported[88]. Other studies have found that the fresh-food PPT has good sensitivity for carrot, celery, cherry, apple, tomato, orange and peach[89]. The main difficulty with any estimation of specific IgE is that the high epitope homology between different plant foods leads to false positive test results, and can mean that testing with standard panels of foods could lead to positive results with no clinical relevance[90,91]. Figure 7.1 shows two patients who have undergone PPT with a panel of foods and pollens. The results show that both are highly sensitised to apple and tree nuts, but only one has reported reactions to those foods. This demonstrates the importance of distinguishing between sensitisation and allergy to a food, and only testing to foods with reported symptoms. Many birch-, grass- and latex-sensitised individuals will have positive PPT to foods, but this does not mean they are allergic unless they report symptoms to that food.

PPT can also be used with good effect to diagnose primary food allergy, although if there are severe reactions reported then it may be more prudent to undertake serum specific IgE measurements in the first instance. The difficulty with using PPT with fresh foods for diagnosis is a lack of standardisation of the material used and the fact that different varieties of fruits elicit different levels of reaction. Until recently this has been the only method available, but the sequencing of allergens has now led to the development of purified allergen reagents (recombinant allergens).

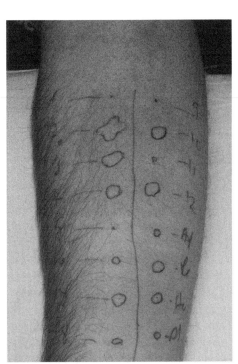
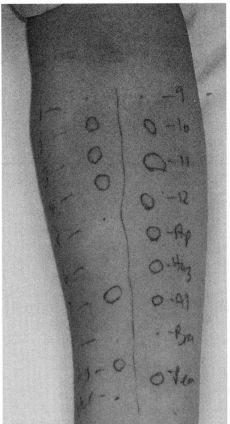

Figure 7.1   Do they both have oral allergy syndrome?

It has been suggested that these single-allergen reagents will enable a component-based diagnosis of OAS/PFS to be made; recombinant Bet v 1 and Bet v 2 allergens can be used to assess likely sensitisation to Bet v 1 and Bet v 2 homologues[2]. At present, although there are a number of pollen, aeroallergen, nut and legume recombinants available, the numbers for fruits and vegetables are much lower, although they do include Bet v 1 homologues for kiwi, celery, peach and apple, and the peach nsLTP Pru p 3, which could be used as a marker of sensitisation to nsLTP in selected patients.

When skin tests or IgE tests do not confirm the history, an oral food challenge is the next step. Double-blind placebo-controlled food challenges (DBPCFC) using fruits and vegetables are difficult to perform, as the materials are hard to disguise or find a matching placebo for. With some foods, the peel contains more allergen than the pulp, and so peeling the fruit in order to disguise it can remove much of the allergen present[92]. European guidelines suggest that if PFS is suspected then it is acceptable to perform an open challenge[93]. Studies suggest that a good method for PFS is to undertake a labial challenge followed by asking patients to chew and disgorge a small piece of the raw fruit or vegetable with the peel for 30–60 seconds[10,88]. Since PFS symptoms are usually immediate, a 15-minute wait period may be sufficient in most cases to effect a diagnosis.

In addition to evaluating sensitivity to food allergens, it will also be useful to establish the presence or absence of pollen and/or latex sensitisation using SPT. Sensitisation to one or more pollens, especially a combination of birch, grass and other trees, is strongly linked to the likelihood of the person having PFS[94]. If particular foods such as carrot or celery or spices are reported to cause symptoms, then mugwort should also be tested. Although it is possible to ascertain the presence or absence of hay-fever symptoms, linked to the reported food symptoms, not all sensitised individuals will have clinical symptoms, and PFS symptoms to foods may occur in people who do not have seasonal hay fever; therefore skin prick testing for pollen allergens will be useful.

7.5 Management

For primary allergy to fruits and vegetables, sufferers need to be advised to avoid the food in all of its forms, raw, cooked, juiced, canned, dried and crystallised. Although there may be some cross-reactivity between foods if the patient is sensitised to nsLTP, most primary allergies to these foods will occur to the single food, unlike OAS, where multiple foods could be reported to cause symptoms in people with PFS or latex–food syndrome. Unfortunately there may be some misunderstanding about how serious these allergies can be; people with severe systemic reactions to fruits or vegetables may be thought to be mistaken in their belief that a particular food causes the reaction. People often assume only peanuts can precipitate such severe responses. However, it is because of severe reported reactions that celery is one of the allergens required by the EU to be labelled if it has been added to a product. This is important, as celery spice may be used quite often and would be difficult to detect otherwise.

The reactions in PFS can also be viewed as so mild that there is no need for the sufferer to avoid the food, and many will opt to continue to consume the food, despite the symptoms. A survey of North American allergy clinics showed that because of the perception that OAS is characterised by mild non-systemic symptoms, practitioners may not advocate any avoidance of trigger foods[43]. Little is known about the development of tolerance or of increasingly severe reactions in those who do not avoid OAS-provoking foods. It is also still unknown whether the continued consumption of Bet v 1 homologues by someone with a diagnosed reaction to one particular Bet v 1 homologue will perpetuate sensitivity. There is speculation that symptom-free consumption of pollen-related food allergens may have implications for the pollen-specific immune response of allergic individuals[46].

However, even for mild reactions, the current advice is to avoid the food which precipitates symptoms, although advice with regard to tree nuts may need to be given on an individual basis depending on reported symptoms, since some nuts which cross-react with pollen still provoke symptoms even if cooked. However, patients are normally also advised that cooked or canned foods will not elicit symptoms, and many advocate peeling fruit and/or microwaving it for short periods, as this will also reduce the allergen load[92,95]. Different varieties of fruits and vegetables may affect people differently: for example, some apple types such as Granny Smith, Cox's Orange and Golden Delicious are more likely to cause a problem[96]. The peels of different apples can also contain different amounts of nsLTP allergens, with one study examining 10 apple varieties showing that Starking apples contained the most protein and precipitated the largest SPT wheals in sensitised patients, while Royal Gala appeared to be the least allergenic[97]. Storage of foods may also affect the amount of allergen they contain. A study looking at apples showed that levels of Mal d 1 increased during the storage of the fruit, suggesting that stored apples are more likely to precipitate PFS reactions than those freshly picked[98].

Although avoidance is currently the only option for treatment, several studies have looked at whether immunotherapy with birch pollen will also reduce or eliminate the reactions to cross-reacting foods. Results have been mixed, with immunotherapy to birch pollen reported to give protection against the development of symptoms to apple, although this effect is often negated once immunotherapy is stopped, and other studies have not reported similar findings[99–101]. More recently it was shown that successful sublingual immunotherapy (SLIT) with birch pollen did not effectively reduce concomitant allergy to apple because the immune response to Mal d 1 was not significantly altered. The authors concluded that combining pollen and related food allergens in a vaccine may be the way forward[102].

It is often supposed that for those with reported reactions to fruits or vegetables, nutritional consequences due to avoidance are highly unlikely. However, it is known that people experiencing PFS reactions may often remove all fruits and associated vegetables from their diets, in the mistaken belief that this is required. There are also some people who are genuinely symptomatic on consuming a whole range of raw fruits and vegetables. Such restrictions may lead to serious nutritional deficiencies in isolated cases, with one case report of a male with OAS who was found to be suffering from the clinical manifestation of scurvy due to a lengthy avoidance of all fruits and vegetables in his diet[103].

References

1. Breiteneder H, Mills ENC. Molecular properties of food allergens. *J Allergy Clin Immunol* 2005; **115**: 14–23.
2. Mari A, Ballmer-Weber BK, Veiths S. The oral allergy syndrome: improved diagnostic and treatment methods. *Curr Opin Allergy Clin Immunol* 2005; **5**: 267–73.
3. Pastorello EA, Ortalani C. Oral allergy syndrome. In: Metcalfe DD, Sampson HJ, Simon RA, eds. *Food Allergy: Adverse Reactions to Foods and Food Additives*. Oxford: Blackwell, 2003: 425–37.
4. Eriksson NE, Formaren H, Svenonius E. Food hypersensitivity in patients with pollen allergy. *Allergy* 1982; **37**: 437–43.
5. Steinke M, Fiocchi A, Kirchlechner V *et al*. Perceived food allergy in children in 10 European nations: a randomised telephone survey. *Int Arch Allergy Immunol* 2007; **143**: 290–5.
6. Zuberbier T, Edenharter G, Worm M *et al*. Prevalence of adverse reactions to food in Germany: a population study. *Allergy* 2004; **59**: 338–45.

7. Eriksson NE, Möller C, Werner S *et al*. Self-reported food hypersensitivity in Sweden, Denmark, Estonia, Lithuania and Russia. *J Investig Allergol Clin Immunol* 2004; **14**: 70–9.

8. Cuesta-Herranz J, Lazaro M, de las Heras M *et al*. Peach allergy pattern: experience in 70 patients. *Allergy* 1998; **53**: 78–82.

9. Ballmer-Weber B, Wüthrich B, Wangorsch A *et al*. Carrot allergy: double-blinded, placebo-controlled food challenge and identification of allergens. *J Allergy Clin Immunol* 2001; **108**: 301–7.

10. Ballmer-Weber BK, Vieths S, Luttkopf D, Heuschmann P, Wüthrich B. Celery allergy confirmed by double-blind, placebo-controlled food challenge. *J Allergy Clin Immunol* 2000; **106**: 373–8.

11. Lucas JSA, Lewis SA, Hourihane J. Kiwi fruit allergy: a review. *Pediatr Allergy Immunol* 2003; **14**: 420–8.

12. Alemán A, Sastre J, Quirce S, *et al*. Allergy to kiwi: a double-blind, placebo-controlled food challenge study in patients from a birch-free area. *J Allergy Clin Immunol* 2004; **113**: 543–50.

13. Sicherer SH, Sampson HA. Food allergy. *J Allergy Clin Immunol* 2006; **117**: S470–5.

14. Falcão H, Lunet N, Lopes C, Barros H. Food hypersensitivity in Portuguese adults. *Eur J Clin Nutr* 2004; **58**: 1621–5.

15. Osterballe M, Hansen TK, Mortz CG, Høst A, Bindslev-Jensen C. The prevalence of food hypersensitivity in an unselected population of children and adults. *Pediatr Allergy Immunol* 2005; **16**: 567–73.

16. Vierk KA, Koehler KM, Fein SB, Street DA. Prevalence of self-reported food allergy in American adults and use of food labels. *J Allergy Clin Immunol* 2007; **119**: 1504–10.

17. Venter C, Pereira B, Voigt K *et al*. Prevalence and cumulative incidence of food hypersensitivity in the first three years of life. *Allergy* 2008; **63**: 354–9.

18. Pereira B, Venter C, Grundy J *et al*. Prevalence of sensitization to food allergens, reported adverse reaction to foods, food avoidance, and food hypersensitivity among teenagers. *J Allergy Clin Immunol* 2005; **116**: 884–92.

19. Schäfer T, Böhler E, Ruhdorfer S *et al*. Epidemiology of food allergy/food intolerance in adults: associations with other manifestations of atopy. *Allergy* 2001; **56**: 1172–9.

20. Hoffmann-Sommergruber K, Radauer C. Bet v 1-homologous allergens. In: Mills ENC, Shewry PR, eds. *Plant Food Allergens*. Oxford: Blackwell, 2004: 125–40.

21. Dreborg S. Allergy in pollen-sensitive patients. *Ann Allergy* 1988; **64**: 41.

22. Veiths S, Scheurer S, Ballmer-Weber B. Current understanding of cross-reactivity of food allergens and pollen. *Ann N Y Acad Sci* 2002; **964**: 47–68.

23. Bauchau V, Durham SR. Prevalence and rate of diagnosis of allergic rhinitis in Europe. *Eur Respir J* 2004; **24**: 758–64.

24. Mothes N, Westritschnig K, Valenta R. Tree pollen allergens. In: Lockey RF, Bukantz S, Bousquet J, eds. *Allergens and Allergen Immunotherapy*. New York, NY: Informa Health Care, 2004: 165–84.

25. Royal College of Physicians Working Party. *Allergy: the Unmet Need*. London: Royal College of Physicians, 2003.

26. Breiteneder H, Radauer C. A classification of plant food allergens *J Allergy Clin Immunol* 2004; **113**: 821–30.

27. Radauer C, Breiteneder H. Evolutionary biology of plant food allergens. *J Allergy Clin Immunol* 2007; **120**: 518–25.

28. Vaughan JG, Geissler CA. *The New Oxford Book of Food Plants*. Oxford: Oxford University Press, 1997.

29. Radauer C, Hoffmann-Sommergruber K. Profilins. In: Mills ENC, Shewry PR, eds. *Plant Food Allergens*. Oxford: Blackwell, 2004: 105–24.

30. Breiteneder H. Thaumatin-like proteins: a new family of pollen and fruit allergens. *Allergy* 2004; **59**: 479–81.

31. Salcedo G, Sanchez-Monge R, Diaz-Perales A, Garcia-Casado G, Barber D. Plant non-specific lipid transfer proteins as food and pollen allergens. *Clin Exp Allergy* 2004; **34**: 1336–41.

32. Asero R, Mistrello G, Roncarolo D, Amato S. Relationship between peach lipid transfer protein specific IgE levels and hypersensitivity to non-Rosaceae vegetable foods in patients allergic to lipid transfer protein. *Ann Allergy Asthma Immunol* 2004; **92**: 268–72.

33. Fernández–Rivas M, Bolhaar S, González-Moncebo E *et al.* Apple allergy across Europe: how allergen sensitisation profiles determine the clinical expression of allergies to plant foods. *J Allergy Clin Immunol* 2006; **118**: 481–8.

34. Kalogeromitros DC, Makris MP, Gregoriou SG *et al.* Grape anaphylaxis: a study of 11 adult onset cases. *Allergy Asthma Proc* 2005; **26**: 53–8.

35. Schad SG, Trcka J, Vieths S *et al.* Wine anaphylaxis in a German patient: IgE–mediated allergy against a lipid transfer protein of grapes. *Int Arch Allergy Immunol* 2005; **136**: 159–64.

36. Lucas JSA, Nieuwenhuizen NJ, Atkinson RG *et al.* Kiwifruit allergy: actinidin is not a major allergen in the United Kingdom. *Clin Exp Allergy* 2007; **37**: 1340–8.

37. André F, André C, Colin L, Cacaraci F, Cavagna S. Role of new allergens consumption in the increased incidence of food sensitization in France. *Toxicology* 1994; **92**: 77–83.

38. Ballmer-Weber BK, Hoffmann A, Wüthrich B *et al.* Influence of food processing on the allergenicity of celery: DBPCFC with celery spice and cooked celery in patients with celery allergy. *Allergy* 2002; **57**: 228–35.

39. San Miguel-Moncín M, Krail M, Scheurer S *et al.* Lettuce anaphylaxis: identification of a lipid transfer protein as the major allergen. *Allergy* 2003; **58**: 511–17.

40. Palacín A, Cumplido J, Figueroa J *et al.* Cabbage lipid transfer protein Bra o 3 is a major allergen responsible for cross-reactivity between plant foods and pollens. *J Allergy Clin Immunol* 2007; **6**: 1423–9.

41. De Swert LFA, Cadot P, Ceuppens JL. Diagnosis and natural course of allergy to cooked potatoes in children. *Allergy* 2007; **62**: 750–7.

42. Egger M, Mutschlechner S, Wopfner N *et al.* Pollen–food syndromes associated with weed pollinosis: an update from the molecular point of view. *Allergy* 2006; **61**: 461–76.

43. Ma S, Sicherer SC, Nowark-Wegrzyn A. A survey on the management of pollen–food allergy syndrome in allergy practices. *J Allergy Clin Immunol* 2003; **112**: 784–8.

44. Breiteneder H, Ebner C. Molecular and biochemical classifications of plant-derived food allergens. *J Allergy Clinn Immunol* 2000; **106**: 27–36.

45. Sampson H. Update on food allergy. *J Allergy Clin Immunol* 2004; **113**: 805–19.

46. Bohle B. The impact of pollen-related food allergens on pollen allergy. *Allergy* 2007; **62**: 3–10.

47. Mills ENC, Jenkins JA, Shewry PR. The role of common properties in determining plant food protein allergenicity. In: Mills ENC, Shewry PR, eds. *Plant Food Allergens*. Oxford: Blackwell, 2004: 158–70.

48. Osterballe M, Hansen TK, Mortz CG, Bindslev-Jensen C. The clinical relevance of sensitisation to pollen-related fruits and vegetables in unselected pollen-sensitised adults. *Allergy* 2005; **60**: 218–25.

49. Mortz CG, Andersen KE, Bindeslev-Jensen C. Prevalence of peanut sensitisation and the association to pollen sensitisation in a cohort of unselected adolescents: the Odense Adolescence Cohort Study on Atopic Diseases and Dermatitis (TOACS). *Pediatr Allergy Immunol* 2005; **16**: 501–6.

50. Emberlin JC. Grass, tree and weed pollens. In: Kay AB, ed. *Allergy and Allergic Diseases*. Oxford: Blackwell, 1997: 835–57.

51. Enrique E, Cisteró-Bahima A, Bartolomé B *et al. Platanus acerifolia* pollinosis and food allergy. *Allergy* 2002; **75**: 351–6.

52. Hugues B, Didierlaurent A, Charpin D. Cross-reactivity between cypress pollen and peach: a report of seven cases. *Allergy* 2006; **61**: 1241–3.

53. Asero R. Birch and ragweed pollenosis of Milan: a model to investigate the effects of exposure to 2 new airborne allergens. *Allergy* 2002; **57**: 1063–6.

54. Wagner S, Breiteneder H. The latex–fruit syndrome. *Biochem Soc Trans* 2002; **30**: 935–40.

55. Jarolim E, Rumpold H, Endler AT *et al.* IgE and IgG antibodies of patients with allergy to birch pollen as tools to define the allergen profile of *Betula verrucosa*. *Allergy* 1989; **44**: 385–95.

56. Hoffmann-Sommergruber K. Plant allergens and pathogenisis-related proteins. What do they have in common? *Int Arch Allergy Immunol* 2000; **122**: 155–66.

57. Rodriguez-Perez R, Crespo J, Rodruigez J, Salcedo G. Profilin is a relevant melon allergen susceptible to pepsin digestion in patients with oral allergy syndrome. *J Allergy Clin Immunol* 2003; **111**: 634–9.

58. Asero R. Plant food allergies: a suggested approach to allergen-resolved diagnosis in the clinical practice by identifying easily available sensitisation markers. *Int Arch Allergy Immunol* 2005; **138**: 1–11.
59. van Ree RM, Fernandez-Rivas M, Cuevas M, van Wijngaarden M, Aalberse RC. Pollen-related allergy to peach and apple: an important role for profilin. *J Allergy Clin Immunol.* 1995; **95**: 726–34.
60. van Ree R, Aalberse RC. Pollen vegetable food cross-reactivity: serological and clinical relevance of cross-reactive IgE. *J Clin Immunoassay* 1993; **16**: 124–30.
61. Ortolani C, Ispano M, Pastorello E, Bigi A, Ansaloni R. The oral allergy syndrome. *Ann Allergy* 1988; **61**: 47–52.
62. Etesamifar M, Wüthrich B. IgE-vermittelte Nahrungsmittelallergie bei 383 Patienten unter Berücksichigung des oralen Allergie-Syndroms. *Allergologie* 1998; **21**: 451–7.
63. Jensen-Jarolim E, Leitner A, Hirschwehr R *et al.* Characterization of allergens in Apiaceae spices: anise, fennel, coriander and cumin. *Clin Exp Allergy* 1997; **27**: 1299–306.
64. Moneret-Vautrin DA, Morisset M , Lemerdy P , Croizier A, Kanny G. Food allergy and IgE sensitization caused by spices: CICBAA data (based on 589 cases of food allergy). *Allerg Immunol (Paris)* 2002; **34**: 135–40.
65. Chiu AM, Zacharisen MC. Anaphylaxis to dill. *Ann Allergy Asthma Immunol* 2000; **84**: 559–60.
66. Bock SA. Anaphylaxis to coriander: a sleuthing story. *J Allergy Clin Immunol* 1993; **91**: 1232–3.
67. Kleiber-Janke T, Crameri R, Scheurer S, Veiths S, Becker WM. Patient-tailored cloning of allergens by phage display: peanut (*Arachis hypogaea*) profilin, a food allergen derived from a rare mRNA. *J Chromatogr B Biomed Sci Appl* 2001; **756**: 295–305.
68. Mittag D, Akkerdass J, Ballmer-Weber B *et al.* Ara h 8, a Bet v 1-homologous allergen from peanut, is a major allergen in patients with combined birch pollen and peanut allergy. *J Allergy Clin Immunol* 2004; **114**: 1410–17.
69. Pastorello EA, Vieths S, Pravettoni V *et al.* Identification of hazelnut major allergens in sensitive patients with positive double-blind, placebo-controlled food challenge results. *J Allergy Clin Immunol* 2002; **109**: 563–70.
70. Raulf-Heimsoth M, Rihs HP, Rozynek P *et al.* Quantitative analysis of immunoglobulin E reactivity profiles in patients allergic or sensitised to natural rubber latex (*Hevea brasiliensis*) *Clin Exp Allergy* 2007; **37**: 1657–67.
71. Wagner S, Breiteneder H. *Hevea brasiliensis* latex allergens: current panel and clinical relevance. *Int Arch Allergy Immunol* 2005; **136**: 90–7.
72. Ibero M, Castilio M, Pineda F. Allergy to cassava: a new allergenic food with cross-reactivity to latex. *J Investig Allergol Clin Immunol* 2007; **17**: 409–12.
73. Pereira C, Tavares B, Loureiro G, Lundberg M, Chieira C. Turnip and zucchini: new foods in the latex–fruit syndrome. *Allergy* 2007; **62**: 452–3.
74. Ho MHK, Hill DJ. White button mushroom food hypersensitivity in a child. *J Paediatr Child Health* 2006; **42**: 555–6.
75. Senti G, Leser C, Lundberg M, Wüthrich B. Allergic asthma to shiitake and oyster mushroom. *Allergy* 2000; **55**: 975–6.
76. Aalto-Korte K, Susitaival P, Kaminska R, Mäkinen-Kiljunen S. Occupational protein contact dermatitis from shiitake mushroom and demonstration of shiitake-specific immunoglobulin E. *Contact Dermatitis* 2005; **53**: 211–13.
77. Levy AM, Kita H, Phillips SF *et al.* Eosinophilia and gastrointestinal symptoms after ingestion of shiitake mushrooms. *J Allergy Clin Immunol* 1998; **101**: 613–20.
78. Dauby PAL, Whisman BA, Hagan L Cross-reactivity between raw mushroom and molds in a patient with oral allergy syndrome. *Ann Allergy Asthma Immunol* 2002; **89**: 319–21.
79. Herrera I, Moneo I, Caballero ML *et al.* Food allergy to spinach and mushroom. *Allergy* 2002; **57**: 261–2.
80. Koivikko A, Savolainen J. Mushroom allergy. *Allergy* 1988; **43**: 1–10.
81. Helbling A, Gayer F, Pichler WJ, Brander KA. Mushroom (Basidiomycete) allergy: diagnosis established by skin test and nasal challenge. *J Allergy Clin Immunol* 1998; **102**: 853–8.

82. Airola K, Petman L, Mäkinen-Kiljunen S. Clustered sensitivity to fungi: anaphylactic reactions caused by ingestive allergy to yeasts. *Ann Allergy Asthma Immunol* 2006; **97**: 294–7.

83. Fernandez-Rivas M, Miles S. Food allergies: clinical and psychosocial perspectives. In: Mills ENC, Shewry PR, eds. *Plant Food Allergens*. Oxford: Blackwell, 2004: 1–23.

84. Schimek EM, Zwölfer B, Brize P *et al.* Gastrointestinal digestion of Bet v 1-homologous food allergens destroys their mediator-releasing, but not T-cell activating, capacity. *J Allergy Clin Immunol* 2005; **116**: 1327–33.

85. Bohle B, Zwölfer B, Heratizadeh A *et al.* Cooking birch pollen-related food: divergent consequences for IgE- and T cell-mediated reactivity in vitro and in vivo. *J Allergy Clin Immunol* 2006; **118**: 242–9.

86. Dreborg S, Foucard T. Allergy to apple, carrot and potato in children with birch pollen allergy. *Allergy* 1983; **38**: 167–72.

87. Helm RM. Food allergy: in-vivo diagnostics including challenge. *Curr Opin Allergy Clin Immunol* 2001; **1**: 255–9.

88. Anhøj C, Backer V, Nolte H. Diagnostic evaluation of grass- and birch-allergic patients with oral allergy syndrome. *Allergy* 2001; **56**: 548–52.

89. Ortolani C, Ispano M, Pastorello EA, Ansaloni R, Magri GC. Comparison of results of skin prick tests (with fresh foods and commercial food extracts) and RAST in 100 patients with oral allergy syndrome. *J Allergy Clin Immunol* 1989; **83**: 683–90.

90. Sicherer SH. Clinical implications of cross-reactive food allergens. *J Allergy Clin Immunol* 2001; **108**: 881–90.

91. Crespo JF, Rodriguez J, James JM *et al.* Reactivity to potential cross-reactive foods in fruit-allergic patients: implications for prescribing food avoidance. *Allergy* 2002; **57**: 946–9.

92. Fernandez-Rivas M, Cuevas M. Peels of Rosaceae fruits have a higher allergenicity than pulps. *Clin Exp Allergy* 1999; **29**: 1239–47.

93. Bindslev-Jensen C, Ballmer-Webber BK, Bengtsson U *et al.* Standardisation of food challenges in patients with immediate reactions to foods: position paper from the European Academy of Allergology and Clinical Immunology. *Allergy* 2004; **59**: 690–7.

94. Asero R, Massironi F, Velati C. Detection of prognostic factors for oral allergy syndrome in patients with birch pollen hypersensitivity. *J Allergy Clin Immunol* 1996; **2**: 611–16.

95. Sloan D, Sheffer A. Oral allergy syndrome. *Allergy Asthma Proc* 2001; **22**: 321–5.

96. Veiths S, Jankiewicz A, Schöning B, Aulepp H. Apple allergy: the IgE-binding potency of apple strains is related to the occurrence of the 18-kDa allergen. *Allergy* 1994; **49**: 262–71.

97. Carnés J, Ferrer A, Fernández-Caldas E. Allergenicity of 10 different apple varieties. *Ann Allergy Asthma Immunol* 2006; **96**: 564–70.

98. Sancho AI, Foxall R, Browne T *et al.* Effect of postharvest storage on the expression of the apple allergen Mal d 1. *J Agric Food Chem* 2006; **54**: 5917–23.

99. Assero R. How long does the effect of birch pollen injection SIT on apple allergy last? *Allergy* 2003; **58**: 435–8.

100. Hansen KS, Khinchi MS, Skov PS *et al.* Food allergy to apple and specific immunotherapy with birch pollen. *Mol Nutr Food Res* 2004; **48**: 441–8.

101. Bucher X, Pichier WJ, Dahinden CA, Heibling A. Effect of tree pollen specific subcutaneous immunotherapy on the oral allergy syndrome to apple and hazelnut. *Allergy* 2004; **59**: 1272–6.

102. Kinaciyan T, Jahn-Schmid B, Radakovics A *et al.* Successful sublingual immunotherapy with birch pollen has limited effects on concomitant food allergy to apple and the immune response to the Bet v 1 homolog Mal d 1. *J Allergy Clin Immunol* 2007; **119**: 937–43.

103. des Roches A, Paradis L, Paradis J, Singer S. Food allergy as a new risk factor for scurvy. *Allergy* 2006; **61**: 1487–8.

8 Peanuts, Legumes, Seeds and Tree Nuts

Ruth Towell

8.1 Peanuts

8.1.1 Prevalence

Peanuts are one of the eight common foods known to cause up to 90% of all food reactions[1], and peanut allergy (PA) has become increasingly common in recent years. Many studies have demonstrated that the prevalence of PA has doubled in the last 10 years, and it is now estimated to be somewhere between 1.3% and 1.5%[2–7]. The UK adult prevalence is estimated to be 0.5%[2], whilst in children peanut allergy is more prevalent, at 1 in 70 (1.4%)[3]. Two UK studies have corroborated a clinical history with diagnostic testing, reporting an increase in peanut allergy prevalence in children from 0.5% to 1.5% between 1994 and 2000[3,4]. There is geographical variation in the prevalence of peanut allergy in children. It is relatively common in the UK, France, Switzerland and North America, whereas in Israel it is only the fourth most common food allergy seen in infants (under 2 years of age), and it is rarely seen in Italy and Singapore[8].

Peanuts have historically been shown to be responsible for the majority of all reported food-induced fatal anaphylaxis in both the UK and the USA (59% and 19% respectively)[9–11]. Other nuts such as cashew nut, however, can also cause anaphylaxis[12]. The culprit of these life-threatening reactions is the Ara h 1 allergen, which prompts an immediate IgE-mediated allergic reaction in susceptible individuals. A study in 1997 found that the commonest age of onset of peanut allergy was 2 years[13], a finding confirmed by a 2003 study which showed that the mean age of onset was between 1 and 3 years[14]. The onset of any nut allergy in adults is thought to be rare, with one study showing only 8% of nut allergy developing in teenagers or older people[15].

It was once assumed that peanut allergy was an allergy for life, but a study in 1998 found that 9.6% of subjects were no longer peanut-allergic, with 5 years of age being the median for passing of an oral peanut challenge in those with previously diagnosed peanut allergy[16]. A 2001 study in the USA confirmed that around 20% of children will outgrow their peanut allergy by 5 years of age[17].

8.1.2 Foods and allergens involved

Peanuts are part of the botanical family known as Fabaceae or Leguminosae (Chapter 7, Table 7.1) and so are classified as a legume. Despite being in the same family as other legumes such as peas, beans and lentils, cross-reactivity with these foods is relatively rare[14,18,19]. A peanut is 26% protein and contains nine known allergens, Ara h 1 to Ara h 9. Everyone with a peanut allergy will be sensitised to Ara h 2, making it the allergen involved in the majority of allergic reactions to peanuts, but it is Ara h 1 that causes the severe reactions. Ara h 1 is also protected from protease breakdown by the presence of Ara h 2, which may help to explain why peanuts can so easily cause severe reactions[20]. These allergens do not fall within the same allergen superfamily: Ara h 1 is within the vicilin superfamily, while Ara h 2 falls within a superfamily similar to the albumin seed storage proteins within the prolamins (see Chapters 4 and 7, Tables 7.2 and 7.3). As with other plant food allergens, it is the classification of the allergens within the superfamilies that tends to dictate cross-reactivity between legumes, seeds and tree nuts, rather than their botanical classification.

There is a co-reactivity between soya protein, other legumes and peanuts that is purely immunological in nature and probably due to epitopes on soya protein being homologous to those found within peanut protein[21]. This has been confirmed by a study looking at the development of peanut allergy and confounding factors, in which it was found that there was an association between soya protein and peanut allergy[14]. However this link does not translate into clinical cross-reactivity, as peanut-allergic individuals in this study were not found to be soya-allergic. This finding agreed with two earlier studies on children where only 0.8% of children with atopic dermatitis had an allergy to both peanut and soya bean[18], and only 3% of peanut-allergic children had a soya-bean allergy[19].

The fact that it is epitope homology rather than botanical classification which is responsible for cross-reactivity is exemplified by the cross-reactivity between peanuts and tree nuts, even though they are from different botanical families. In practice this means that people with a peanut allergy are at a greater risk (about a 1 in 5 chance) of having a tree-nut allergy[15,22,23]. A study of 784 children showed that by the age of 2 years 2% of peanut-allergic children were multiple-nut-allergic to Brazil, almond, hazel and walnut[24].

Many allergens are affected by heat treatments and processing, which may either increase or decrease the allergen's potency. It is the conformational epitopes, where the amino acids are found on two different chains of the peptide sequence, which are thought to be more susceptible to thermal destruction, with the linear epitopes being more likely to be susceptible to hydrolysis processes (see also Chapter 4). Frying and boiling peanuts has been shown to significantly reduce the amount of Ara h 1, thus reducing the peanuts' allergenicity[25]. In contrast, roasting peanuts has been found to increase the Ara h 1 and Ara h 2 allergens' ability to bind to the IgE antibodies by 90-fold, thus making roasted peanuts more allergenic than raw peanuts[21]. Refining peanut oils reduces the allergenicity, as virtually all of the protein is removed, and refined peanut oil is therefore safe for virtually all peanut allergy sufferers[26].

8.1.3 Diagnosis

As with all medical diagnosis, a good clinical history is paramount when investigating peanut allergy. However, diagnostic tools such as skin prick tests (SPT) and specific IgE measurement within blood are very helpful in corroborating clinical history. In children SPT has been shown to have an excellent negative predictivity and specificity for peanut allergy diagnosis. Sporik and colleagues showed that SPT ≥ 8 mm was 100% predictive of peanut allergy in children (median age 3 years), i.e. a negative reaction to peanut did not occur[27]. For children of less than 2 years of age the required diameter was only ≥ 4 mm to ensure 100% specificity in peanut allergy diagnosis. In a study of children with atopic dermatitis the SPT wheal size required was ≥ 6 mm for peanut, giving a 95% predictive probability of peanut allergy diagnosis[28].

Similar work has investigated the diagnostic use of specific IgEs in children and adolescents (mean age 5.2 years)[29]. It has been shown that a specific IgE greater than 15 kU_A/L has a 95% predictive probability for diagnosing peanut allergy and a value of less than 0.35 kU_A/L has a 85% predictive probability for ruling out peanut allergy. Both these studies were carried out on highly atopic and high-risk children, so caution needs to be exercised in using these values in the general paediatric population. However, this work means that there are now clear cut-off diagnostic decision points for both specific IgE and SPTs that, together with a good clinical history, can be used for a confident diagnosis of the presence or absence of peanut allergy in children. Unfortunately no such data exist for adults, where clinicians have to rely more heavily on a good clinical history and cautiously interpret SPTs and IgEs for a diagnosis of peanut allergy.

When SPT and IgE tests return equivocal results which do not corroborate the clinical history then an oral challenge with peanut is required. Depending upon the likely severity and immediacy of an allergic reaction this may need to take place under strict medical supervision within a hospital unit, or it may be carried out safely at home under professional advice. In the case of children an open challenge, where all parties know that peanut is being used, is generally adequate, but with an older population – and especially if subjective symptoms are expected – then a blinded challenge will be required. This means that the person being challenged is unaware of which food the peanut is hidden in, so a placebo as well as a peanut 'meal' is used. The main hurdle with a blind peanut challenge is the strong taste and smell of peanut products and thus the difficulty of putting peanut in a meal undetected.

More detailed information on the tests available for diagnosing a food allergy can be found in Chapter 3.

8.1.4 Management

Dietary avoidance is currently the only proven safe and effective management of peanut allergy. At present peanut allergy cannot be treated, although as previously mentioned it is now thought that about one in five children will outgrow their peanut allergy by 5 years of age[17,19].

Treatments

There are currently a few treatment options undergoing clinical trials, including immunotherapy, herbal remedies and epitope alteration, but the common use of desensitisation and other treatments in day-to-day clinical practice is still a long way off.

Dietary avoidance

In order to ensure that no accidental reaction to peanut occurs, avoidance of all peanut-containing food and drinks must be complete. In addition, all tree nuts should be avoided due to the 1-in-5 risk of cross-reactivity[15] and the contamination risks. In addition, there seems to be an inability, especially in children, to easily distinguish one nut from another: a recent study found that 27% of children were unable to correctly distinguish which nut(s) they were allergic to[30].

Degree of avoidance

It is essential that peanut and tree-nut avoidance is total because of the IgE-mediated nature of the reaction to these allergens and the immediacy and possible severity of a reaction.

Practical tips for avoidance

Peanut is one of allergens required by EU labelling law to be clearly stated on the label of a packaged product, no matter how small the quantity (see Chapter 4). It is therefore extremely important that those with a peanut allergy learn how to read and interpret the labels, and which words to look out for that may indicate the presence of peanut. Peanuts can be listed in a variety of ways:

- peanuts;
- nuts;
- ground nuts;
- earth nuts;
- monkey nuts;
- arachis oil;
- *Arachis hypogaea*;
- groundnut oil;
- peanut oil;
- peanut flour;
- peanut butter.

Other foods which may contain peanuts, and which must be avoided, are listed in Table 8.1.

Manufacturers now generally use refined peanut oil within products, and this has been found to be safe for peanut allergy sufferers due to the lack of protein remaining after refinement[26]. The product, however, must state 'refined' peanut oil

Table 8.1   Common foods which may contain peanuts.

Food type	Examples
Spreads	Peanut butter, other nut butters
Snacks	Peanut snacks, trail mix, rice crackers, chocolate-covered peanuts, cereal bars
Cakes and biscuits	Cookies, brownies
Ice creams	Nut toppings
Vegetarian meals	Nut roast, veggie burgers
Sauces	Satay sauce, salad dressings (may contain unrefined peanut oil)
Breakfast cereals	Anything with crunchy nut or honey nut, muesli and other fruit and nut cereals
Meals out	Indonesian, Malaysian, Thai and Chinese meals often contain peanuts; Indian food may also contain peanuts, although other nuts are more likely

rather than just peanut oil, which is unsafe as it has not gone through this refinement process. If in doubt, avoidance is always the safe option.

Tips on eating out and take-away meals

Fatality registries suggest that adolescents and young adults are at greatest risk, with delayed injection of adrenaline during anaphylaxis as an influencing factor, when they are no longer under strict parental supervision and no longer carry their adrenaline 'pens' with them, e.g. at friends' houses or in bars or restaurants[9–11]. One study showed that only 29% of anaphylaxis fatalities registered were at home, and 54% occurred when eating out or from a take-away[11]. Unfortunately, accidental ingestion is fairly common, as demonstrated by a review amongst Canadian schoolchildren which saw an annual reported incidence rate of 14.3%[31].

Peanut allergy sufferers who wish to eat out should be advised always to speak to the chef, and if this is not possible they should choose not to eat in that establishment. Most restaurants clearly label the meals that are nut-free, and allergy sufferers must always ask how strict this criterion is. Commonly child-friendly meals are nut-free. When ordering take-away meals, allergy sufferers should try to use the same place once they are sure about its safety. It is very important that the chef is aware of the seriousness of using peanuts/nuts and the implications of cross-contamination and changing the ingredients. Asian meals are the most likely to contain nuts, so extra caution is needed, especially as many 'authentic' Asian food establishments will use unrefined peanut oil in their cooking. For further information on lifestyle issues of food hypersensitivity, see Chapter 12.

Contamination

Many manufacturers are still using the blanket label of 'may contain traces of nuts', which means that these products should be avoided as the risk of potential contamination is unknown. The Food Standards Agency (FSA) has produced guidance on food labelling of allergens for manufacturers, but this is not compulsory. There are, however, a few manufacturers using nut-free factories, who guarantee that all their products are peanut-free:

- Fabulous Bakin' Boys (www.bakinboys.co.uk);
- It's Nut Free (www.itsnutfree.com);
- Kinnerton Confectionery (www.kinnerton.com).

The Anaphylaxis Campaign (www.anaphylaxis.org.uk) is currently working with manufacturers to get more stringent labelling in general usage with regards to allergens within products and the measured risk of contamination.

Accidental exposure via contamination is a real risk for the peanut-allergic individual. For example, it has been found that Ara h 1 remains in the saliva for up to 1 hour after ingestion and that 1 ml of saliva can contain up to 1,110 mg Ara h 1[32]. People who are peanut-allergic, and their families and friends, need to be advised about hand washing with soap and water, and cleaning cooking and eating surfaces effectively using soap and water, as it has been found that water alone and some antibacterial hand wipes do not remove the allergen[33].

Nutritional issues

Within the general population the avoidance of peanuts and other nuts should not pose a risk of a nutritional deficiency. Special consideration, however, needs to be paid to those who are strict vegetarians and vegans, as these groups are more likely to use peanut and other nuts as a major source of protein. For such at-risk individuals, dietary advice from a specialised healthcare professional such as a registered dietitian is required, to ensure that the diet has sufficient protein and is nutritionally adequate. For further details of nutritional issues surrounding the avoidance of specific foods, see Chapter 11.

8.2   Other legumes

8.2.1   Prevalence

Soya allergy appears to be more prevalent in infants and children than in adults. As already mentioned, it is the second most prevalent legume allergy worldwide (after peanut)[34]. There is significant geographical variation in legume prevalence and type. For example, in India lentils and chickpeas are a major cause of allergy due to their predominance in cooking[35], and there have even been reports of fenugreek allergy[36]. In Spain legume allergy is the fifth most prevalent food allergy within children[37], and allergy to lentils is more common than allergy to peanuts[38]. Lupin allergy has become more common as the seed flour is now being used in wheat flour (up to 10%) in France, and adverse reactions to the lupin flour have been reported[39,40]. Soya allergy appears to be a predominantly transient childhood allergy much like egg and milk. However, in contrast to egg and milk allergy, researchers and clinicians are still unsure how common it is for children to outgrow this allergy, or at what age this is most likely to occur. A study of children diagnosed with food-protein-induced enteropathy found that one-quarter of the soya-allergic children were no longer soya-sensitive by 25 months of age[41]. Other legume allergies such as lentil and chickpea are, unlike soya allergy, more prevalent in adults.

8.2.2   Foods and allergens involved

Legumes are dicotyledonous plants belonging to the order Fabales. In addition to the peanut, other legumes classified in the botanical family of Fabaceae (Leguminosae) are soya, runner, French, Goa, haricot, butter, lima, mung and faba beans; chickpea and pigeon pea; pea; lupin; lentils; tamarind; guar, acacia and tragacanth gum; fenugreek and liquorice. The most significant allergenic food after peanut is the soya bean, which alongside peanuts is one of the eight foods causing 90% of all food allergies[1]. There have, however, been numerous case reports of severe reactions to guar gum, tragacanth and lupin, and both chickpeas and lentils are significant allergens in some countries where they are a staple food.

Many of the major allergens in legumes can be found in the vicilin superfamily, including the soya allergen Gly m Bd 60k, the lentil allergen Len c 1 and the Ara h 1 peanut epitope. Again, the similarity of allergen structures appears to dictate cross-reactivity between legumes, and many studies have shown *in vitro* cross-sensitivity between members of the legume family. Clinical cross-reactivity, however, appears to be extremely rare. In children there appears to be a link between soya exposure and peanut allergy[14], but this sensitisation rarely translates into clinical cross-reactivity[18,19]. However, cross-reactivity has been demonstrated between lentils and chickpeas, with one study showing that 70% of children who suffer from lentil allergy are also allergic to chickpeas[37]. A recent upsurge in lupin flour usage has led to research into the cross-reactivity potential between peanut and lupin flour, with one study reporting 44% cross-reactivity between these two legumes[42]. In 1997 lupin flour was accepted as a permissible addition to wheat flour (up to 10%) in France, and its high protein content (40%) has helped it to be a potent allergen.

As with all food allergens, processing can affect allergenicity, but it cannot be assumed that heating always destroys allergens. Highly refined soya oil (like peanut oil) appears not to induce an allergic reaction in those with soya allergy, suggesting that the refining process removes all protein within the soya bean, ensuring its safety[43]. However, soya fermentation does not reduce allergenicity, so soya sauce is as allergenic as soya-bean products[44].

8.2.3   Diagnosis

Researchers have tried to provide predictive SPT wheal diameters and specific IgE levels for soya allergy diagnosis in children, as they have done for other common allergens, e.g. peanut. To date, however, they have found that SPT wheal-diameter cut-off points are unreliable and cannot accurately predict soya allergy[28]. Furthermore, specific IgE level ≥ 65 kU$_A$/L was only 50% predictive and thus also unreliable in diagnosing soya allergy[29]. Diagnosing soya allergy in both adults and children therefore relies heavily on a good clinical history, and a hospital-based oral food challenge may need to be performed if clinical history is inconclusive.

8.2.4 Management

Complete dietary avoidance of the offending allergen is currently the only proven safe and effective management of any legume allergy. There appears to be no consistent evidence to date that avoidance of all legumes is necessary; only the specific legume known to trigger the allergic reaction (for example soya bean) needs to be avoided. If the allergic reaction to the legume is known to be IgE-mediated, then complete avoidance is imperative. A reaction that is non-IgE mediated may mean that trace amounts of the legume will not trigger a reaction, so complete avoidance may not be necessary.

Soya beans and lupin are the only two legumes that fall within the 2005 EU allergen labelling list for packaged foods, and thus for all other legumes extra-careful reading of labels is essential. Many different products are likely to contain legumes: see Table 8.2 for some examples.

Nutritional issues

As with peanut and tree-nut avoidance, strict vegetarians and vegans are likely to be at nutritional risk when avoiding legumes, especially soya bean, due to their need for protein from this food group. However, if only one legume needs to be avoided, as is usually the case, then the nutritional risk is minimal. Soya-bean avoidance is

Table 8.2 Foods likely to contain legumes.

Legume	Foods involved
Soy	Textured vegetable protein (TVP), vegetable burgers, tofu (soya-bean curd), tempeh, tamari, miso, soy sauce, pre-packaged Chinese meals, soya milks, soya yoghurts, soya desserts
Lupin	Lupin flour is often used in mainland Europe in pastries, breads and pizza bases, and lupin seeds are sometimes used in seeded breads
Chickpeas	Indian dishes, especially vegetarian, e.g. chana dhal; added as flour to some French breads, hummus
Lentils	Gram flour, chappatis, puri, dhal, vegetarian dishes
Tragacanth	Used as a thickening agent and stabilizer in food products, e.g. salad dressings, ice cream; used medicinally for digestive disorders (laxative effect) and coughs, so may be found within cough syrups and lozenges
Guar (E412)	Used as a thickener and emulsifier in foods, e.g. yoghurts, fruit juice drinks, ice creams, salad dressings
Fenugreek	Curry powder

the most likely to cause nutritional difficulties, as soya is the only non-animal source of high-biological-value protein, and thus a major food source for vegetarians and vegans. Vegetarians and vegans will therefore need additional dietetic help and advice if they have a soya allergy, to ensure that their diet is nutritionally adequate.

8.3 Seeds

8.3.1 Prevalence

Hypersensitivity reactions to sunflower seed, cottonseed and linseed were recorded as early as 1906, 1929 and 1930 respectively[45–49]. There has even been a report of anaphylaxis to dye made from the annatto seed[50]. Although allergy to these seeds is extremely rare, anaphylaxis has been reported, and consequently any suspicion of an allergic reaction must be taken seriously and investigated thoroughly.

Sesame-seed allergy was first reported in 1950, but it is a recent phenomenon within North America and Europe. This may be due to an increase in the consumption of sesame seeds and products as part of the 'health food' drive. The increasing consumption of sesame seeds, sesame products and sesame oil has been mirrored by an increase in reporting of serious reactions to sesame, especially in children, where serious allergic reactions including anaphylaxis have been reported[51–53]. In Australia, sesame-seed allergy in infants is more common (0.42%) than tree-nut allergy and is the fourth most prevalent food allergy in this age group behind eggs, milk and peanuts[54]. In Israel, sesame is a major cause of immediate IgE allergy, and it is the third commonest cause of IgE-mediated food allergy. It is more prevalent than peanut allergy and is the second highest cause of anaphylaxis behind cow's-milk allergy in infants under 2 years of age[8]. In Israel the mean age of those found to be sesame-allergic was 10.5 months, with six of the 14 cases of anaphylaxis being caused by sesame allergy[8]. Little research has been carried out on resolution of sesame-seed allergy, so it is still not known whether the allergy is outgrown.

In France, mustard seed is a major allergen in children, being the fourth most prevalent[8], with an estimated prevalence of 1.1% in children and a prevalence of 0.84% in adults[55]. It is for this reason that mustard seed is one of the 12 allergens included in the EU food labelling laws list.

8.3.2 Foods and allergens involved

Seeds come from plants with differing botanical classifications. For example, sesame is a member of the family Pedaliaceae, while the sunflower is in the family Compositae (Asteraceae). Allergic reactions have been reported to a variety of different seeds: sesame, linseed (flaxseed), poppy seed, cottonseed, mustard seed, annatto seed and sunflower seed. The allergens within these seeds are spread amongst many different superfamilies, with the potent sesame allergen Ses i 2 being classed within the prolamin superfamily and Ses i 3 within the vicilin superfamily along with the previously mentioned peanut and cashew-nut allergens (Ara h 1 and

Ana o 1). Researchers are continually discovering new allergens within seeds: for example, linseed has now been found to have five different allergen epitopes.

Unlike peanut oil, which is typically consumed as highly refined oil with the protein removed, sesame oil is cold-pressed and traces of the protein are still found within the oil. Thus sesame oil may be even more allergenic than the whole seeds. A case report suggested that a sesame-allergic individual's symptoms were most severe when the sesame was in the form of oil, with the severity decreasing according to whether the sesame was ground, cooked whole and raw[53]. This may be due to the fact that some allergen epitopes are hidden within the whole seed, making them unavailable if the seed is eaten whole. There are different varieties of sesame seeds, e.g. black and white, which have varying amounts of protein and thus allergen, white seeds having six times more protein than black seeds[56].

8.3.3 Diagnosis

A clear clinical history is vital when diagnosing most seed allergies, as the other diagnostic tools available such as SPT and specific IgE are fairly difficult to interpret, with no predictive levels yet reported. Diagnosing sesame allergy without clear clinical history is difficult due to the unreliability of the SPT commercial extracts, and using natural sesame extract appears to be more accurate[8,57]. As with other allergens, an SPT ≥ 3 mm is considered to be a positive result. However, unlike some food allergens, e.g. peanut, there are no 95% predictive SPT cut-off levels for sesame allergy diagnosis in children, and SPT cannot be used alone as a definitive diagnostic test[58-60] (see Chapter 3). Where there is real discordance between history and test results an oral food challenge may be required to confirm or refute diagnosis.

8.3.4 Management

Complete dietary avoidance of the known seed allergen is currently the only proven safe and effective management of any seed allergy, especially as the risk of anaphylaxis appears to be high for this particular food group. There appears to be no reason to avoid all seeds, only the specific seed known to trigger the allergic reaction. Sesame is more widely available now in foods, and children in particular are more commonly being found to have sesame allergy, so vigilance is necessary.

Practical tips for avoidance

Only sesame and mustard seed are required by the EU to be listed on packaged food. Other seeds such as sunflower, poppy and linseed do not have to be listed by law. Typically, seeds are found within breads, cakes, biscuits, crackers and muffins (Table 8.3). Frequently food labels will just list 'seeds'. Linseed is also known as flaxseed and is frequently sold as a dietary supplement. Many Middle Eastern countries use sesame seeds and poppy seeds within their foods, so Iranian and Lebanese restaurants, as well as Greek and Turkish restaurants, may be better avoided.

Table 8.3 Foods commonly containing seeds.

Seed	Foods involved
Sesame	Sesame oil, tahini (sesame paste), halvah (Turkish sweet), gomashio, hummus, aqua libra, vegetarian burgers, speciality seeded breads and burger baps, Asian foods cooked using sesame oil, Greek and Turkish pastries such as baklava
Poppy	Speciality breads, pastries, especially those from eastern Europe
Mustard	Curry powder, pizza, ready-prepared sauces
Sunflower	Seeded breads, sunflower cooking oil; unspecified vegetable oils may be made from sunflower
Linseed (flaxseed)	Seeded breads, food supplements, e.g. linseed oil

As with peanuts and tree nuts, there are manufacturers who guarantee their food to be sesame-free (see list in Section 8.1.4, above).

Unlike peanuts, sesame seeds and seeds in general are easy to wash off surfaces, so accidental contamination is less likely. However, sesame seed oil may be an issue in places where it is added to common dishes and the same serving utensils are used, such as in a Chinese restaurant.

Nutritional issues

Generally, seeds do add major nutritional value to the human diet, and thus avoidance of seeds should not put anyone at nutritional risk.

8.4 Tree nuts

8.4.1 Prevalence

The overall prevalence of tree-nut allergy in the USA appears to be constant, but in children it is apparently increasing. In both 1997 and 2002, a telephone survey found that 0.4% of the general population reported a tree-nut allergy, with walnut being the most common[7]. When this was subdivided into adults (over 18 years old) and children the rate for children rose from 0.2% in 1997 to 0.6% in 2002.

There is geographical variation in the prevalence of tree-nut allergy. In the USA the commonest tree-nut allergies are walnut, almond and pecan[7], whereas in the UK the tree-nut allergies most commonly seen are Brazil, almond and hazelnut[15]. In Australia, Brazil and almond allergy are rarely seen, and cashew-nut allergy is the most common nut allergy in infants affecting 0.33%, with hazelnut as the second most common (0.18%) and walnut third (0.16%)[54]. The prevalence of cashew-nut allergy in the USA is estimated to be 0.5%, affecting 41% of those reporting an allergy to tree nuts[7].

This American study also investigated the mean age of first allergic reaction to cashew nut, finding it to be at 2 years old with only one in five having had a history of previous exposure[7]. Cashew-nut allergy appears to show a similar clinical history to peanut allergy; two recent studies have shown that serious reactions (cardiovascular symptoms, wheezing and even anaphylaxis) from cashew-nut allergy are now more common than those from peanuts[12,61]. One of these studies, following children retrospectively, found that 74% of cashew-nut allergy sufferers had experienced an anaphylaxis reaction, compared to 31% of peanut allergy sufferers[61]. Other nuts can also cause severe reactions, with one UK study reporting that, together with peanut, Brazil, almond, hazel and walnut produced 86% of the 'worst reactions' seen[62].

A further complicating factor with tree-nut allergy is that tree nuts, especially hazelnuts, are commonly associated with the phenomenon known as oral allergy syndrome (OAS: see Chapter 7). Therefore it is important that diagnosis of true tree-nut allergy occurs rather than assumptions being made, as is often the case in adults with hazelnut allergy, that this is part of the OAS. It has been shown that 78% of those with hazelnut allergy symptoms had a true food allergy[63]. Another study also found that nut-allergy onset among teenagers or adults was only 8%, confirming that true nut allergy usually starts in childhood[15].

It is estimated that only 9% of tree-nut allergies are outgrown, in contrast to 20% of peanut allergy[64]. At present it appears that cashew-nut allergy is rarely outgrown (9%); however, as with peanut allergy, this may be amended as the natural history of such allergies is investigated further over the next few years.

8.4.2 Foods and allergens involved

Tree nuts include cashew, almond, Brazil, hazelnut, chestnut, pistachio, pecan, walnut, macadamia, pine nut and coconut. Some tree nuts fall into the same botanical families as fruits such as mango, dates, and palm hearts (see Chapter 7, Table 7.1). From an allergy perspective, the absence of a botanical link between the different tree nuts does not mean that someone with one tree-nut allergy will not cross-react to other nuts.

As with legumes and seeds, it is the plant food superfamily classification of the allergens involved in tree-nut allergy which is more important with regard to cross-reactivity (Chapter 7, Tables 7.2, 7.3). Like peanuts, many tree nuts have both major and minor allergens in different superfamilies; for example cashew nut has allergens in the vicilin (Ana o 1), legumin (Ana o 2) and 2S-albumin (Ana o 3) superfamilies. Allergens from different tree nuts fall into the same superfamilies. For example, the walnut allergen Jug r 2 and the cashew-nut allergen Ana o 1 are both vicilins, the same superfamily as the peanut allergen Ara h 1. The 2S-albumin-type allergen within cashew nut (Ana o 3) shares great similarities with one of the walnut allergens, Jug r 1, which may explain the known cross-reactivity between cashew nut and walnut for allergy sufferers[65]. A study looking at the allergens within three different tree nuts, walnut (Jug r 4), cashew (Ano o 4) and hazelnut (Cor a 9), all of which are legumins, concluded that their epitope homology may be the reason for the frequently seen multiple tree-nut cross-reactivity, which is independent of the tree nuts being within the same botanical classification[66].

Studies have shown a strong clinical cross-reactivity between tree nuts and peanuts within allergic individuals. Studies have estimated that 23–50% of atopic patients are allergic to both peanut and tree nuts[7,13,15,67,68], and in one 1996 UK study up to 31% of children with confirmed peanut allergy also had a confirmed tree-nut allergy[15]. In the general population, however, this risk of having both a peanut and tree-nut allergy may be as little as 2.5%[67].

The level of co-sensitisation will vary depending on the tree nut involved. A French study in 2003, looking at the clinical history of cashew-nut allergy, found that although the allergens Ana o 1 (cashew nut) and Ara h 1 (peanut) are both found within the vicilin superfamily they showed no epitope homology, which may explain why no co-sensitisation between cashew nut and peanut allergy was seen[69]. However, this same study did find an increased likelihood (33%) of cross-reactivity between cashew and pistachio, nuts which do share a botanical relationship as they are both in the Anacardiaceae family. Thus the combination of the allergen and botanical classifications, and their influence on clinical cross-reactivity, creates a complex picture where generalisations cannot be made.

As with all food allergens, wet or dry thermal processing and proteolysis can alter the protein structure and thus allergenicity of the food. Epitopes may be destroyed or their IgE-binding capacity reduced, or even increased, the peanut epitope is increased on roasting. However, it is also possible that due to protein reconfiguration new epitopes could be formed; these are known as neoallergens[70]. In pecan nuts these are known to occur on heating, and in fact anaphylaxis to these neoallergens has been reported[71]. Neither blanching nor roasting appears to reduce the allergen content of almonds[72]. Roasting appears to decrease the allergenicity of hazelnuts[73], especially for those sensitive to the epitopes Cor a 1 and Cor a 2, but for those people with OAS roasted nuts can still cause a reaction on challenge.

OAS can often be triggered by tree nuts, and it can be confused with a true allergy to the nut in question (see Chapter 7). The commonest cross-reactivity occurs between allergens from almond, hazelnut and walnut and antibodies to the main birch-pollen allergen Bet v 1. Similar cross-reactivity can also occur between latex and some tree nuts.

8.4.3 Diagnosis

In hazelnut allergy diagnosis, skin prick tests and specific IgE tests have demonstrated a reasonable sensitivity and positive predictive value but a very low specificity and negative predictive value, thus implying that these tests should not be used to validate the diagnosis of hazelnut allergy[63]. When the clinical history and SPT and IgE results are contradictory an oral food challenge may be more common and necessary in tree-nut allergy diagnosis because predictive values for SPTs and IgEs are so far unavailable for both adults and children. As with peanut food challenges, blinding of tree nuts into a 'meal' is difficult due to the strong smell and taste of the nuts. Thus expertise in carrying out oral food challenges is needed.

8.4.4   Management

Dietary avoidance is currently the only proven safe and effective management of any tree nut allergy. Given the risk (1 in 5) of cross-reactivity between tree nuts and peanuts, and also cross-reactivity within the tree nuts, avoidance of all nuts is necessary unless safe toleration of a particular nut is certain and contamination can be ruled out. Because of the IgE-mediated nature of tree-nut allergy, avoidance must be complete, as even traces of the allergen can trigger an immediate life-threatening reaction, as seen with cashew-nut allergy.

Practical tips for avoidance

All tree nuts are included within the list of allergens specified by EU law that must be labelled on packaged foods which contain them, however small the amount (chestnut and pine nut are not considered tree nuts and are therefore not on this list). For safety reasons, and to ensure low risk of contamination, all tree nuts should be avoided as well as peanuts (see Section 8.1, above). Some nuts have alternative names, and it is important that those with a confirmed diagnosis are aware of all the different words which indicate the presence of nuts (Table 8.4).

For a list of manufacturers who guarantee their food to be nut-free refer to Section 8.1.4, above. For more details see Table 8.5.

Table 8.4   Alternative names for some nuts.

Nut	Alternative names
Hazelnut	Filbert, cob nut
Macademia	Queensland nut, candle nut
Pecan	Hickory nut

Table 8.5   Foods likely to contain tree nuts.

Food Type	Examples
Spreads	Chocolate hazelnut spread
Snacks and sweets	Cereal bars, mixed nuts, praline, nougat, Turkish delight, marzipan
Cakes and biscuits	Cookies, brownies, fruit cake, anything with marzipan, almond croissants
Ice creams	Nut toppings, pistachio ice cream, kulfi
Vegetarian meals	Nut roast, veggie burgers
Sauces	Almond essence, nut oils
Breakfast cereals	Anything with crunchy nut or honey nut, muesli and other fruit and nut cereals
Meals out	Indian food may contain almonds and pistachio nuts; Chinese food may contain cashew nuts; nut-flavoured liqueurs, e.g. amaretto

Nutritional issues

The avoidance of tree nuts may only affect the nutritional status of those who are following a strict vegetarian or vegan diet, where nuts form a major part of the diet in their role as a non-animal source of protein. It is important that this group gets the necessary dietary advice from an appropriate healthcare professional such as a registered dietitian, to help them ensure that their diet has sufficient protein and is nutritionally adequate. Avoidance of the products containing the wording 'may contain traces of nuts' can also lead to major dietary restrictions, as unfortunately this statement is placed on many products, thus reducing the nut-allergic individual's range of foods to eat.

References

1. Food and Agriculture Organization (FAO). *Report of the FAO Technical Consultation on Food Allergies*. Rome: FAO, 1995.
2. Emmett SE, Angus FJ, Fry JS, Lee PN. Perceived prevalence of peanut allergy in Great Britain and its association with other atopic conditions and with peanut allergy in other household members. *Allergy* 1999; **54**: 380–5.
3. Grundy J, Matthews S, Bateman B, Dean T, Arshad SH. Rising prevalence of allergy to peanut in children: Data from 2 sequential cohorts. *J Allergy Clin Immunol* 2002; **110**: 784–9.
4. Munoz-Furlong A. Patient's perspective and public policy regarding anaphylaxis. *Novartis Found Symp* 2004; **257**: 265–74.
5. Tariq SM, Stevens M, Matthews S *et al*. Cohort study of peanut and tree nut sensitisation by age of 4 years. *BMJ* 1996; **313**: 514–17.
6. Kanny G, Moneret-Vautrin DA, Flabbee J *et al*. Population study of food allergy in France. *J Allergy Clin Immunol* 2001; **108**: 133–40.
7. Sicherer SH, Muñoz-Furlong A, Sampson HA. Prevalence of peanut and tree nut allergy in the United States determined by means of a random digit dial telephone survey: a 5-year follow-up study. *J Allergy Clin Immunol* 2003; **112**: 1203–7.
8. Dalal I, Binson R, Reifen Z *et al*. Food allergy is a matter of geography after all: sesame as a major cause of severe IgE-mediated food allergic reactions among infants and young children in Israel. *Allergy* 2002; **57**: 362–5
9. Bock SA, Muñoz-Furlong A, Sampson HA. Fatalities due to anaphylactic reactions to foods. *J Allergy Clin Immunol* 2001; **107**: 191–3.
10. Bock SA, Muñoz-Furlong A, Sampson HA. Further fatalities caused by anaphylactic reactions to food, 2001–2006. *J Allergy Clin Immunol* 2007; **119**: 1016–18.
11. Pumphrey RS, Gowland MH. Further fatal allergic reactions to food in the United Kingdom, 1999–2006. *J Allergy Clin Immunol* 2007; **119**: 1018–19.
12. Davoren M, Peake J. Cashew nut allergy is associated with a high risk of anaphylaxis *Arch Dis Child* 2005; **90**: 1084–5
13. Hourihane JO, Kilburn SA, Dean P, Warner JO. Clinical characteristics of peanut allergy. *Clin Exp Allergy* 1997; **27**: 634–9.
14. Lack G, Fox D, Northstone K, Golding J. Factors associated with the development of peanut allergy in childhood. *N Engl J Med* 2003; **348**: 977–85
15. Ewan PW. Clinical study of peanut and nut allergy in 62 consecutive patients: new features and associations. *BMJ* 1996; **312**: 1074–8.
16. Hourihane JO, Roberts SA, Warner JO. Resolution of peanut allergy: a case–control study. *BMJ* 1998; **316**: 1271–5.
17. Skolnick HS, Conover-Walker MK, Koerner CB *et al*. The natural history of peanut allergy. *J Allergy Clin Immunol* 2001; **107**: 367–74.
18. Sampson HA, McCaskill CC. Food hypersensitivity and atopic dermatitis: evaluation of 113 patients. *J Pediatr* 1985; **107**: 669–75.

19. Bock SA, Atkins FM. The natural history of peanut allergy. *J Allergy Clin Immunol* 1989; **83**: 900–4.
20. Maleki SJ, Chung SY, Champagne T, Raufman JP. The effects of roasting on the allergenic properties of peanut proteins. *J Allergy Clin Immunol* 2000; **106**: 763–8.
21. Barnett D, Bonham B, Howden MEH. Allergenic cross-reactions among legume foods: an in vitro study. *J Allergy Clin Immunol* 1987; **79**: 433–8.
22. Ewan PW, Clark AT. Long-term prospective observational study of patients with peanut and nut allergy after participation in a management plan. *Lancet* 2001; **357**: 111–15.
23. Hourihane JO, Dean TP, Warner JO. Peanut allergy in relation to heredity, maternal diet, and other atopic diseases: results of a questionnaire survey, skin prick testing, and food challenges. *BMJ* 1996; **313**: 518–21.
24. Clark AT, Ewan PW. The development and progression of allergy to multiple nuts at different ages. *Pediatr Allergy Immunol* 2005; **16**: 507–11.
25. Beyer K, Morrow E, Li XM *et al.* Effects of cooking methods on peanut allergenicity. *J Allergy Clin Immunol* 2001; **107**: 1077–81.
26. Hourihane JO, Bedwani SJ, Dean TP, Warner JO. Randomised, double blind, crossover challenge study of allergenicity of peanut oils in subjects allergic to peanuts. *BMJ* 1997; **314**: 1084–8.
27. Sporik R, Hill DJ, Hosking CS. Specificity of allergen skin testing in predicting positive open food challenges to milk, egg and peanut in children. *Clin Exp Allergy* 2000; **30**: 1540–6.
28. Eigenmann PA, Sampson HA. Interpreting skin prick tests in the evaluation of food allergy in children. *Pediatr Allergy Immunol* 1998; **9**: 186–91.
29. Sampson HA, Ho DG. Relationship between food-specific IgE concentrations and the risk of positive food challenges in children and adolescents. *J Allergy Clin Immunol* 1997; **100**: 444–51.
30. Ferdman RM, Church JA. Mixed-up nuts: identification of peanuts and tree nuts by children. *Ann Allergy Asthma Immunol* 2006; **97**: 73–7.
31. Yu JW, Kagan R, Verreault N *et al.* Accidental ingestions in children with peanut allergy. *J Allergy Clin Immunol* 2006; **118**: 466–72.
32. Maloney JM, Chapman MD, Sicherer SH. Peanut allergen exposure through saliva: assessment and interventions to reduce exposure. *J Allergy Clin Immunol* 2006; **118**: 719–24.
33. Perry TT, Conover-Walker MK, Pomés A, Chapman MD, Wood RA. Distribution of peanut allergen in the environment. *J Allergy Clin Immunol* 2004; **113**: 973–6.
34. Bernhisel-Broadbent J, Sampson HA. Cross allergenicity in the legume botanical family in children with food hypersensitivity. *J Allergy Clin Immunol* 1989; **83**: 435–40.
35. Patil SP, Niphadkar PV, Bapat MM. Chickpea: a major food allergen in the Indian subcontinent and its clinical and immunochemical correlation. *Ann Allergy Asthma Immunol* 2001; **87**: 140–5.
36. Patil SP, Niphadkar PV, Bapat MM. Allergy to fenugreek (*Trigonella foenum graecum*). *Ann Allergy Asthma Immunol* 1997; **78**: 297–300.
37. Ibáñez MD, Martínez M, Sánchez JJ, Fernández-Caldas E. Legume cross-reactivity: *Allergol Immunopathol (Madr)* 2003; **31**: 151–61.
38. Crespo JF, Pascual C, Burks AW, Helm, RM, Esteban MM. Frequency of food allergy in a pediatric population from Spain. *Pediatr Allergy Immunol* 1995; **6**; 39–43.
39. Hefle SL, Lemanske RF, Bush RK. Adverse reaction to lupine-fortified pasta. *J Allergy Clin Immunol* 1994; **94**: 167–72.
40. Romano C, Ferrara A, Tarallos S. Allergic reaction to lupine seed (*Lupinus albus*). *Allergy* 1997; **52**: 113–14.
41. Sicherer SH, Eigenmann PA, Sampson HA. Clinical features of food protein-induced enterocolitis syndrome. *J Pediatr* 133: 214–19.
42. Moneret-Vautrin DA, Guérin L, Kanny G *et al.* Cross-allergenicity of peanut and lupine: The risk of lupine allergy in patients allergic to peanuts. *J Allergy Clin Immunol* 1999; **104**: 883–8.
43. Taylor SL, Nordlee JA, Sicherer SH *et al.* Soybean oil is not allergenic to soybean-allergic individuals. *J Allergy Clin Immunol* 2004; **113**: S99.
44. Hefle SL, Lambrecht DM, Nordlee JA. Soy sauce retains allergenicity through the fermentation production process. *J Allergy Clin Immunol* 2005; **115**: S32.

45. Alonso L, Marcos ML, Blanco JG. Anaphylaxis caused by linseed (flaxseed) intake. *J Allergy Clin Immunol* 1996; **98**: 469–70.
46. Lezaun A, Fraj J, Colas C *et al.* Anaphylaxis from linseed. *Allergy* 1998; **53**: 105–6.
47. Atkins FM, Wilson M, Bock SA. Cottonseed hypersensitivity: new concerns over an old problem. *J Allergy Clin Immunol* 1998; **82**: 242–50.
48. Noyes JH, Boyd GK, Settipane GA. Anaphylaxis to sunflower seed. *J Allergy Clin Immunol* 1979; **63**: 242–4.
49. Axelsson IG, Ihre E, Zetterstrom O. Anaphylactic reactions to sunflower seed. *Allergy* 1994; **49**: 517–20.
50. Nish WA, Whisman BA, Goetz DW, Ramirez DA. Anaphylaxis to annatto dye: a case report. *Ann Allergy* 1991; **66**: 129–31.
51. Malish D, Glovsky MM, Hoffman DR, Ghekiere L, Hawkins JM. Anaphylaxis after sesame seed ingestion. *J Allergy Clin Immunol* 1981; **67**; 35–8.
52. Levy Y, Danon YL. Allergy to sesame seed in infants. *Allergy* 2001; **56**: 193–4.
53. Chiu JT, Haydik IB. Sesame seed oil anaphylaxis. *J Allergy Clin Immunol* 1991; **88**: 414–15.
54. Hill DJ, Hosking CS, Chen YZ *et al.* The frequency of food allergy in Australia and Asia. *Environ Toxicol Pharmacol* 1997; **4**: 101–10.
55. Morisset M, Moneret-Vautrin DA, Maadi F *et al.* Prospective study of mustard allergy: first study with double-blind placebo-controlled food challenge trials (24 cases). *Allergy* 2003; **58**: 295–9.
56. Fremont S, Zitouni N, Kanny G *et al.* Allergenicity of some isoforms of white sesame proteins. *Clin Exp Allergy* 2002; **32**; 1211–15.
57. Kanny G, de Hauteclocque C, Moneret-Vautrin DA. Sesame seed and sesame seed oil contain masked allergens of growing importance. *Allergy* 1996; **51**: 952–7.
58. Dreborg S, Frew A. Allergen standardisation and skin tests. *Allergy* 1993; **47** (Suppl 14): 48–82.
59. Bock SA, Buckley J, Holst A, May CD. Proper use of skin tests with food extracts in diagnosis of hypersensitivity to food in children. *Clin Allergy* 1997; **7**: 375–83.
60. Bock SA, Sampson HA, Atkins FM *et al.* Double-blind, placebo-controlled food challenge (DBPCFC) as an office procedure: a manual. *J Allergy Clin Immunol* 1988; **82**: 986–97.
61. Clark AT, Anagnostou K, Ewan PW. Cashew nut causes more severe reactions than peanut: case matched comparison in 141 children. *Allergy* 2007; **62**; 913–16.
62. Clark AT, Ewan PW. Interpretation of tests for nut allergy in one thousand patients, in relation to allergy or tolerance. *Clin Exp Allergy* 2003; **33**: 1041–5.
63. Ortolani C, Ballmer-Weber BK, Skamstrup Hansen K *et al.* Hazelnut allergy: a double-placebo-controlled food multicenter study. *J Allergy Clin Immunol* 2000; **105**: 577–81.
64. Fleishcher D, Conover-Walker M, Matsui E, Wood R. The natural history of tree nut allergy. *J Allergy Clin Immunol* 2005; **116**: 1087–93.
65. Robotham JM, Wang F, Seamon V *et al.* Ana o 3, an important cashew nut (*Anacardium occidentale* L.) allergen of the 2S albumin family. *J Allergy Clin Immunol* 2005; **115**: 1284–90.
66. Wallowitz ML, Teuber S, Beyer K *et al.* Cross-reactivity of walnut, cashew, and hazelnut legumin proteins in tree nut allergic patients. *J Allergy Clin Immunol* 2004; **113**: S156.
67. Sicherer SH, Furlong TJ, Muñoz-Furlong A, Burks AW, Sampson HA. Prevalence of peanut and tree nut allergy in the United States of America determined by a random digit dial telephone survey. *J Allergy Clin Immunol* 2001; **103**: 559–62.
68. Sicherer SH, Burks AW, Sampson HA. Clinical features of acute allergic reactions to peanut and tree nuts in children. *Pediatrics* 1998; **102**: e6.
69. Rancé F, Bidat E, Bourrier T, Sabouraud D. Cashew allergy: observations of 42 children without associated peanut allergy. *Allergy* 2003; **58**: 1311–14.
70. Shridhar K, Sathe SK, Teuber SS, Roux KH. Effects of food processing on the stability of food allergens. *Biotechnol Adv* 2003; **23**; 423–9.
71. Malanin K, Lundberg M, Johansson SGO. Anaphylactic reaction caused by neoallergens in heated pecan nut. *Allergy* 1995; **50**: 988–91.
72. Venkatachalam M, Teuber SS, Roux KH, Sathe SK. Effects of roasting, blanching, autoclaving, and microwave heating on antigenicity of almond (*Prunus dulcis* L.) proteins. *J Agric Food Chem* 2002; **50**: 3544–8.
73. Hansen KS, Ballmer-Weber BK, Lüttkopf D *et al.* Roasted hazelnuts: allergenic activity evaluated by double blind, placebo-controlled food challenge. *Allergy* 2003; **58**: 132–8.

9 Food Hypersensitivity Involving Cereals

9.1 Coeliac disease

Norma McGough, Emma Merrikin and Emily Kirk

9.1.1 Introduction

Coeliac disease (CD) is a permanent autoimmune inflammatory condition of the small intestinal mucosa[1], for which there is a clearly-defined pathology and diagnostic process. The pathological changes observed in CD result from the interaction between 'gluten' and immune, genetic and environmental factors[2]. A number of toxic protein fractions, found in the endosperm of certain cereals, have been identified in CD. *Gluten* is established as a general term used to cover the alcohol-soluble prolamins: gliadins in wheat, hordeins in barley, secalins in rye[2]. Research suggests that the alcohol-insoluble prolamins called glutenins may also have a role to play, although further research is needed to understand this better[3]. People with CD are diagnosed at different stages of the disease process. In addition, CD is a spectrum, in the wide variation and degree of severity of symptoms, antibody serology and degree of damage to the small intestine.

9.1.2 Prevalence and onset

Screening studies indicate that CD affects 1% of the population[4,5], making CD one of the most common small bowel disorders to affect Western populations[6] and the most common cause of malabsorption in the UK[7]. Despite this, under-diagnosis, late diagnosis and misdiagnosis of CD are all significant problems; evidence suggests that only 1 in 8 cases is currently diagnosed[8]. A research project commissioned by Coeliac UK and undertaken by the Health Economics Unit, University of Oxford, found that the average time for an individual to be diagnosed with CD after initial reporting of symptoms is 13 years (A. Gray, unpublished data).

CD affects different ethnic groups, and is common not just in Europe but also in southern Asia, the Middle East, north, west and east Africa and South America[9]. Whilst the most common age for diagnosis of CD is between 40 and 50 years[10], it can present at any age after introduction of gluten-containing cereals or later on in life. There is evidence to suggest that more women are diagnosed than men[11].

Environmental triggers

Environmental factors such as pregnancy, childbirth, gastroenteritis or surgery may 'trigger' CD in some patients.

Genetic susceptibility

CD is genetically determined, with an increased prevalence of 10% amongst first-degree relatives and 2% amongst second-degree relatives of those with the disease[12]. Although there are no firm guidelines on the issue, if relatives of those with CD also have or develop symptoms of CD, they should be considered for screening.

In those diagnosed with CD, 95% are human leucocyte antigen (HLA) DQ2- or DQ8-positive. Studies looking at twins have found concordance levels of 75–90%[13]. A significant proportion (39.5%) of the general population are HLA DQ2/DQ8-positive and do not go on to develop CD[14,15], so other unspecified genetic factors are also involved.

HLA-DQ typing is not a substitute for an intestinal biopsy or serological test. However, HLA typing may play a complementary role in excluding CD in challenging circumstances such as discrepancies in serological and histopathological results, or continuing symptoms despite a gluten-free (GF) diet[16].

9.1.3   Clinical presentation

CD is a multi-system disorder that can present with non-specific symptoms that may be overlooked[17–19] (Table 9.1). Symptoms range from mild to severe and vary between individuals. A common misdiagnosis of CD is irritable bowel syndrome (IBS)[20]. NICE guidelines for the diagnosis of IBS recommend that CD should be excluded before a diagnosis of IBS is made[21].

Table 9.1   Symptoms of coeliac disease, adapted from CREST guidelines[19].

Gastrointestinal due to	Diarrhoea, steatorrhoea, abdominal cramps, bloating, excessive flatus, weight loss
Gastrointestinal due to dysmotility	Constipation, epigastric pain, heartburn
Haematological	Any combination of iron, B_{12}, folic-acid deficiency
Liver	Abnormal liver biochemistry
Skin and mucous membrane	Dermatitis herpetiformis (DH), hair loss, aphthous mouth ulcers
Rheumatological	Arthralgia (joint pain)
Bone	Osteoporosis, defective tooth enamel
Gynaecological	Late menarche, early menopause, infertility, recurrent miscarriage
Neurological	Ataxia, partial seizures, peripheral neuropathy
Other	Short stature, chronic fatigue, depression

Although often cited as common symptoms, evidence shows that less than half of newly diagnosed patients have symptoms of diarrhoea, and even fewer show signs of weight loss[22]. The stereotypical presentation of the underweight patient therefore no longer applies; research has found a significant proportion of patients are of normal weight or overweight at diagnosis[23].

Infants can present after weaning onto gluten with symptoms such as failure to thrive, diarrhoea, vomiting, abdominal distention, constipation, muscle wasting and irritability. Symptoms in older children vary as in adults, and can include poor growth, anaemia and recurrent mouth ulcers. The practice for introducing gluten to a baby is important, since exposure to gluten is believed to be a trigger for CD.

9.1.4   Diagnosis

Active case-finding strategies in primary care have been shown to improve diagnosis rates of CD[24].

Serological antibody tests

Increasing recognition of CD is attributed to the use of serological antibody tests: immunoglobulin A (IgA) class of anti-tissue transglutaminase (tTG) and/or endomysial antibody (EMA)[25]. The approximate sensitivity and specificity of both antibodies is regarded as over 90%[26], although there are studies which indicate that the sensitivity of the tests declines with lesser degrees of gut damage[27,28].

Immunoglobin A (IgA) deficiency occurs in 2% of people with CD compared to 0.2% of the general population[26]. Since the usual antibody tests (tTG/EMA) are IgA-dependent, IgA deficiency could cause a false negative result, even if a gluten-containing diet is maintained. On an initial screening blood test, total IgA count should be measured. If this is low or negative, IgG class of tTG/EMA can be used as an alternative, although these are less specific and sensitive than the IgA class of antibody[29].

The prevalence of seronegative CD is 6.4–9.1% of all diagnosed cases[30]. Therefore patients with suspicious symptoms, positive family history and/or presence of other autoimmune disease should be referred for bowel biopsy investigations, regardless of the serological test results[31]. This strategy can help to ensure that the number of cases of CD missed is minimised[32].

Intestinal biopsy

A small intestinal biopsy is mandatory in all cases to confirm a diagnosis of CD in adults[19,33] and children[34].

In CD, immune responses to toxic proteins promote an inflammatory reaction, characterised by infiltration of the lamina propria and the epithelium with chronic inflammatory cells and villous atrophy. This response is mediated by both the innate and adaptive immune systems[35] (see Chapter 13). The typical mucosal changes start to occur within 4–6 hours of exposure to the toxic peptide[36]. This mucosal damage may lead to clinical malabsorption of nutrients. Individual clinical and mucosal responses can occur; varying degrees of gut damage are classified by Marsh (Table 9.2)[37,38].

Table 9.2 Classification of gut damage in coeliac disease.

Grade	Gut damage
0	Normal
I	Increased intraepithelial lymphocytes (> 30 per 100 enterocytes)
II	Intraepithelial lymphocytes plus increase in crypt depth (crypt hypertrophy)
III	Above plus villous atrophy: the 'classic' coeliac lesion
IV	Atrophic lesion without lymphocytes: rare, typically unresponsive to GFD; can be associated with enteropathy-associated T-cell lymphoma

Although responses may be variable and dependent on a range of factors not yet clearly identified, if gluten is reintroduced at a later stage, mucosal damage will reoccur.

Diagnosis in children

The diagnostic pathway of a serological test, followed by a small bowel biopsy, applies to both adults and children. If the initial diagnosis is uncertain in children under the age of 2, a gluten challenge (where gluten is reintroduced into the diet: see below for further details) to confirm diagnosis is recommended at age 6–7 or after pubertal growth[34].

Preparation for diagnostic tests

For CD to develop, and for serology and biopsy results to be meaningful, it is essential that the patient is eating gluten. Patients should not be advised to start a GF diet until diagnosis of CD is established[39]. Therapeutic trials of a GF diet are not warranted if CD is suspected; clinical response to either withdrawal or reintroduction of gluten alone has no role in the diagnosis of CD[40]. If gluten has been removed from the diet it should be reintroduced for approximately 6 weeks at a level of around four slices of bread per day[41]. If the GF diet has been imposed for a significant period, this should be seen as an absolute minimum; guidelines from Northern Ireland recommend 3 months on a gluten-containing diet[19]. Children may refuse obvious gluten-containing foods if they associate them with being unwell. In this instance, foods that may be better tolerated such as biscuits or rusks should be encouraged. Different approaches can be used to ensure an adequate gluten intake during the diagnostic process without disruption to the diet.

9.1.5 Associated conditions

Dermatitis herpetiformis (DH)

DH is the skin manifestation of CD, affecting 1 in 10,000 people[42]. The symptoms are red, raised patches, often with blisters that burst on scratching, accompanied by severe stinging and itching. Any area of skin can be affected, although areas typically affected include elbows, knees and buttocks. The presentation of DH is characteristically symmetrical in pattern, e.g. both elbows. DH is diagnosed by a skin biopsy, which involves removing a small sample of skin (from an unaffected area) and testing for the presence of IgA antibodies.

Although people with DH may not experience typical gut symptoms, most people with DH have some degree of mucosal damage that is consistent with CD[43], so patients should be referred for small-bowel biopsy investigations. Once the GF diet has commenced, further investigations regarding diagnosis of CD may be inconclusive. It is therefore necessary to delay diet therapy until all diagnostic tests for CD have been completed.

Although the treatment for DH is a GF diet, medications such as dapsone (a sulphonamide antibacterial drug) may also be necessary in the short term to help alleviate symptoms. The GF diet can take as many as 4 years to be effective in some cases[44]. The lowest effective dose of medication should be used, as side effects are relatively common and can include haemolytic anaemia, nerve damage, depression and headaches. The drug treatment will suppress the skin symptoms, but it will not treat the mucosal damage in the small intestine. The GF diet is therefore an essential part of treatment for DH.

As DH is a skin manifestation of CD, those with the condition are just as susceptible to the long-term complications associated with untreated CD, including lymphoma[45].

Other autoimmune diseases

There is increased prevalence of CD among patients with other autoimmune disorders (Table 9.3). CD is also more common among people with Down's syndrome than in the general population[51].

Type 1 diabetes

A diagnosis of CD can precede that of type 1 diabetes, but in most cases (about 90%) diabetes is diagnosed first[52]. Unstable diabetes, growth failure and symptoms associated with malabsorption in those with type 1 diabetes may indicate the presence of CD[53]. Screening studies of those with type 1 diabetes have found that significant numbers of those subsequently diagnosed with CD are clinically

Table 9.3 Prevalence of coeliac disease (CD) in those with other autoimmune disorders.

Disorder	Prevalence of CD
Type 1 diabetes mellitus	3–6%[46]
Autoimmune thyroid disease	4%[47]
Primary biliary cirrhosis	3%[48]
Sjögren's syndrome	3.3%[49]
Addison's disease	5.9%[50]

asymptomatic[54], or have atypical features only recognised in retrospect[55]. This may have been an issue regarding compliance to the GF diet.

Blood glucose levels must be monitored closely following diagnosis of CD, as insulin levels often need to be altered due to improved absorption of carbohydrate and other nutrients which affect glycaemic control. In children with type 1 diabetes who are diagnosed with CD and follow a GF diet, improvements in growth (weight, body mass index)[56] and blood glucose control (HbAlc)[57] have been demonstrated. There is a lack of similar evidence in adults with CD[58].

Research has shown that the glycaemic index (GI) of GF substitute foods such as breads and pasta is comparable to that of their gluten-containing equivalents[59], so a GF diet should not necessarily be compromised in terms of GI.

Other pathology

Once gluten-related causes of ongoing symptoms have been excluded, additional pathology can be considered. Pancreatic insufficiency[60], small intestinal bacterial overgrowth[61], microscopic (lymphocytic or collagenous) colitis[62], lactose intolerance and refractory coeliac disease[63] have all been reported as possible causes of ongoing symptoms in patients with CD. There are also reports of fructose intolerance.

Refractory coeliac disease

Refractory coeliac disease (RCD) is defined as continuing villous atrophy with crypt hyperplasia and intra-epithelial lymphocytes, despite adherence to a strict GF diet for at least a year[64,65]. Refractory coeliac disease is a diagnosis of exclusion, so other possible causes which may lead to persistence of clinical and histological features should be excluded by necessary investigations[66].

Two categories of RCD are recognised, grouped immunologically according to the presence of abnormal T cells in the intestinal mucosa on biopsy:

- type 1 RCD: without aberrant (abnormal) T lymphocytes;
- type 2 RCD: with aberrant T lymphocytes.

Type 1 RCD is usually treatable with immunosuppressive treatment, whereas type 2 RCD is usually resistant to medical therapies and is closely associated with development of enteropathy-associated T-cell lymphoma (EATL).

Lactose intolerance

Lactose intolerance (LI) is a secondary intolerance which can be associated with undiagnosed CD. Symptoms of lactose intolerance include bloating, wind and diarrhoea, which can easily be confused with symptoms of CD (see Chapter 5).

In undiagnosed CD, the typical mucosal damage can result in a reduction in the enzyme activity which in turn results in a failure to digest lactose. Once established on a GF diet the mucosal damage is able to heal and lactose digestion returns to normal[67,68]. Hence LI is usually temporary, and adherence to the GF diet means most people with CD do not have additional problems with LI.

Osteoporosis

Untreated CD is related to a significant risk of decreased bone mineral density (osteopenia)[69] and osteoporosis[70]. Research shows that even years after diagnosis there is an increased risk of hip fracture in those with CD[71]. A systematic review using data from a total of 20,955 patient years confirms a significant association between bone fractures and CD[72]. The association of CD and osteoporosis is thought to be largely related to a chronic malabsorption of calcium as a result of mucosal damage prior to diagnosis[73], as well as a reduced dietary intake of calcium[74]. In addition, bone loss is regulated by various mediators of the immune system, so the chronic inflammatory process in CD may also play a role[75].

Adherence to the GF diet in people with CD optimises absorption of nutrients; it has been shown to minimise bone loss and can help to normalise or improve bone mass[76]. A more recent review of osteoporosis in CD provides an insight into the possible mechanisms and complexity of osteoporosis in CD[77]. Other risk factors for developing osteoporosis include excessive alcohol consumption, smoking and being underweight.

Current guidelines recommend that adult patients newly diagnosed with CD should have a DEXA (dual x-ray absorptiometry) scan to assess bone mineral density, and that this should be repeated at the menopause, over the age of 55 years for men, or at any age should a fragility fracture occur. How often DEXA scanning should be repeated is a matter of debate, and depends on the individual case.

Because of the increased risk of osteoporosis and osteopenia in those with CD, adults are advised to aim for an increased calcium intake (1,000 mg for those over 18 years and 1,200 mg for postmenopausal women and men over the age of 55 years)[78]. This compares to a calcium recommendation for the general population without CD of 700 mg per day. Dietary supplements should be recommended on an individual basis and their use monitored against clinical and biochemical markers.

There is no increased requirement for calcium in children with CD. This is because there is the potential for absorption of calcium and other nutrients to normalise in time. Children and young adults who adhere to their GF diet should therefore be able to attain peak bone mass in their lifetime, so minimising the risk of developing osteopenia and osteoporosis in the future[79].

Malignancy

CD is associated with an increased risk of a number of malignancies such as non-Hodgkin's lymphoma, oropharyngeal cancer and oesophageal cancer, although the risk of developing all types of malignancy for people with CD is reduced to that of the general population after 5 years on a GF diet[80].

CD is associated with an increased risk of enteropathy-associated T-cell lymphoma (EATL)[81]. However, prevalence is low and more recent research suggests the increased risk is lower than previously thought[82]. The development of EATL is closely associated with refractory CD. The prognosis for EATL is poor: one study shows a 5-year survival rate of only 8% in those with CD who developed EATL[65].

A decreased risk of breast and lung cancer has been described in patients with CD, although the aetiology behind this has not yet been explained[83].

9.1.6   Dietary management

A lifelong GF diet is currently the only treatment available for patients with CD.

Adherence to the GF diet is known to be variable, both in children[84] and in adults[85]. Following a GF diet may sound very straightforward, but there are many factors that are important to take into consideration when managing patients with CD.

The GF diet

The GF diet is restrictive as it requires complete avoidance of the cereals wheat, barley, rye and their associated staple products and ingredients from the diet.

The most obvious sources of gluten in the diet are breads, flour, pasta, pizza bases, biscuits, cakes and pastries. However, gluten-containing cereals may also be used as ingredients in soups, sauces, ready meals and other processed foods such as sausages.

GF foods can be considered as three distinct categories: those which are naturally GF, processed foods that happen to be GF, and GF 'substitute' foods (products manufactured to replace staples like bread, pasta and other foods made from flour).

Naturally GF foods

There are many foods which are naturally GF and suitable for people with CD, such as fresh meat, fish, eggs, poultry, cheese, milk, pulses (peas, beans and lentils), rice, corn (maize), potatoes, fruit and vegetables. A more extensive list is included in Table 9.4.

Processed GF foods

Processed foods which are GF are listed in Coeliac UK's Food and Drink Directory.

Manufactured GF 'substitute' foods

Specially manufactured GF 'substitute' foods, including bread, pasta, pizza bases and flours, are available in health-food shops, supermarkets, via the internet or mail order, and on prescription. Some substitute GF products may be made of naturally GF ingredients.

Toxicity of oats

Historically oats have been considered unsafe for people with CD, and it is only re-cently that it has become accepted practice for patients to include pure uncontaminated

Table 9.4 Gluten-free and gluten-containing foods.

Gluten-free	Check products	Gluten-containing
Cereals and flour Corn, corn flour, rice, rice flour, arrowroot, amaranth, buckwheat, millet, teff, quinoa, sorghum, soya flour, potato starch, modified starch, potato flour, gram flour	Flavoured savoury rice products, cereal bars	Wheat, bulgar wheat, durum wheat, wheat bran, wheatgerm, wheat starch, semolina, couscous, barley, malt, malted barley, rye, triticale, kamut, spelt
Meat, poultry, fish, cheese, eggs All fresh meats, poultry, fish, shellfish, smoked meats and fish, cured pure meats, smoked, fish in oil/brine, cheese, eggs	Meat and fish pastes, pates, sausages, burgers, fish in sauce	Meat, poultry, fish cooked in batter or bread-crumbs, faggots, rissoles, haggis, breaded ham
Milk and milk products Fresh, UHT, dried, condensed, evaporated, goat's, sheep's milk, fresh and soured cream, buttermilk, crème frâiche	Coffee and tea whiteners, oat milk, flavoured yoghurt and fromage frais	Milk with added fibre, artificial cream, yogurt and fromage frais containing muesli or cereals
Fats and oils Butter, margarine, lard, cooking oils, ghee, low fat spread	Suet	
Fruits and vegetables All fresh, frozen, canned and dried pure fruits and vegetables	Oven, microwave and frozen chips, instant mash, fruit pie fillings, waffles	Vegetables and potatoes in batter, breadcrumbs or flour, potato croquettes
Savoury snacks Plain potato crisps, homemade popcorn	Flavoured crisps	Snacks made from wheat, rye, barley and oats, pretzels
Soups, sauces and pickles Tomato and garlic puree, individual herbs and spices, vinegars, mixed herbs and spices, ground pepper	Gravy, stock cubes, soups, sauces, mixes, tamari, mustard, mayonnaise, salad cream, dressings, pickles, chutney, blended seasoning, curry powder	Shoyu (Chinese soy sauce), stuffing mix
Preserves and spreads jam, conserves, honey, golden syrup, treacle, marmalade, peanut and other nut butters	Mincemeat, lemon curd	
Drinks Tea, coffee, fruit juice, squash, clear fizzy drinks, cocoa, wine, spirits, cider, sherry, port	Drinking chocolate, cloudy drinks	Malted milk drinks, barley waters/squash, beer, lager, ales, stouts
Miscellaneous Gelatine, bicarbonate of soda, cream of tartar, yeast, artificial sweeteners	Tofu, cake decorations, marzipan, baking powder, ready to use icings	Ice cream cones and wafers

oats as part of a balanced GF diet. Studies have shown that most children[86,87] and adults[88] with CD can tolerate the avenins found in oats. However, most available oat and oat products are contaminated with wheat, rye, barley or a mixture of these cereals during processes such as milling, which makes them unsuitable for people with CD[89].

Systematic reviews assessing the evidence on the issue have concluded that while most patients with CD can tolerate the avenins found in oats, some may still be sensitive to them[90], and that people with CD should be followed up by their health-care team to assess tolerance to avenins[91]. In practice, advice on inclusion of oats in a GF diet varies. Pure uncontaminated oats may be introduced gradually into the diet with monitoring from the healthcare team, by clinical assessment, serology and possibly follow-up small-bowel biopsy[92].

Including pure, uncontaminated oats in the GF diet has been shown to add welcome variety, satiety and improved bowel function in those with CD[93]. Oats are also a useful source of soluble fibre, which can help in controlling blood glucose in those with diabetes and help in managing hypercholesterolaemia[94], and so should not be discouraged unless there is good clinical reason. It is essential that patients ensure they choose oat products that are pure and uncontaminated.

The Codex standard for those intolerant to gluten

The Codex standard for gluten is an international standard used to guide producers on the accepted levels of gluten in food products. The Codex standard for those intolerant to gluten was established in 1981 at the level of up to 200 mg gluten/kg or 200 parts per million (ppm)[95].

In November 2007, there was agreement to lower this standard[96]. The changes introduce a dual Codex standard with two categories:

- foods containing less that 20 ppm gluten;
- foods containing between 20 and 100 ppm gluten.

The European Commission is developing legislation under the Foods for Particular Nutritional Uses ('PARNUTS') Directive 89/398/EEC[97], based on this new Codex standard. When the EC regulation comes into force, only foods that contain less than 20 ppm of gluten will be labelled as 'gluten-free'. This labelling term will also apply for pure, uncontaminated oat products with a gluten level of less than 20 ppm. Specialist substitute GF products (such as breads and flour mixes) that con-tain Codex wheat starch with a gluten level of 20–100 ppm will be labelled as 'very low gluten'.

The precise timetabling of the introduction of the legislation based on the new Codex standard has not yet been finalised, although it is expected to be adopted at the end of 2008. There will be a 3-year period from the time the regulation is introduced to enable the manufacturers to make all necessary changes to product ranges and labels.

Codex wheat starch

Codex wheat starch is a highly processed ('washed') wheat starch which has a level of gluten within the Codex standard. Codex wheat starch is used by some manufacturers who produce GF food for prescription sales to try and improve the taste and texture of the food. It must appear in an ingredients list if it has been used. The term 'gluten-free' implies no gluten, but in practice a gluten level of zero is impossible to achieve, since even naturally GF cereals such as rice, which are not toxic to people with CD, can contain up to 20 ppm of gluten[98].

Evidence suggests that although some patients with CD do show mucosal recovery consuming products up to 200 ppm[99], other studies have observed varying clinical responses in patients with CD to smaller gluten levels[100].

In addition to this, patients with CD consume variable amounts of GF substitute products[101], so another factor to consider is the likely additive effect on the total amount of daily gluten consumed, as well as an individual's tolerance level.

A systematic review of the evidence base surrounding gluten thresholds concludes that what is most important is the total amount of gluten ingested rather than just the concentration of gluten in food products alone[102]. The amount of gluten eaten depends both on the concentration and on the volume of food products consumed. Some more sensitive people with CD can experience symptoms on consuming Codex wheat starch products. If this is the case, they may need to choose products currently labelled as 'wheat-free, gluten-free'.

Barley malt, malt extract and malt vinegar

Foods with barley malt or barley flour content (e.g. malted drinks or barley squashes) should be avoided by patients with CD. Malt extract and malt-extract flavourings are most commonly prepared from barley, although they can be produced from other grains. Barley malt extract is widely used in small amounts in the food industry as part of the flavouring, for example in some rice- and corn-based breakfast cereals. Products containing barley malt extract in low levels that meet the Codex standard for gluten can be tolerated by most people with CD. Products that contain barley malt extract have to be labelled as such in line with Allergen labelling (2003/89 EC are highlighted where the information is available from the manufacturer).

Barley malt vinegar is found in pickles, chutneys and condiments such as sauces. In line with food allergen labelling legislation, manufacturers must list the word 'barley' on the ingredients list. Its manufacturing process means there is only a trace amount of gluten in the end product, which is well below the Codex standard for gluten. It is therefore suitable for most people with CD to include in their GF diet.

Prescriptions of GF food

In the UK, people with medically diagnosed CD are eligible for GF products on prescription. The products available are generally staples in the diet such as bread and pasta rather than foods which can be considered luxury items, such as confectionery.

The GF foods that are prescribable are agreed by the Advisory Committee on Borderline Substances (ACBS). At present, in England, Scotland and Northern Ireland, people with CD must pay for their prescriptions, unless they are exempt from charges for other reasons (such as age, income and other conditions). Prescriptions in Wales are currently free of charge. To assist healthcare professionals to prescribe reasonable amounts of GF products, guidelines that suggest a minimum monthly requirement of GF foods are available[103].

Allergen labelling

EU-wide allergen labelling directive 2003/89/EC became mandatory on 25 November 2005 and applies to all pre-packaged foods. It is a legal requirement for manufacturers to declare any food allergen included in a food as a deliberate ingredient (see Chapter 4). Gluten-containing cereals are one of the 14 allergens included in this legislation, and must therefore be listed in the ingredients, regardless of how much has been used[104]. The manufacturer must name the specific grain used, e.g. wheat, rye, barley, oats, triticale, kamut, spelt.

The use of an allergen advice box, e.g. 'contains (wheat) gluten', is recommended, although this is not compulsory. Therefore patients should check the ingredients list of a product, and not just the allergy advice box (if used). The European Commission has worked with the European Food Safety Authority (EFSA) to develop a list of ingredients that are exempt from this allergen labelling legislation.

The following ingredients are safe for people with CD, as the level of processing has removed any allergenic protein:

- glucose syrups derived from wheat or barley, including dextrose;
- wheat-based maltodextrins;
- distilled ingredients made from gluten-containing cereals, for example alcoholic spirits.

Allergen labelling and oats
Currently oats are listed as a gluten-containing cereal in allergen labelling directive 2003/89/EC. For this reason, consumers may see an allergen advice box 'contains (oat) gluten' on oats and oat products, even though they may be suitable for them, i.e. they are pure, uncontaminated oats. The proposed EC regulation based on the new Codex standard for gluten, which will allow pure oats to be labelled as 'gluten-free', is expected to lead to a review of how oats fit into the allergen labelling directive.

Cross-contamination with gluten

Cross-contamination of GF foods can be a major problem for patients with CD. For example certain GF cereals, such as buckwheat, and related products such as flours, have a high risk of contamination during processing, e.g. milling.

The Food Standards Agency has produced guidance for food manufacturers on best practice on allergen management, including assessment of contamination risk and the use of appropriate advisory labelling. Manufacturers generally invest in having procedures in place that ensure quality control so that contamination is not an issue[105]. Quality control within the food industry should incorporate traceability of ingredients and the risk of contamination.

Manufacturers may put an advisory statement such as 'may contain gluten' on a food product if they have identified that there is a risk of cross-contamination with gluten.

Patients should be advised to take sensible steps to prevent cross-contamination with gluten when preparing food at home, for example:

- using a separate toaster, toaster bags or clean foil on the grill when toasting GF bread;
- using a separate breadboard for handling GF bread;
- keeping all utensils separate during preparation and cooking, and washing thoroughly between uses;
- using separate tubs of spreads (margarine, butter etc) and jam, marmalade and pickles;
- avoiding frying food in oil which has been previously used for foods which contain gluten.

Nutritional adequacy of the GF diet

The main priority after diagnosis of CD is to maintain the GF diet, to allow the mucosal damage to heal. However, following a balanced GF diet is an important long-term goal to promote good health and prevent health problems. A GF diet should meet individual nutritional requirements and dietary reference nutrient intakes (RNIs) as per the general population[106].

Ensuring nutritional adequacy of the diet is important, especially since anaemia is a frequent finding in those with CD, and can be the sole presenting symptom in many cases[107]. The anaemia may be secondary to iron deficiency but may also be multi-factorial in aetiology[108]. Folate deficiencies have also been identified in undiagnosed people with CD, as well as vitamin B_{12} deficiency[109].

There is evidence that despite good clinical response on a GF diet mucosal damage does not completely return to normal in some cases, even after many years[110]. The clinical significance of this is not known, but it may have implications for meeting nutritional requirements on the GF diet. One study concludes that those treated with a GF diet for 8–12 years show signs of poor vitamin status[111].

There are reports that GF cereals and substitute products made from them do not contain as much iron, fibre, folate, thiamine, riboflavin and niacin as their gluten-containing equivalents[112,113], which may put those with CD at risk of developing nutritional deficiencies. There is also evidence that patients with CD eat less than recommended amounts of calcium, iron and fibre[114,115] as well as folate and vitamin B_{12}[116].

Weight gain leading to obesity after diagnosis of CD is now recognised[23] and may in the long term contribute to morbidity associated with obesity. Obesity increases the risk of a number of medical conditions, including coronary heart disease and type 2 diabetes, so appropriate follow-up is important to identify issues which may impact on dietary intake.

General healthy eating guidelines can also be applied to those with CD, e.g. regular meals, consuming plenty of fruit and vegetables, limiting saturated fat, sugar and salt, drinking plenty of fluids and consuming alcohol in moderation[117,118].

9.1.7   Follow-up

After initial assessment, patients should be reviewed after 3 and 6 months[119]. If otherwise well, patients should be reviewed annually[33]. Annual IgA antibody tests can be a useful tool in the monitoring process[119], although antibody titres do not always correlate with improved histology[30,120].

In addition to the serological coeliac test, an annual review blood test may include markers of nutritional deficiency (particularly if present before diagnosis). Table 9.5 shows suggested aspects of monitoring patients with CD.

Current guidelines recommend repeating the small-bowel biopsy between four and six months[33], although in practice this may not be indicated in all patients[121].

Ongoing symptoms

Non-responsive CD, either where the patient fails to respond to the GF diet initially after diagnosis or where a patient who has previously responded to gluten exclusion becomes non-responsive to therapy, is estimated to affect 7–30% of patients with CD[122].

The most common cause of ongoing symptoms is continued gluten ingestion[63,123], whether deliberate or inadvertent, so reviewing specific aspects of the GF diet, such as intake of oats, Codex wheat starch, barley malt extract, and the patient's knowledge of allergen labelling, should always be reviewed. Every patient with CD has a different level of sensitivity, so this should be considered on an individual basis. It is entirely possible that a patient's sensitivity could change over time.

Sometimes making the necessary changes to a GF diet can dramatically change a patient's intake of dietary fibre, whether increasing it by eating more fruits, vegetables and pulses, or decreasing it by eating less bread and pasta. Any sudden change in fibre intake can contribute to gastrointestinal symptoms such as bloating and wind, but these should resolve promptly as the body adjusts to the change.

Table 9.5   Suggested monitoring for follow-up of coeliac disease.

Anthropometry	Height, weight and BMI (body mass index)
Symptoms	Comparison with symptoms prior to diagnosis
Haematological tests	Haemoglobin, folate, ferritin, albumin, alkaline phosphatase Calcium, vitamin D, vitamin B_{12} IgA endomysial antibodies (EMA) and/or tissue transglutaminase antibodies (tTGA)

9.1.8 Dietary considerations in particular groups

Pregnancy

There are no specific guidelines for pregnant women who have CD. Pregnancy is a particularly important time for patients with CD to be reviewed, in terms of compliance to the GF diet, and assessment for nutritional adequacy[119]. All women are recommended to take 400 µg of folic acid per day prior to conception and until the twelfth week of pregnancy to protect against neural tube defects[124].

Weaning

Care taken in weaning an infant is important, since exposure to gluten is a trigger for CD. Exclusive breast-feeding is favourable in all babies[125], and has been shown to confer some protection against development of CD, although it is not clear whether the effect is to delay the onset of symptoms, or permanent protection[126].

Breast milk and all infant formulas are gluten-free, so weaning is the first challenge. It is advised that weaning is delayed until the baby is 4–6 months old, and it is recommended that no food containing gluten should be given before 6 months of age. From 6 months, gluten-containing foods may be introduced gradual, ideally while the baby is still receiving breast milk[127]. It is sensible not to delay weaning onto gluten; there is no evidence to suggest that this is of any benefit.

First-stage weaning foods such as pureed vegetables and baby rice are naturally gluten-free, so in practice it is not normally until the baby is 7–9 months of age that gluten-containing cereals are a regular part of the diet. Where a family history of CD exists, the introduction of gluten should be carefully monitored for symptoms of CD. If an infant does develop symptoms of CD, gluten intake should be maintained and the child should be put forward for diagnostic investigations. A GF diet should not be initiated until diagnostic tests have been completed.

9.1.9 Resources

Coeliac UK is the national charity that supports people diagnosed with CD and the healthcare professionals involved in diagnosis and managing patients with CD. Professional membership of Coeliac UK is free of charge. The Coeliac UK website (www.coeliac.org.uk) has a dedicated area for healthcare professionals with fully referenced information. The telephone number is 0870 444 8804. A prescribing guide for gluten-free products is available at bspghan.org.uk/document/gluten-free_foods.pdf.

References

1. Ferenci DA. Celiac disease. In: Altschuler SM, Liacouras CA, eds. *Clinical Pediatric Gastroenterology*. Philadelphia, PA: Churchill Livingstone 1998: 143–58.
2. Green P, Cellier C. Celiac disease. *N Engl J Med* 2007; **357**: 1731–43.
3. Howdle PD. Gliadin, glutenin or both? The search for the Holy Grail in coeliac disease. *Eur J Gastroenterol Hepatol* 2006; **18**: 703–6.

4. West J, Logan RFA, Hill PG *et al.* Seroprevalence, correlates and characteristics of unde-tected coeliac disease in England. *Gut* 2003; **52**: 960–5.

5. Bingley PJ, Williams AJ, Norcross AJ *et al.* Avon longitudinal study of parents and children study team. *BMJ* 2004; **328**: 322–3.

6. Thomas PD, Forbes A, Green J *et al.* Guidelines for the investigation of chronic diarrhoea, 2nd edition. *Gut* 2003; **52** (Suppl V): v1–15.

7. Goddard AF, James MW, McIntyre AS, Scott BB. Guidelines for the management of iron deficiency anaemia. British Society of Gastroenterology, 2005. www.bsg.org.uk.

8. van Heel D, West J. Recent advances in coeliac disease. *Gut* 2006; **55**: 1037–46.

9. Cataldo F, Montalto G. Celiac disease in the developing countries: a new and challenging public health problem. *World J Gastroenterol* 2007; **13**: 2153–9.

10. Hin H, Bird G, Fisher P, Mahy N, Jewell D. Coeliac disease in primary care: case finding study. *BMJ* 1999; **318**: 164–7.

11. Bardella MT, Fredella C, Saladino V *et al.* Gluten intolerance: gender- and age-related differ-ences in symptoms. *Scand J Gastroenterol* 2005; **40**: 15–19.

12. Hogberg L, Fälth-Magnusson K, Grodzinsky E, Stenhammar L. Familial prevalence of coeliac disease: a twenty year follow-up study. *Scand J Gastroenterol* 2003; **38**: 61–5.

13. Greco L, Romino R, Coto I *et al.* The first large population based twin study of coeliac disease. *Gut* 2002; **50**: 624–8.

14. Book L, Zone JJ, Neuhausen SL. Prevalence of celiac disease among relatives of sib pairs with celiac disease in US families. *Am J Gastroenterol* 2003; **98**: 377–81.

15. Gudjónsdóttir AH, Nilsson S, Ek J, Kristiansson B, Ascher H. The risk of celiac disease in 107 families with at least two affected siblings. *J Pediatr Gastroenterol Nutr* 2004; **38**: 338–42.

16. Hadithi M, von Blomberg BM, Crusius JB *et al.* Accuracy of serological and HLA typing for diagnosing celiac disease. *Ann Intern Med* 2007; **147**: 294–302.

17. Hopper AD, Hadjivassiliou M, Butt S, Sanders S. Adult coeliac disease. *BMJ* 2007; **335**: 558–62.

18. Ravikumara M, Tuthill DP, Jenkins HR. The changing clinical presentation of coeliac dis-ease. *Arch Dis Child* 2006; **91**: 969–71.

19. Clinical Resource Efficiency Support Team (CREST) (Northern Ireland). Guidelines for the diagnosis and management of coeliac disease in adults. 2006. www.crestni.org.uk.

20. Shahbazkhani B, Forootan M, Merat S *et al.* Coeliac disease presenting with symptoms of irritable bowel syndrome. *Aliment Pharmacol Ther* 2003; **18**: 231–5.

21. National Institute for Health and Clinical Excellence. *Irritable Bowel Syndrome in Adults: Diagnosis and Management of Irritable Bowel Syndrome in Primary Care.* NICE Clinical Guideline 61. London: NICE, 2008.

22. Green PHR, Jabri B. Coeliac disease. *Lancet* 2003; **362**: 383–92.

23. Dickey W, Kearney N. Overweight in celiac disease: prevalence, clinical characteristics, and effect of a gluten-free diet. *Am J Gastroenterol* 2006; **101**: 2356–9.

24. Catassi C, Kryszak D, Louis-Jacques O *et al.* Detection of celiac disease in primary care: a multicenter case-finding study in America. *Am J Gastroenterol* 2007; **102**: 1–7.

25. Fasono A, Catassi C. Current approaches to diagnosis and treatment of celiac disease: an evolving spectrum. *Gastroenterology* 2001; **120**: 636–51.

26. Lewis N, Scott B. Systematic review: the use of serology to exclude or diagnose coeliac dis-ease (a comparison of the endomysial and tissue transglutaminase antibody tests). *Aliment Pharmacol Ther* 2006; **24**: 47–54.

27. Roston A, Dubé C, Cranney A *et al.* The diagnostic accuracy of serologic tests for celiac disease: a systematic review. *Gastroenterology* 2005; **128**: S38–46.

28. Abrams JA, Diamond B, Rotterdam H, Green PH. Seronegative celiac disease: increased prevalence with lesser degrees of villous atrophy. *Dig Dis Sci* 2004; **49**: 546–50.

29. Karponay-Szabo IR, Dahlbom I, Laurila K *et al.* Elevation of IgG antibodies against tissue transglutaminase as a diagnostic tool for coeliac disease in selective IgA deficiency. *Gut* 2003; **52**: 1567–71.

30. Collin P, Kaukinen K, Vogelsang H, *et al.* Antiendomysial and antihuman recombinant tissue transglutaminase antibodies in the diagnosis in the diagnosis of coeliac disease:

a biopsy-proven European multicentre study. *Eur J Gastroenterol Hepatol* 2005; **17**: 85–91.

31. Hopper A, Cross SS, Hurlstone DP *et al.* Pre-endoscopy serological testing for coeliac disease: evaluation of a clinical decision tool. *BMJ* 2007; **334**: 729.

32. Esteve M, Rosinach M, Fernández-Bañares F *et al.* Spectrum of gluten-sensitive enteropathy in first-degree relatives of patients with coeliac disease: clinical relevance of lymphocytic enteritis. *Gut* 2006; **55**: 1739–45.

33. British Society of Gastroenterology (BSG). Guidelines for the management of patients with coeliac disease. BSG, 2002. www.bsg.org.uk.

34. Coeliac Working Group of British Society of Paediatric Gastroenterology Hepatology and Nutrition (BSPGHAN). *Guideline for the Diagnosis and Management of Coeliac Disease in Children.* London: BSPGHAN, 2006.

35. Brandtzaeg P. The changing immunological paradigm in coeliac disease. *Immunol Lett* 2006; **105**: 127–39.

36. Fraser JS, Engel W, Ellis HJ *et al.* Coeliac disease: in vivo toxicity of the putative immuno-dominant epitope. *Gut* 2003; **52**: 1698–702.

37. Marsh MN. Gluten, major histocompatibility complex, and the small intestine. *Gastroenterology* 1992; **102**: 330–54.

38. Whitehead R. *Gastrointestinal and Oesophageal Pathology.* Hong Kong: Churchill Livingstone, 1995.

39. Midhagen G, Aberg AK, Olcén P *et al.* Antibody levels in adult patients with coeliac disease during gluten-free diet: a rapid initial decrease of clinical importance. *J Intern Med* 2004; **256**: 519–24.

40. Campanella J, Biagi F, Bianchi P *et al.* Clinical response to gluten withdrawal is not an indicator of coeliac disease. *Scand J Gastroenterol* 2008 Jun 13. [Epub ahead of print]

41. Wahab PJ, Crusius JB, Meijer JW, Mulder CJ. Gluten challenge in borderline gluten-sensitive enteropathy. *Am J Gastroenterol* 2001; **96**: 1464–9.

42. Smith JB, Tullock JE, Meyer LJ, Zone JJ. The incidence and prevalence of dermatitis herpetiformis in Utah. *Arch Dermatol* 1992; **128**: 1608–10.

43. Zone J. Skin manifestations of celiac disease. *Gastroenterology* 2005; **128** (4 Suppl 1): S87–91.

44. Garioch JJ, Lewis HM, Sargent SA, Leanord JN and Fry LL (1994) 25 years' experience of a gluten-free diet in the treatment of dermatitis herpetiformis. *Br J Dermatol* 1994; **131**: 541–5.

45. Hervonen K, Vornanen M, Kautiainen H, Collin P, Reunala T. Lymphoma in patients with dermatitis herpetiformis and their first-degree relatives. *Br J Dermatol* 2005; **152**: 82–6.

46. Holmes G. Coeliac disease and type 1 diabetes mellitus: the case for screening. *Diabet Med* 2001; **18**: 169–77.

47. Cuoco L, Certo M, Jorizzo RA *et al.* Prevalence and early diagnosis of celiac disease in autoimmune thyroid disorders. *Ital J Gastroenterol Hepatol* 1999; **31**: 283–7.

48. Kingham JGC, Parker DR. The association between biliary cirrhosis and coeliac disease: a study of relative prevalences. *Gut* 1998; **42**: 120–2.

49. Collin P, Reunala T, Pukkala E *et al.* Coeliac disease: associated disorders and survival. *Gut* 1994; **35**: 1215–18.

50. Biagi F, Campanella J, Soriani A, Vailati A, Corazza GR. Prevalence of celiac disease in Italian patients affected by Addison's Disease. *Scand J Gastroenterol* 2006; **41**: 302–5.

51. Uibo O, Teesalu K, Metskula K *et al.* Screening for celiac disease in Down's syndrome patients revealed cases of subtotal villous atrophy without typical for celiac disease HLA-DQ and tissue transglutaminase antibodies. *World J Gastroenterol* 2006; **12**: 1430–4.

52. Barera G, Bianchi C, Calisti L *et al.* Screening of diabetic children for coeliac disease with antigliadin antibodies and HLA typing. *Arch Dis Child* 1991; **66**: 491–4.

53. Holmes GKT. Screening for coeliac disease in type 1 diabetes. *Arch Dis Child* 2002; **87**: 495–8.

54. De Vitis I, Ghirlanda G, Gasbarrini G. Prevalence of coeliac disease in type 1 diabetes: a multicentre study. *Acta Paediatr Suppl* 1996; **412**: 56–7.

55. Not T, Tommasini A, Tonini G *et al.* Undiagnosed celiac disease and risk of autoimmune disorders in subjects with type 1 diabetes mellitus. *Diabetologia* 2001; **44**: 151–5.

56. Saadah O, Zacharin M, O'Callaghan A, Oliver M, Catto-Smith A. Effect of gluten-free diet and adherence on growth and diabetic control in diabetics with celiac disease. *Arch Dis Child* 2004; **89**: 871–6.

57. Amin R, Murphy N, Edge J *et al.* A longitudinal study of the effects of a gluten-free diet on glycaemic control and weight gain in subjects with type 1 diabetes and celiac disease. *Diabetes Care* 2002; **25**: 1117–22.

58. Depczynski B. Coeliac disease and its relation to glycaemic control in adults with type 1 diabetes mellitus. *Diabetes Res Clin Pract* 2008; **79**: e10.

59. Packer SC, Dornhorst A, Frost GS. The glycaemic index of a range of gluten-free foods. *Diabet Med* 2000; **17**: 657–60.

60. Leeds J, Hopper A, Hurlstone D *et al.* Is exocrine pancreatic insufficiency in adult coeliac disease a cause for persisting symptoms? *Aliment Pharmacol Ther* 2006; **25**: 265–71.

61. Rubio-Tapia A, Barton SH, Rosenblatt JE, Murrary JA. Prevalence of small intestine bacterial overgrowth diagnosed by quantitative culture of intestinal aspirate in celiac disease. *J Clin Gastrol* 2008 Aug 20. [Epub ahead of print]

62. Nyhlin N, Bohr J, Eriksson S, Tysk C. Microscopic colitis: a common and an easily overlooked cause of chronic diarrhoea. *Eur J Intern Med* 2008; **19**: 181–6.

63. Leffler DA, Dennis M, Hyett B *et al.* Etiologies and predictors of diagnosis in non-responsive celiac disease. *Clin Gastroenterol Hepatol* 2007; **5**: 445–50.

64. Abdallah H, Leffler D, Dennis M, Kelly CP. Refractory celiac disease. *Curr Gastroenterol Rep* 2007; **9**: 401–5.

65. Al-Toma A, Verbeek WHM, Hadithi M, von Blomberg BME, Mulder CJJ. Survival in refractory coeliac disease and enteropathy-associated T-cell lymphoma: retrospective evaluation of single-centre experience. *Gut* 2007; **56**: 1373–8.

66. Daum S, Cellier C, Mulder C. Refractory coeliac disease. *Best Pract Res Clin Gastroenterol* 2005; **19**: 413–24.

67. Murphy MS, Sood M, Johnson T. Use of the lactose H2 breath test to monitor mucosal healing in coeliac disease. *Acta Paediatr* 2002; **91**: 141–4.

68. Ojetti V, Nucera G, Migneco A *et al.* High prevalence of celiac disease in patients with lactose intolerance. *Digestion* 2005; **71**: 106–10.

69. Bianchi ML, Bardella MT. Bone and celiac disease. *Calcif Tissue Int* 2002; **71**: 465–71.

70. Kemppainen T, Kröger H, Janatuinen E *et al.* Osteoporosis in adult patients with celiac disease. *Bone* 1999; **24**: 249–55.

71. Ludvigsson JF, Michaelsson K, Ekbom A, Montgomery MS. Coeliac disease and the risk of fractures – a general population based cohort study *Aliment Pharmacol Ther* 2007; **25**: 273–85.

72. Olmos M, Antelo M, Vazquez H *et al.* Systematic review and meta-analysis of observational studies on the prevalence of fractures in coeliac disease. *Dig Liver Dis* 2008; **40**: 46–53.

73. Walters JRF. Bone mineral density in coeliac children. *Gut* 1994; **35**: 150–1.

74. McFarlane XA, Marsham J, Reeves D, Dalla AK, Robertson DAF. Subclinical nutritional deficiency in treated coeliac disease and nutritional content of the gluten-free diet. *J Hum Nutr Diet* 1995; **8**: 231–7.

75. Tilg H, Moschen AR, Kaser A, Pines A, Dotan I. Gut, inflammation and osteoporosis: basic and clinical concepts. *Gut* 2008; **57**: 684–94.

76. Valdimarsson T, Löfman O, Toss G, Ström M. Reversal of osteopenia with diet in adult coeliac disease. *Gut* 1996; **38**: 322–7.

77. Bianchi ML, Bardella MT Bone in celiac disease. *Osteoporos Int* 2008 [Epub ahead of print].

78. Lewis NR, Scott BB for the British Society of Gastroenterology. Guidelines for osteoporosis in coeliac disease and inflammatory bowel disease. London: BSG, 2007. www.bsg.org.uk

79. Mora S. Celiac disease in children: impact on bone health. *Rev Endocr Metab Disord* 2008; **9**: 123–30.

80. Holmes GKT, Prior P, Lane MR, Pope D, Allan RN. Malignancy in coeliac disease: effect of a gluten free diet. *Gut* 1989; **30**: 333–8.

81. Catassi C, Fabiani E, Corrao G *et al.* Risk of non-Hodgkin lymphoma in celiac disease. *JAMA* 2002; **287**: 1413–19.

82. Card TR, West J, Holmes GK. Risk of malignancy in diagnosed coeliac disease: a 24 year prospective, population based, cohort study. *Aliment Pharmacol Ther* 2004; **20**: 769–75.

83. West J, Logan RFA, Smith CJ, Hubbard RB, Card TR. Malignancy and mortality in people with coeliac disease: population based cohort study. *BMJ* 2004; **329**: 716–18.

84. Jadresin O, Misak Z, Sanja K, Sonicki Z, Zizic V. Compliance with gluten-free diet in children with coeliac disease. *J Pediatr Gastroenterol Nutr* 2008; **47**: 344–8.

85. Leffler D, Edwards-George J, Dennis M *et al*. Factors that influence Adherence to a gluten-free diet in adults with celiac disease. *Dig Dis Sci* 2008; **53**: 1573–81.

86. Holm K, Maki M, Vuolteenaho N *et al*. Oats in the treatment of childhood coeliac disease: a 2-year controlled trial and a long-term clinical follow-up study. *Aliment Pharmacol Ther* 2006; **23**: 1463–72.

87. Hogberg L, Laurin P, Fälth-Magnusson K *et al*. Oats to children with newly diagnosed coeliac disease: a randomised double blind study. *Gut* 2004; **53**: 649–54.

88. Janatuinen EK, Kemppainen TA, Julkunen R *et al*. No harm from five year ingestion of oats in coeliac disease. *Gut* 2002; **50**: 332–5.

89. Hernando A, Mujico J, Mena M, Lombardia M, Mendez E. Measurement of wheat gluten and barley hordeins in contaminated oats from Europe, the United States and Canada by Sandwich R5 ELISA. *Eur J Gastroenterol Hepatol* 2008; **20**: 545–54.

90. Garsed K, Scott BB. Can oats be taken in a gluten-free diet? A systematic review. *Scand J Gastroenterol* 2007; **42**: 171–8.

91. Haboubi NY, Taylor S, Jones S. Coeliac disease and oats: a systematic review. *Postgrad Med J* 2006; **82**: 672–8.

92. Dickey W. Making oats safer for patients with coeliac disease. *Eur J Gastroenterol Hepatol* 2008; **20**: 494–5.

93. Storsrud S, Hulthen LR, Lenmer RA. Beneficial effect on oats in the gluten-free diet of adults with special reference to nutrient status, symptoms and subjective experiences. *Br J Nutr* 2003; **90**: 101–7.

94. Varady KA, Jones PJH. Combination diet and exercise interventions for the treatment of dyslipidemia: an effective preliminary strategy to lower cholesterol levels? *J Nutr* 2005; **135**: 1829–35.

95. Codex Alimentarius Commission (CAC). Codex Standard for 'Gluten-Free Foods'. Codex stan 118-1981 (amended 1983).

96. Codex Alimentarius Commission (CAC). Report of the 29th Session of the Codex Committee on Nutrition and Food for Special Dietary Uses (ALINORM 08/31/26). Rome: CAC, 2007.

97. Food Standards Agency. Draft Commission Regulation foods suitable for people intolerant to gluten (England). London: FSA, 2008. http://www.food.gov.uk/consultations/consulteng/2008/regulationglutenfreefoods. Accessed September 2008.

98. Collin P, Thorell L, Kaukinen K, Maki M. The safe threshold for gluten contamination in gluten-free products. Can trace amounts be accepted in the treatment of coeliac disease? *Aliment Pharmacol Ther* 2004; **19**: 1277–83.

99. Peraaho M, Kaukinen K, Paasikivi K, Sievanen H, Lohiniemi S, Maki M *et al*. Wheat-starch-based gluten-free products in the treatment of newly detected coeliac disease: prospective and randomized study. *Aliment Pharmacol Ther* 2003; **17**: 587–94.

100. Catassi C, Fabiani E, Iacono G *et al*. A prospective, double-blind, placebo-controlled trial to establish a safe gluten threshold for patients with coeliac disease. *Am J Clin Nutr* 2007; **85**: 160–6.

101. Gibert A, Espadaler M, Canela MA *et al*. Consumption of gluten-free products: should the threshold value for trace amounts of gluten be at 20, 100 or 200 ppm? *Eur J Gastroenterol Hepatol* 2006; **18**: 1187–95.

102. Akobeng AK, Thomas AG. Systematic review: tolerable amount of gluten for people with coeliac disease. *Aliment Pharmacol Ther* 2008; **27**: 1044–52.

103. British Society of Paediatric Gastroenterology Hepatology and Nutrition (BSPGHAN). Gluten-free foods: a prescribing guide. London: BSPGHAN, 2004.

104. European Union. Commission Directive 2007/68/EC of 27 November 2007 amending Annex IIIa to Directive 2000/13/EC of the European Parliament and of the Council as regards certain food ingredients. *Official Journal of the European Union* 2007; **L310**: 11–14.

105. Food Standards Agency. *Guidance on Allergen Management and Consumer Information: Best Practice Guidance on Managing Food Allergens with Particular Reference to Avoiding Cross-Contamination and Using Appropriate Advisory Labelling (e.g. 'May Contain' Labelling)*. London: FSA, 2006.

106. Department of Health. *Dietary Reference Values for Food Energy and Nutrients for the United Kingdom*. Report on Health and Social Subjects 41. London: HMSO, 1991.

107. Bottaro G, Cataldo F, Rotolo N, Spina M, Corazza GR. The clinical pattern of subclinical/silent coeliac disease: an analysis on 1026 consecutive cases. *Am J Gastroenterol* 1999; **94**: 691–6.

108. Harper JW, Holleran SF, Ramakrishnan R, Bhagat G, Green PH. Anemia in celiac disease is multifactorial in etiology. *Am J Hematol* 2007; **82**: 996–1000.

109. Tikkakoski S, Savilahit E, Kolho KL. Undiagnosed coeliac disease and nutritional deficiencies in adults screened in primary health care. *Scand J Gastroenterol* 2007; **41**: 60–5.

110. Lee SK, Lo W, Memeo L, Rotterdam H, Green P. Duodenal histology in patients with celiac disease after treatment with a gluten-free diet. *Gastrointest Endosc* 2003; **57**: 187–91.

111. Hallert C, Grant C, Grehn S *et al*. Evidence of poor vitamin status in coeliac patients on a gluten-free diet for 10 years. *Aliment Pharmacol Ther* 2002; **16**: 1333–9.

112. Thompson T. Thiamin, riboflavin and niacin contents of the gluten-free diet: is there cause for concern? *J Am Diet Assoc* 1999; **99**: 858–62.

113. Thompson T. Folate, iron, and dietary fiber contents of the gluten-free diet. *J Am Diet Assoc* 2000; **100**: 1389–96.

114. Thompson T, Dennis M, Higgins LA, Lee AR, Sharrett MK. Gluten-free diet survey: are Americans with coeliac disease consuming recommended amounts of fibre, iron, calcium and grain foods? *J Hum Nutr Diet* 2005; **18**: 163–9.

115. Kinsey L, Burden ST, Bannerman E. A dietary survey to determine if patients with coeliac disease are meeting current healthy eating guidelines and how their diet compares to that of the British general population. *Eur J Clin Nutr* 2007 Aug 15. [Epub ahead of print]

116. Grehn S, Fridell K, Lilliecreutz M, Hallert C. Dietary habits of Swedish adult coeliac patients treated by a gluten-free diet for 10 years. *Scand J Nutr* 2001; **45**: 178–82.

117. Food Standards Agency. *Eat Well. Your Guide to Healthy Eating: Eight Tips for Healthier Choices*. London: FSA, 2005.

118. Food Standards Agency. *The Balance of Good Health: Information for Educators and Communicators*. London: FSA, 2001.

119. Primary Care Society for Gastroenterology. *The Management of Adults with Coeliac Disease in Primary Care*. Rickmansworth: PCSG, 2006.

120. Tursi A, Brandimarte G, Girogetti GM. Lack of usefulness of anti-transglutaminase antibodies in assessing histologic recovery after gluten-free diet in celiac disease. *J Clin Gastroenterol* 2003; **37**: 387–91.

121. Rostami K, Danciu M. Endoscopy and small-bowel biopsy in celiac disease: indications and implications. *Endoscopy* 2007; **39**: 573.

122. O'Mahony S, Howdle PD, Losowsky MS. Management of patients with non-responsive coeliac disease. *Aliment Pharmacol Ther* 1996; **10**: 671–80.

123. Abdulkarim AS, Burgart LJ, See J, Murray JA. Etiology of nonresponsive celiac disease: results of a systematic approach. *Am J Gastroenterol* 2002; **97**: 2016–22.

124. Committee on Medical Aspects of Food and Nutrition Policy (COMA). Folic acid and the prevention of disease: report of the Committee on Medical Aspects of Food and Nutrition Policy. London: COMA, 2000.

125. Department of Health. *Infant Feeding Recommendation*. London: DoH, 2003. www.dh.gov.uk/en/Publicationsandstatistics/Publications/PublicationsPolicyAndGuidance/DH_4097197. Accessed October 2007.

126. Akobeng A, Ramanan A, Buchan I, Heller R. Effect of breast feeding on risk of coeliac disease: a systematic review and meta-analysis of observational studies. *Arch Dis Child* 2006; **91**: 39–43.

127. Agostoni C, Decsi T, Fewtrell M *et al*. Complementary feeding: a commentary by the ESPGHAN Committee on Nutrition. *Pediatr Gastroenterol Nutr* 2008; **46**: 99–110.

9.2   Allergy to wheat and other cereals

Isabel Skypala

9.2.1   Introduction

There are a number of immune responses to wheat[1], including cutaneous and gastrointestinal (coeliac disease) cell-mediated reactions, IgE-mediated reactions, inhalation reactions and a particular type of wheat allergy known as wheat-dependent exercise-induced anaphylaxis (WDEIA; see Chapter 10). Coeliac disease is discussed in section 1 of this chapter, and allergy to wheat and other cereals in section 2. Wheat is often also cited as a precipitating factor of irritable bowel syndrome (IBS), with 15% of subjects in one study reporting symptoms to wheat[2], although the mechanisms involved are not clear. The foods involved in IBS are fully discussed in Chapter 2 and therefore will not be covered here.

9.2.2   Onset, prevalence and natural history

The most common foods to cause food hypersensitivity reactions are milk, egg, peanuts, tree nuts, fish and shellfish[3]. However, there is a paucity of information on the prevalence of diagnosed wheat hypersensitivity. Wheat is commonly reported to cause food hypersensitivity (FHS), but as there is known to be a big discrepancy between reported and actual FHS, the actual prevalence of wheat allergy is unclear. It is thought to be quite low, though more common in children, with 0.4% of children in the USA reported to be allergic to wheat[3]. Children who are sensitised to wheat, milk, egg and soya through the gastrointestinal tract will usually lose this sensitivity as they get older, except in the case of WDEIA[4].

In 6-year-old children in the UK, wheat was shown to be an important allergen in those whose reported symptoms were confirmed by oral food challenge[5]. Interestingly, another study of 11- and 15-year-olds from the same population group showed that although wheat was reported to cause a problem for 4% of 11-year-olds and 8% of 15-year-olds, it was only confirmed to be a problem in the older age group[6].

In adults wheat allergy is thought to be infrequent, and more commonly associated with WDEIA[7]. In a study of self-reported allergy in five Baltic countries, only 9% of the total numbers of reported food reactions were to wheat, with other foods being much more common causes of reported reactions[8]. However, there is variation between countries: there were no reported reactions to wheat in a Portuguese study of adults with FHS[9], compared to 4.7% of those with reported reactions and concordant positive skin prick test (SPT) to wheat in a German population study[10].

Only a limited number of studies have undertaken double-blind placebo-controlled food challenge (DBPCFC) to confirm diagnosis of wheat allergy in adults. There was a very low prevalence of wheat allergy in a Danish study, with only one reported reaction to wheat, which was not confirmed through challenge[11]. Although food allergy in adults is not thought to be common, a study investigating wheat allergy in a cohort of Danish and Italian adults with a reported wheat allergy showed that more than 50% of the subjects had their symptoms confirmed by DBPCFC[12].

Occupational allergy can also involve wheat. One study showed cereals were the main sensitising agent involved in the occupational asthma of 75% of bakers and 66% of farmers, although alpha-amylase, soya beans and storage mites can also cause this condition[13].

The prevalence of reported or confirmed allergic reactions to other cereals is less well documented. Rice is not known to be a major cause of FHS in the UK, although with patterns of consumption greatly altered in the last two decades this may change in the future. In countries where rice is the main carbohydrate staple of the diet, sensitisation and reported allergy to rice is high. Thirty per cent of Malaysian patients with clinical symptoms of rhinitis had a positive skin prick test to rice[14]. In India, of 1,200 patients screened using a standard questionnaire, 165 presented with history of rice allergy[15]. Of these, 20 (12.1%) patients had positive skin prick test and 13 raised specific IgE to rice, although rice allergy was only confirmed in 6 of the 10 patients who underwent a DBPCFC. More recently, rice allergy has been confirmed in Italian patients sensitised to the non-specific lipid transfer proteins (nsLTPs)[16] (see Chapter 7).

The prevalence of maize allergy is unknown, although it has been reported to cause severe reactions, thought to be linked to the main maize allergen, which is an nsLTP[17,18]. However, where maize is the staple starchy food, maize allergy may be more prevalent. A Mexican study showed that 8.5% of an adult cohort had reported symptoms to maize which were confirmed by positive cutaneous testing[19]. There are no reported cases of oat allergy in the literature, although it has been shown that children with atopic dermatitis using oat-based emollient creams were more likely to be sensitised to oats[20]. Barley has been linked to case reports of urticaria and anaphylaxis to beer and malt, but the prevalence of allergy to barley is unknown[21,22].

Although it is not a cereal, buckwheat is used to make dishes which are usually made with wheat flour, such as noodles, in Japan and Korea. Buckwheat is the commonest food cause of anaphylaxis in Korea, and it has been estimated that 5% of Koreans have positive skin prick tests to buckwheat[23,24]. However, the consumption of buckwheat is also likely in parts of Europe: for example buckwheat pancakes, known as *galettes*, are a speciality of the Brittany region of France. There have also been case reports of buckwheat allergy in the USA[25] and Germany[26]. However, sensitisation to buckwheat can come through the use of buckwheat pillows. Buckwheat hulls, also known as sobakawa hulls or sobagara husks, have been used in pillows for over 600 years, and there have been case reports of buckwheat pillow-induced asthma and allergic rhinitis[27].

9.2.3   Foods and allergens involved

Most cereal allergens are found in the prolamin family of plant allergens and include cereal α-amylase and protease inhibitors, cereal prolamins and nsLTPs (see

Chapter 4). Cereal α-amylase inhibitors are produced by barley, wheat, rice, corn and rye and interfere with the digestion of plant starches and proteins by impeding insect gut enzymes. Sensitisation is through ingestion or inhalation, and they can therefore precipitate both inhalant allergy and IgE-mediated food allergy[18]. Studies have shown that α-amylase inhibitor allergens are among the most important wheat allergens in food allergy and may also play a role in WDEIA[28].

Cereal prolamins are thought to be involved in both IgE-mediated wheat allergy and coeliac disease. The glutenins and gliadins in wheat, secalins in rye and hordeins in barley are major storage proteins in the endosperm of cereal grains. The highest IgE reactivity is to glutenin, and glutenin subunits in the gluten fraction may also be important in primary food allergy to wheat as they are resistant to heat[28]. Although alpha gliadin and gamma gliadin also have high IgE reactivity, it is omega-5 gliadin which may be the most important allergen in young children with immediate reaction to ingested wheat. It has been suggested that detection of omega-5-gliadin-specific IgE is a useful comparator to wheat-specific IgE when diagnosing wheat allergy in children[29]. Levels of this allergen may also be higher in those who have more severe symptoms, including anaphylaxis[30]. It is also known that omega-5 gliadin is the main allergen involved in eliciting WDEIA, and serum levels increase in accordance with allergic symptoms in patients with this condition[31,32]. Omega-5 gliadin cross-reacts with gamma-70 and gamma-35 secalins from rye and with gamma-3 hordein from barley, which may mean these foods can also cause symptoms in patients with WDEIA[33].

The other important allergens are the nsLTPs. The main LTP in wheat is Tri a 14, and this has been shown to be a major allergen linked to occupational asthma caused by wheat, with 60% of patients having specific IgE against this allergen[34]. However another study concluded that LTPs in wheat were only major allergens in Italian patients and may not be a universally important allergen[16]. The important allergens in rice, maize and barley are also thought to be nsLTPs. Three cases of rice-induced anaphylaxis have been reported to be caused by a rice nsLTP, and it may also be involved in other manifestations of rice allergy[16,35]. The major allergen of maize, Zea m 14, is an LTP with a molecular weight of 9 kDa, which maintains its structure after cooking at high temperatures and is highly homologous with the peach nsLTP allergen Pru p 3[17,36]. There are several different allergens in barley, with two being identified as the causative agents in beer allergy, an nsLTP and a second barley protein[37]. Other studies have also identified barley allergens in beer, and shown that patients sensitised to the nsLTP in beer can also cross-react with other nsLTPs in foods such as corn, but this may extend to nsLTPs in botanically unrelated foods such as apples, peaches and nuts[21,22,37,38]. Barley is the main allergen in beer, but wheat beer is becoming increasingly common, and anaphylaxis to wheat beer has been reported[39]. A relatively new group of allergens, thioredoxins, have been identified in both wheat and maize. They are cross-reactive allergens that studies suggest might contribute to the symptoms of baker's asthma and could also be related to grass-pollen allergy[18].

9.2.4 Diagnosis

Although history is always useful when trying to diagnose a wheat allergy, it may be more difficult than with other foods to ascertain that wheat is the symptom trigger. One study looking at retrospective diagnosis found that only 30% of subjects diagnosed with a wheat allergy had a suggestive or convincing history, compared with over 85% for peanut or fish allergy and 65% for milk and egg[40]. When making the diagnosis it is important to consider the age of the patient: wheat allergy is much more common in childhood, and in adults is very infrequent and most commonly associated with WDEIA (see Chapter 10)[7]. In adults, an allergy to cereals may be more likely linked to nsLTP, and therefore may manifest as isolated allergic reactions to foods such as beer (barley) and malt (barley).

Presenting symptoms can be cutaneous, such as atopic dermatitis, but studies suggest that in the case of children half of those presenting with an allergy to wheat will have severe symptoms including urticarial rash, laryngeal oedema, and anaphylaxis – which may often occur as the first manifestation[41]. Presenting symptoms in adults range from erythema and pruritis, through to more severe angio-oedema and anaphylaxis, the latter more associated with WDEIA[4,12].

A retrospective study has shown that diagnostic skin prick and *in vitro* tests measuring sensitisation against water/salt-soluble wheat proteins have poor predictive values[12]. The positive predictive value of wheat skin prick test and serum specific IgE estimation were considerably less than 50%, although the values of the blood test increased to 85% if grass-pollen patients were excluded from the result[12]. Another study showed that a serum specific IgE level of 26 kU$_A$/L was 90% predictive of a positive challenge to wheat, but a level of 100 kU$_A$/L was required for a 95% predictive probability, the recommendation from the author being that only subjects with a level greater than 80 kU$_A$/L will not require a food challenge to establish the presence or absence of wheat allergy[40]. A similar study could not establish predictive probabilities for wheat as there was no specific IgE level at which all of the children had a positive DBPCFC. The positive predictive value for wheat in this study was 41%[42]. The other difficulty with interpreting wheat test results is co-sensitisation to grass pollen. Many patients with a grass allergy often have significant levels of specific IgE to wheat and other cereals, but are usually able to tolerate cereal products without ill effect; many positive specific IgE tests to wheat in grass-sensitised individuals have no clinical significance[6]. It is therefore very important to establish the presence or absence of grass-pollen allergy when undertaking the estimation of specific IgE antibodies to wheat.

For children, it may be helpful to consider the level of specific IgE as being predictive of the severity of symptoms, with one study reporting higher levels linked to an increased risk of anaphylaxis[41]. Other studies in children have also found the measurement of specific IgE antibodies to omega-5 gliadin to be a useful predictor of the presence or absence of wheat allergy, and again levels may also predict severity[30,43]. The epitope-binding domains of the gliadins may also differ depending on the type of symptoms elicited by wheat. Those with WDEIA, anaphylaxis and urticarial reactions to wheat recognise sequential epitopes on gliadins, whereas those suffering from atopic dermatitis related to wheat recognise conformational epitopes[44] (see Chapter 4).

There are no reports in the literature on the predictive values of tests for maize, rice, barley or buckwheat.

9.2.5 Management

It is important to distinguish between wheat allergy, coeliac disease and non-allergic hypersensitivity to wheat. Patients allergic to wheat cannot eat many gluten-free products as they are not wheat-free and may contain wheat starch. Any patient with a diagnosed allergy to wheat will need expert advice about diet modification, because wheat is the main staple food in many countries. Wheat contains important nutrients, and bread may also be fortified with other nutrients not naturally present in wheat. A wheat-free diet will put the patient at risk of suboptimal intakes of thiamine, riboflavin, iron, calcium and energy. It may also adversely affect protein intake. Therefore for all patients it is important that appropriate wheat substitutes are incorporated into the diet, and that the patient also increases his or her intake of other starchy staple foods. Given the cross-reactivity between the nsLTPs, patients must not be advised to take a wheat substitute which may also cause reactions. One study showed that barley was often positive on challenge in patients with a known wheat allergy, but the same clinical reactivity was not shown to corn or rice despite sensitisation to those foods[45]. Appropriate substitutes for wheat will therefore usually be corn, rice and potato, although other non-cereal foods may also be useful substitutes, such as cassava, sago, chickpea and lentil (gram) flour.

Wheat is found in a wide range of foods including bread, cereals, cakes, biscuits, pasta, noodles, thickeners, pastries, pies, couscous, semolina, cheesecake, soups, pizza and bottled sauces. There are many wheat-free substitutes for some or all of these foods readily available in supermarkets and health-food shops. The advent of bread machines has made it easier for people with a wheat allergy to prepare home-baked wheat-free bread products. People with a wheat allergy are not necessarily entitled to gluten-free products on prescription, but in any case many such products will not be suitable due to the presence of wheat starch.

For other grains, corn is present in breakfast cereals, corn snacks and tortilla chips, polenta, corn crackers, cornflour – which may be found in custard and gravy mixes – and some foods use corn starch and corn syrup, although this is more common in the USA. Barley is not a very common food ingredient, but it is present in beer, malt, and malt-containing foods such as granary bread, breakfast cereals, malt drinks and milky drinks. Wholemeal bread may also have malt or barley added. Rice may be present in foods as rice flour or ground rice, and is also found in rice cakes, rice pudding, rice noodles, breakfast cereals and edible rice paper, which may be found on macaroons etc. Buckwheat is used to make noodles and pancakes.

European Union food labelling laws require that all food products containing wheat, oats, barley or rye declare these on the label (see Chapter 4). There is no such requirement for corn or rice at present.

References

1. Bock SA. Prospective appraisal of complaints of adverse reactions to foods in children during the first 3 years of life. *Pediatrics* 1987; **79**: 683–8.
2. Monsbakken KW, Vandvik PO, Farup PG. Perceived food intolerance in subjects with irritable bowel syndrome – aetiology, prevalence and consequences. *Eur J Clin Nutr* 2006; **60**: 667–72.
3. Sicherer SH, Sampson HA. Food allergy. *J Allergy Clin Immunol* 2006; **117**: S470–5.
4. Chapman JA, Bernstein IL, Lee RE *et al*. Food allergy: a practice parameter. *Ann Allergy Asthma Immunol* 2006; **96**: S1–68.
5. Venter C, Pereira B, Grundy J *et al*. Prevalence of sensitization reported and objectively assessed food hypersensitivity amongst six-year-old children: a population-based study. *Pediatr Allergy Immunol* 2006; **17**: 356–63.
6. Pereira B, Venter C, Grundy J *et al*. Prevalence of sensitization to food allergens, reported adverse reaction to foods, food avoidance, and food hypersensitivity among teenagers. *J Allergy Clin Immunol* 2005; **116**: 884–92.
7. Crespo JF, Rodriguez J. Food allergy in adulthood. *Allergy* 2003; **58**: 98–113.
8. Eriksson NE, Möller C, Werner S *et al*. Self-reported food hypersensitivity in Sweden, Denmark, Estonia, Lithuania and Russia. *J Investig Allergol Clin Immunol* 2004; **14**: 70–9.
9. Falcão H, Lunet N, Lopes C, Barros H. Food hypersensitivity in Portuguese adults. *Eur J Clin Nutr* 2004; **58**: 1621–5.
10. Zuberbier T, Edenharter G, Worm M *et al*. Prevalence of adverse reactions to food in Germany: a population study. *Allergy* 2004; **59**: 338–45.
11. Osterballe M, Hansen TK, Mortz CG, Bindslev-Jensen C. The clinical relevance of sensitization to pollen-related fruits and vegetables in unselected pollen-sensitized adults. *Allergy* 2005; **60**: 218–25.
12. Scibilia J, Pastorello EA, Zisa G *et al*. Wheat allergy: a double-blind, placebo-controlled study in adults. *J Allergy Clin Immunol* 2006; **117**: 433–9.
13. Alvarez MJ, Tabar AI, Quirce S *et al*. Diversity of allergens causing occupational asthma among cereal workers as demonstrated by exposure procedures. *Clin Exp Allergy* 1996; **26**: 147–53.
14. Gendeh BS, Murad S, Razi AM *et al*. Skin prick test reactivity to foods in adult Malaysians with rhinitis. *Otolaryngol Head Neck Surg* 2000; **122**: 758–62.
15. Kumar R, Srivastava P, Kumari D *et al*. Rice (*Oryza sativa*) allergy in rhinitis and asthma patients: a clinico-immunological study. *Immunobiology* 2007; **212**: 141–7.
16. Asero R, Amato S, Alfieri B, Folloni S, Mistrello G. Rice: another potential cause of food allergy in patients sensitized to lipid transfer protein. *Int Arch Allergy Immunol* 2007; **143**: 69–74.
17. Pastorello EA, Farioli L, Pravettoni V *et al*. The maize major allergen, which is responsible for food-induced allergic reactions, is a lipid transfer protein. *J Allergy Clin Immunol* 2000; **106**: 744–51.
18. Weichel M, Glaser AG, Ballmer-Weber BK, Schmid GP, Crameri R. Wheat and maize thioredoxins: a novel cross-reactive cereal allergen family related to baker's asthma. *J Allergy Clin Immunol* 2006; **117**: 676–81.
19. Valencia-Zavala MP, Vega-Robledo GB, Sánchez-Olivas MA, Duarte-Diaz RJ, Oviedo-Cristóbal L. Maize (*Zea mays*): allergen or toleragen? Participation of the cereal in allergic disease and positivity incidence in cutaneous tests. *Rev Alerg Mex* 2006; **53**: 207–11.
20. Boussault P, Léauté-Labrèze C, Saubusse E *et al*. Oat sensitization in children with atopic dermatitis: prevalence, risks and associated factors. *Allergy* 2007: **62**: 1251–6.
21. Curioni A, Santucci B, Cristaudo A *et al*. Urticaria from beer: an immediate hypersensitivity reaction due to a 10-kDa protein derived from barley. *Clin Exp Allergy* 1999; **29**: 407–13.
22. Figueredo E, Quirce S, del Amo A *et al*. Beer-induced anaphylaxis: identification of allergens. *Allergy* 1999; **54**: 630–4.
23. Yang MS, Lee SH, Kim TW *et al*. Epidemiologic and clinical features of anaphylaxis in Korea. *Ann Allergy Asthma Immunol* 2008; **100**: 31–6.

24. Sohn MH, Lee SY, Kim KE. Prediction of buckwheat allergy using specific IgE concentrations in children. *Allergy* 2003; **58**: 1308–10.

25. Stember RH. Buckwheat allergy. *Allergy Asthma Proc* 2006; **27**: 393–5.

26. Oppel T, Thomas P, Wollenberg A. Cross-sensitization between poppy seed and buckwheat in a food-allergic patient with poppy seed anaphylaxis. *Int Arch Allergy Immunol* 2006; **140**: 170–3.

27. Fritz SB, Gold BL. Buckwheat pillow-induced asthma and allergic rhinitis. *Ann Allergy Asthma Immunol* 2003; **90**: 355–8.

28. Pastorello EA, Farioli L, Conti A *et al*. Wheat IgE-mediated food allergy in European patients: alpha-amylase inhibitors, lipid transfer proteins and low-molecular-weight glutenins. Allergenic molecules recognized by double-blind, placebo-controlled food challenge. *Int Arch Allergy Immunol* 2007; **144**: 10–22.

29. Palosuo K. Update on wheat hypersensitivity. *Curr Opin Allergy Clin Immunol* 2003; **3**: 205–9.

30. Shibata R, Nishima S, Kohno K *et al*. Specific IgE antibodies to omega-5 gliadin: indicator of wheat anaphylaxis and its tolerance in wheat sensitised children. *J Allergy Clin Immunol* 2007; **119** (1 Suppl 1): S120.

31. Matsuo H, Morita E, Tatha AS *et al*. Identification of the IgE-binding epitope in omega-5 gliadin, a major allergen in wheat-dependent exercise-induced anaphylaxis. *J Biol Chem* 2004; **279**: 12135–40.

32. Matsuo H, Morimoto K, Akaki T *et al*. Exercise and aspirin increase levels of circulating gliadin peptides in patients with wheat-dependent exercise-induced anaphylaxis. *Clin Exp Allergy* 2005; **35**: 461–6.

33. Palosuo K, Alenius H, Varjonen E, Kalkkinen N, Reunala T. Rye gamma-70 and gamma-35 secalins and barley gamma-3 hordein cross-react with omega-5 gliadin, a major allergen in wheat-dependent, exercise-induced anaphylaxis. *Clin Exp Allergy* 2001; **31**: 466–73.

34. Palacin A, Quirce S, Armentia A *et al*. Wheat lipid transfer protein is a major allergen associated with baker's asthma. *J Allergy Clin Immunol* 2007; **120**: 1132–8.

35. Enrique E, Ahrazem O, Bartra J *et al*. Lipid transfer protein is involved in rhinoconjunctivitis and asthma produced by rice inhalation. *J Allergy Clin Immunol* 2005; **116**: 926–8.

36. Pastorello EA, Pompei C, Pravettoni V *et al*. Lipid-transfer protein is the major maize allergen maintaining IgE-binding activity after cooking at 100 degrees C, as demonstrated in anaphylactic patients and patients with positive double-blind, placebo-controlled food challenge results. *J Allergy Clin Immunol* 2003; **112**: 775–83.

37. García-Casado G, Crespo JF, Rodríguez J, Salcedo G. Isolation and characterization of barley lipid transfer protein and protein Z as beer allergens. *J Allergy Clin Immunol* 2001; **108**: 647–9.

38. Asero R, Mistrello G, Roncarolo D, Amato S, van Ree R. A case of allergy to beer showing cross-reactivity between lipid transfer proteins. *Ann Allergy Asthma Immunol* 2001; **87**: 65–7.

39. Herzinger T, Kick G, Ludolph-Hauser D, Przybilla B. Anaphylaxis to wheat beer. *Ann Allergy Asthma Immunol* 2004; **92**: 673–5.

40. Sampson HA. Utility of food-specific IgE concentrations in predicting symptomatic food allergy. *J Allergy Clin Immunol* 2001; **107**: 891–6.

41. Pourpak Z, Mansouri M, Mesdaghi M, Kazemnejad A, Farhoudi A. Wheat allergy: clinical and laboratory findings. *Int Arch Allergy Immunol* 2004; **133**: 168–73.

42. Celik-Bilgili S, Mehl A, Verstege A *et al*. The predictive value of specific immunoglobulin E levels in serum for the outcome of oral food challenges. *Clin Exp Allergy* 2005; **35**: 268–73.

43. Ito K, Takaoka Y, Futamura M *et al*. Omega-5-gliadin specific IgE as a predictor of wheat allergy in children. *J Allergy Clin Immunol* 2007; **119**: S191.

44. Battais F, Mothes T, Moneret-Vautrin DA *et al*. Identification of IgE-binding epitopes on gliadins for patients with food allergy to wheat. *Allergy* 2005; **60**: 815–21.

45. Pourpak Z, Mesdaghi M, Mansouri M *et al*. Which cereal is a suitable substitute for wheat in children with wheat allergy? *Pediatr Allergy Immunol* 2005; **16**: 262–6.

10 Other Causes of Food Hypersensitivity

Isabel Skypala

10.1 Reactions to food additives

10.1.1 Prevalence

The reported prevalence of food-additive hypersensitivity can be high, especially in paediatric populations. A UK study showed that 26 out of 90 children aged 11 years (29%), and 14 out of 94 children aged 15 years (15%), reported a problem with food additives[1]. In adults, however, the rate appears to be lower, with only 1.3% of adults reporting adverse reactions to additives[2]. A Dutch study showed that food additives and chocolate were the most common foods avoided by adults who thought they had food hypersensitivity[3]. Another study assessing self-reported food hypersensitivity in five countries reported that 19 (range 14–27) of the 1,139 participants (1.7%) reported reactions to additives, a much lower reported prevalence rate which may reflect geographical variation[4]. This appears to be supported by another study on Portuguese adults showing that there were no reported reactions to food additives in a sample of 659 adults[5]. The reported prevalence rate may also vary depending on the food additive implicated. One Australian study cited a 1.3% prevalence rate for reported reactions to artificial colours, but a 6.5% prevalence rate for reported reactions to monosodium glutamate[6].

As with foods, there is a large discrepancy between reported and actual prevalence rates of hypersensitivity to food additives. A study by Young *et al.* estimated the population prevalence of FHS to additives in the UK to be 0.1%[7], and this has been confirmed in a study looking at reported food allergy in a cohort of Danish children and adults[8]. This study showed that 19 of 1,834 subjects (1%) reported an allergy to additives, but hypersensitivity was confirmed by double-blind placebo-controlled food challenge (DBPCFC) in only one adult patient, making the prevalence in the adult cohort 0.1% and in the total cohort 0.05%. A German study in both children and adults conducted investigations for food allergy in 814 of 4,093 subjects who returned a questionnaire; 18 (2.2% of the investigated group) had confirmed reactions to food additives, making the population prevalence 0.4%[9]. These studies suggest that the likelihood of hypersensitivity to food additives is rare, and reviews of the subject support this.

However, prevalence in specific groups could be greater. A study on recurrent chronic idiopathic urticaria showed that sensitivity to food additives may be of the order of 1–3% in this group[10]. Of 838 patients with recurrent idiopathic urticaria,

116 (14%) had positive DBPCFC to mixed challenges containing tartrazine, erythrosine, monosodium benzoate, para-hydroxybenzoate, sodium metabisulphite, monosodium glutamate. However, when DBPCFC using incremental doses of single allergens was performed, only 24 subjects (2.8%) had a positive test to the single food allergens given. It has also been suggested that people with urticaria may have an increased sensitivity to histamine, although the numbers studied were small[11]. People with asthma may also be at increased risk of sensitivity to food additives; in 1979 Weber and colleagues suggested that 2% of asthmatics may be sensitive to food colourings and preservatives[12], but at that time the studies carried out did not use DBPCFC. More robust studies on sodium metabisulphite suggest that 5% of the adult asthmatic population of the USA could be affected by sulphites, even after the 1985 legislation banning sulphites in fresh foods[13-15]. The prevalence is higher in severe asthmatics, ranging from 3.9% in the general asthmatic population to 8.4% in steroid-dependent asthmatics in one study[16,17]. In children, food additives have been especially implicated in hyperactivity disorders (see Chapter 2). A study conducted in 2004 suggested that benzoates and food colourings could adversely affect the behaviour of children[18].

Food additives may also be involved in more severe reactions. In an analysis of 173 food-allergic and anaphylactic events in the USA, 'candy' was cited as a cause of a severe reaction in five cases (3%)[19]. There is no detail about the candy, although gummed sweets are mentioned, which suggests that colours could be involved, although gelatine is also a possible contender. In the UK, a study of severe food-allergic reactions in children also cited food colouring as a cause of two of the 171 non-severe cases (1.2%), but none of the severe reactions[20]. It is possible that these are naturally derived colourings such as carmine or annatto, which may have sufficient traces of allergen to mediate an IgE response.

10.1.2   Foods involved and symptoms elicited

A food additive is defined as 'any substance not normally consumed as a food in itself and not normally used as a characteristic ingredient of food whether or not it has nutritive value, the intentional addition of which to food for a technological purpose in the manufacture, processing, preparation, treatment, packaging, transport or storage of such food results, or may be reasonably expected to result, in it or its by-products becoming directly or indirectly a component of such foods' (Council Directive 89/107/EEC)[21]. The amounts that can be added to foods will be regulated by the type of food and also the amount of additive known to be safe for humans. Thus all additives have an 'acceptable daily intake' (ADI), determined through the establishment of the 'no-observed-adverse-effect level' (NOAEL), which is the maximum level of additive that has no demonstrable toxic effect[22]. The ADI is determined by the joint FAC/WHO Expert Committee on Food Additives and is defined as an estimate of the amount of a food additive, expressed on a body-weight basis, that can be ingested daily over a lifetime without appreciable health risk. It is measured in milligrams per kilogram of body weight[23]. All food additives, whether natural or artificial, have an 'E' number which signifies European Union approval.

The number signifies the function of the additive, so colours, preservatives and flavour enhances will all be in different number ranges. The Food Standards Agency has information on food additives and a comprehensive list of the E numbers used in the UK[24].

There are many hundreds of food additives used, but only a very small number have been implicated in food hypersensitivity and therefore studied in any great detail (Table 10.1). They have been implicated in a wide spectrum of food-hypersensitivity disorders including both immune-mediated and non-allergic conditions. Most additives, except for some natural food colourings, are low-molecular-weight chemicals which are ingested irregularly in very small amounts. In some reactions the dose of allergen may be critical, and there also appears to be a higher likelihood of reactions to additives in people who are atopic and already suffering from an allergic condition such as asthma, rhinitis or atopic dermatitis, who are thus more likely to release histamine after eating certain foods[25].

Most responses to food additives do not involve the production of IgE antibodies, except in a small number of cases where a protein might be involved, such as in allergy to natural food colourings derived from plant or animal sources. However, it has been proposed that some low-molecular-weight additives could bind to a carrier protein and act as a hapten[26]. Delayed type IV hypersensitivity is probably the most common expression of immune involvement in hypersensitivity to food colourings and benzoates, manifesting in eczema/atopic dermatitis (AD) symptoms[25]. Whereas type I hypersensitivity is immediate, type IV reactions are delayed and may involve a type of antigen known as a haptenated protein, where a small organic molecule or hapten becomes covalently attached to proteins in the tissues[27]. Allergic contact dermatitis may involve some food additives such as the antioxidants butylated hydroxytoluene (BHT) or butylated hydroxyanisole (BHA), sorbates or parahydroxy-benzoic acid, but can also involve spices, vitamin E, essential oils and other flavouring agents[25].

For sodium metabisulphite hypersensitivity, several mechanisms have been suggested for reactions, including the inhalation of sulphur dioxide, generated from sulphite-containing foods during the swallowing process. Evidence for an IgE mediation in the sulphite response is mixed, although it has been reported that sulphiting agents could induce mediator release from human mast cells, with a rise in plasma histamine levels demonstrated in one study[28]. Severe reactions, including anaphylaxis, may occur in asthmatics with low levels of sulphite oxidase[13]. Pharmacological mechanisms have also been suggested for some additives, especially those such as tartrazine and sodium benzoate which have similar chemical structures to aspirin. Aspirin can affect the synthesis of prostaglandins and leukotrienes; adverse reactions to aspirin may be caused by the inhibition of cyclooxygenase, which acts as a bronchodilator and inhibits prostaglandin synthesis[25]. In the 1980s it was suggested that food additives such as tartrazine may also have an inhibitory effect on the cyclooxygenase pathway in aspirin-intolerant individuals, but robust studies and reviews of more recent studies have not supported this theory[29,30].

Table 10.1 Main food additives which may be implicated in FHS reactions.

Additive type	Name	E number	Role in food production	Foods most likely to contain additive
Colourings	Tartrazine	E102	Orange food colouring	Coloured soft drinks, sweets, jams, cereals, snack foods, canned fish, packaged soups
	Sunset yellow	E110	Yellow food colouring	Cereals, bakery goods, sweets, snack foods, ice cream, soft drinks, medications
	Annatto	E160b	Naturally derived yellow food colouring	Coloured cheese, butter, margarine, cereals, snack foods
	Cochineal/carmine	E120	Naturally derived red food colouring	Meat, sausages, processed poultry products, marinades, alcoholic drinks, fruit drinks, biscuits, pie fillings, jam, jelly, some varieties of Cheddar cheese, sauces and sweets; sometimes also used in cosmetics.
	Amaranth	E123	Naturally derived red food colouring	Cake mixes, fruit-flavoured fillings, jelly crystals
Preservatives	Sulphites	E220–228	Preservative, and prevent browning	Cider, wine, lager, soft drinks, dried fruit, dried vegetables, lime and lemon juice, frozen potato products, beef burgers, sausages
	Benzoates	E210–219	Prevent yeast and mould growth in acidic foods	Soft drinks (especially orange varieties), salad dressings, jams, pickles and fruit-based products; found naturally in some foods such as cinnamon, cloves, raspberries, cranberries and prunes
Others	Monosodium glutamate	E621	Flavour enhancer	Soups, meat products, sauces, ready meals, dried pasta and noodle snacks, Chinese food

Food colourings

Artificial food colourings have probably attracted the most press with regard to hypersensitivity. In reality, however, reactions are extremely rare, even in high-risk groups such as those with asthma or urticaria, although food colourings have been linked to hyperactivity in non-atopic children (see Chapter 2). It is ironic that concern about artificial colours in foods has led to an increase in the use of natural food colourings, which can retain some protein fragments and have been implicated in IgE-mediated FHS reactions including anaphylaxis.

Natural food colourings

Natural food colourings include cochineal, annatto, turmeric and saffron. Cochineal (E120) is also known as carmine; it is a red dye made from the female bodies of the cactus-eating insect *Dactylopius coccus*. Carmine use was declining until concerns about artificial food colours in the 1980s led to increased demand for natural colorants. Cochineal or carmine is found in many foods, especially sweets, ice lollies, fruit yoghurt, some processed meats, jam, fruit juice etc. There have been several reports in the literature of carmine causing allergic reactions including anaphylaxis[31,32], and it has also been shown that commercial carmine retains insect-derived proteins which are responsible for IgE-mediated carmine allergy[31].

Annatto (E160b), a yellow food colouring, is a carotenoid extracted from the seeds of the tree *Bixa orellana*. It is used in many cheeses such as Cheddar and Red Leicester, but is also found in margarine, butter, smoked fish and custard powder. Although popular literature suggests that annatto is responsible for many allergic reactions, especially in relation to attention-deficit hyperactivity disorder, there have only been a couple of case reports in the scientific literature of an IgE-mediated food allergy to annatto, probably due to contaminating or residual seed proteins[33,34]. Turmeric (E100) is extracted from *Curcuma longa*, a plant from the ginger family. This orange-yellow powder is added to curries and is often part of curry powders. It is also used to colour mustard condiments, and may be added to many orange-coloured foods. Studies of turmeric have not shown that it causes any type of symptoms related to allergic reactions[35], although curcumin, the active ingredient in tumeric, has been reported to cause contact dermatitis in isolated cases[36,37]. Interestingly, curcumin is reported to have antiallergic properties, with Lee *et al.* reporting that it inhibits certain signalling mechanisms in mast cells[38]. Saffron is a red/yellow food dye which is extracted from the bulb *Crocus sativus*. It is traditionally used in rice dishes such as paella, but also in soups, sauces and other foods. Despite its widespread use, there has only been one case report of anaphylaxis to saffron[39].

Artificial food colourings

Artificial food colours include the azo dyes, which are synthetic colours that contain an azo group as part of their structure. There are many azo dyes, but the ones most commonly used in foods in the UK are tartrazine (E102), quinoline yellow (E104), sunset yellow (E110), azorubine or carmoisine (E122), amaranth (E123), ponceau

4R (E124) and allura red (E129). Azo dyes account for approximately 60–70% of all dyes used in food and textile manufacture, as they are very stable and do not fade in sunlight. The azo dye which has been the best studied in connection with food hypersensitivity is tartrazine; its chemical structure is very similar to that of both benzoate and salicylate, the active ingredient in aspirin[25]. It is this chemical similarity which has led many to evaluate whether those who are asthmatic and aspirin-sensitive are more likely to be affected by tartrazine. Although many studies have been carried out the study designs were often limited, and in a large study in 1986 using DBPCFC, Stevenson and colleagues failed to detect tartrazine-induced asthma in any of their 150 subjects[30]. A 2006 best-practice guideline stated that current evidence suggests that although tratrazine may be a rare cause of bronchospasm in asthmatic patients, there is no convincing evidence to support the contention that tartrazine cross-reacts with non-steroidal anti-inflammatory drugs such as aspirin and ibuprofen[29].

Another condition which it has been suggested could be exacerbated by tartrazine is urticaria, with an early study by Juhlin suggesting a very high prevalence of sensitivity to tartrazine amongst those with urticaria[40]. However more recent studies, which have included DBPCFC have not confirmed this. One study of 102 subjects reported that only one patient (1%) had a reaction to a dose of 5 mg tartrazine given by DBPCFC[41], and Di Lorenzo and colleagues showed that out of 838 patients with chronic idiopathic urticaria only 3 (0.4%) had reactions to tartrazine alone[10]. Interestingly, the Di Lorenzo study also assessed reactions to DBPCFC with mixed additives and found that more subjects with urticaria had positive challenges to the mixed challenges than they did to the single challenges. The role of tartrazine has also been evaluated in the aetiology of atopic dermatitis (AD), with tartrazine appearing to be capable of inducing leukotriene release in AD patients with a proven food hypersensitivity, although the same group also found that only a few AD patients reacted to provocation with food additives in a DBPCFC[42,43]. A group of patients with mixed dermatological conditions were studied, and it was shown that although five subjects reacted to a mix of additives including sulphites, benzoates, monosodium glutamate and the colourings amaranth, erythrosine, tartrazine and sunset yellow, the differences in reported reactions between the active and placebo doses were not significant. The conclusion was that these additives at 10% of the ADI do not cause dermatologic reactions or aggravate AD symptoms[44].

The predominant view from experts[45] is that azo dyes are unlikely to precipitate FHS in most people. However, some interesting recent evidence has emerged linking artificial food colours to hyperactivity in children. This link was first proposed in the 1970s by Feingold, who hypothesised that a diet free of additives could help in the treatment or prevention of hyperactivity in children[46]. Although subsequent studies did not appear to support this theory, two studies published in 2004 and 2007 have suggested that a mix of sodium benzoate and food colourings, including tartrazine, could affect behaviour and can increase hyperactivity in some children[18,47]. The publication of these studies has increased pressure on manufacturers to remove artificial colours from foods (see also Chapter 2).

Food preservatives

Benzoates and parabens

These occur naturally, in the form of free acid or salts, in foods such as cinnamon, cloves, tea, prunes and berries such as raspberry and cranberry[48]. Benzoates (E210–219) and in particular sodium benzoate (E211) are added to foods to retard the growth of bacteria, and are typically found in beer, jam, fruit products, pickled foods, yoghurt and salad cream. Parabens are the esters of para-hydroxybenzoic acid and are used as antimicrobial agents mainly in cosmetics and drugs, but they have also been used in foods including fruit juices, pickles, sauces and soft drinks[48]. There have been many studies assessing the involvement of benzoates in chronic urticaria and angio-oedema, and the evidence is very mixed. A study by Ortolani *et al.* in 1984 showed that 3 out of 396 (0.75%) subjects with chronic urticaria and angiooedema had positive DBPCFCs to sodium benzoate alone, but 12 reacted to one or more additives[49]. More recent studies have shown similar results, with one showing that 1 subject out of 47 with urticaria had symptoms induced by sodium benzoate[50]. Another study found that 8 of 838 patients with recurrent chronic idiopathic urticaria (0.95%) had positive DBPCFC with monosodium benzoate[10]. There have also been case reports of sodium-benzoate-induced pruritis in the absence of a skin rash[51]. Benzoates have also been suggested as having a role in both asthma and AD, but the studies have not shown a link, although benzoates have been linked with an increased production of leukotrienes in AD patients[43,48]. Parabens may often cause contact dermatitis when in cosmetics (contact reactions), but rarely cause this problem in the food industry (ingested reaction)[25].

Benzoates have also been proposed to have a role in persistent rhinitis. The evidence was reviewed in 2004 by Asero, who concluded on the basis of previous studies that it is possible that about 5% of patients with non-allergic perennial rhinitis might have additive intolerance[52]. He suggested that those patients who have had perennial rhinitis for more than 6 months, or a diagnosis of allergic rhinitis in the absence of nasal polyps and structural deformities, a normal plain radiograph or scan and no skin prick test reactivity to aeroallergens, should commence an additive-free elimination diet for three weeks. Those who have had a complete and persistent disappearance of their symptoms should undergo an unrestricted diet for three weeks, with those who relapse being challenged by DBPCFC. A study of 226 patients with persistent rhinitis by Pacor and colleagues showed an additive-free diet improved the symptoms of 20 subjects (9%), with 6 being completely symptom-free[53]. On DBPCFC, objective symptoms were shown by 20 subjects (9%) only when challenged with sodium benzoate, although other additives also induced subjective symptoms in 45 patients. Their conclusion was that some patients with chronic vasomotor rhinitis may be intolerant of food additives, but these additives are triggers or aggravating factors rather than aetiological factors. Benzoates have also been linked to behaviour in children, with two studies evaluating the effect of a mix of food colours and benzoates on behaviour and hyperactivity[18,47].

Sodium metabisulphite

Sodium metabisulphite is a multifunctional preservative which is part of the sulphite group of preservatives (E220–228). Sodium metabisulphite (E223) and potassium metabisulphite (E224) are also added to foods to prevent enzymatic and non-enzymatic browning. Sulphites react with the disulphide bonds in proteins, and can also combine with carbohydrates, and therefore will exist in a free or bound form in foods[54]. Free-form sulphite is more likely to cause a reaction than bound sulphite[55]. The main sources of sulphite in the diet will vary according to the type of foods normally consumed and also the amount of sulphites permitted to be added to foods. The maximum permitted level (MPL) of sulphur dioxide, expressed in mg/kg or mg/litre, varies greatly, with dried fruit having an MPL between 600 and 2,000 mg/kg and wine 200 mg/litre (EU Directive 95/2/EC)[56]. The amount added can depend on the raw materials, and so for wine can vary from year to year and from vineyard to vineyard. Wine samples analysed in Italy contained an average of 92 mg/kg, but ranged from undetectable to 198 mg/kg[57]. Wine (especially white wine), cider, lager, frozen chips and roast potatoes, dried foods such as dried fish, onions, apricots and potato products, salads, lemon/lime juice, grape juice, wine vinegar and fruit drinks such as fruit cordial or 'squash' are most likely to cause symptoms in sensitive individuals. The EU Directive adopted in the UK in 2005 (2003/89/EC) requires added sulphites to be listed on the product label if the amount is greater than 10 mg/litre or 10 mg/kg[58]. This considerably simplifies the dietary exclusion of sulphites in the future, but unlabelled foods containing the additive or labelled foods containing less than 10 mg/kg, but consumed in large amounts, could still elicit reactions.

It has been well established through DBPCFCs that sodium metabisulphite mainly affects asthmatic patients, with about 5% of asthmatics being hypersensitive to the chemical, and those with more severe or steroid-dependent asthma being at greater risk[13–17]. The main symptom associated with sulphites is bronchospasm in asthmatic subjects. For many asthmatics, bronchospasm can occur on exposure to less than 1 ppm (1 mg/kg) of sulphur dioxide; however, this is non-progressive and does not require bronchodilator treatment. The bronchoconstriction is not due to the alteration of airway pH, or a response to an irritant (sulphur dioxide) in an asthmatic population more sensitive to airway irritants, since making the lungs more sensitive and hyper-reactive to irritants by challenging the lungs with metha-choline does not lead to an increased reaction when the lungs are then challenged with sulphur dioxide[13,59]. Unlike azo dyes and benzoates, there appears to be no cross-reactivity between aspirin and sulphites, and an aspirin-sensitive asthmatic is unlikely to be at greater risk of having coexisting sulphite sensitivity[28]. Other reactions are less common, although urticaria and angio-oedema have been reported, and anaphylaxis-like events described[60]. There have also been case reports of rhinitis being induced by sodium metabisulphite[61].

Nitrates and nitrites

Nitrates and nitrites (E249–252) are used in processed meats, where they also add flavour and colour. It has been suggested that they can cause urticaria and pruritis in some individuals, and isolated case reports in the literature also suggest they could cause anaphylaxis, although the mechanism is not clear[62–64].

Flavour enhancers

Monosodium glutamate (MSG)

In addition to the four primary tastes, there is a fifth taste called umami, which describes the palatability or deliciousness of food[65]. This taste was characteristic of Asian cuisine, and in 1908 it was discovered that the common amino acid L-glutamate in dried kelp was responsible for the taste[66]. Glutamate is an essential amino acid that occurs naturally, in either a protein-bound or free form, in foods such as tomatoes, Parmesan cheese and soy sauce. Other forms of naturally occurring protein-bound MSG also exist, most notably in yeast extract and hydrolysed vegetable protein. About one-third of the intake of MSG in the UK comes from added MSG (E621), used widely in food manufacturing and restaurants. The average daily intake varies from country to country: figures from the US Food and Drug Administration show that the intake of MSG ranges from up to 0.5 g in the USA to 1.6 g in Korea[66]. MSG appears to produce a variety of symptoms including headache, neck pain, nausea, tingling, flushing and chest heaviness[29] first described by Kwok in 1968 as the 'Chinese restaurant syndrome'[67]. In 1987 Settipane suggested that 'restaurant syndromes' could be precipitated by food allergens, sulphites, MSG, tartrazine, or scombroid poisoning, but described symptoms of burning, pressure, and tightness or numbness in the face, neck, and upper chest following ingestion of Chinese food as likely to be due to a diagnosis of MSG hypersensitivity[68]. However, studies in individuals with reported reactions to MSG have varied. In 1997, a study found that 22 of 61 subjects had reproducible symptoms of headache, muscle tightness, numbness/tingling, general weakness and flushing, with the threshold dose for reactivity being 2.5 gm MSG[69]. In 2000 a larger study of 130 subjects confirmed that large doses of MSG (5 g) given without food may illicit symptoms, but these were not serious or persistent or consistent on re-testing[70].

MSG has been associated with the provocation of symptoms in asthmatic subjects. A study by Allen and colleagues in 1987 showed that 13 of 32 subjects with asthma reacted to doses ranging from 0.5 mg to 5 mg, many with delayed reactions[71]. However, two more recent studies have failed to reproduce these results. One undertook DBPCFC on 12 asthmatics with a history of MSG intolerance over a three-day period, and had no positive responders[72]. A much larger study investigating 100 asthmatics, 30 with a history of oriental restaurant attacks, found that 12 of the 30 had aspirin sensitivity, but none had asthma on challenge with DBPCFC of 2.5 mg MSG[73]. A review by Stevenson in 2000 concluded that the existence of MSG-induced asthma, even in patients with a positive history, has not been established conclusively[74], and this was endorsed by a best-practice review in 2006[29]. MSG has also been linked to urticaria: a study in 2000 found two patients (3%) reacted at a level of 2.5 g MSG but this was not reproduced on DBPCFC[75]. Another study in 2005, looking at multiple additives, reported that only three (0.3%) patients with chronic idiopathic urticaria had reactions to MSG, but the dose was only 0.4 g, which may be considered rather a low dose to elicit a response[10]. Various case reports have suggested that MSG could induce urticaria, and also provoke rhinitis in certain individuals[52,61]. Therefore, although MSG consumption has been linked to many different symptoms, very little evidence from formal studies has shown that MSG in small doses is likely to cause an adverse effect in most people.

Other additives

Various other food additives have been linked with food hypersensitivity, including butylated hydroxytoluene (BHT) and butylated hydroxyanisole (BHA), which are antioxidants used in a large number of foods containing fat. A review suggested that although adverse reactions have been best substantiated in the skin, with a suggested high incidence of intolerance in those with chronic urticaria, a lack of studies using DBPCFC means that the true prevalence of adverse reactions to BHA and BHT is still unclear[76]. Flavourings can sometimes be implicated in allergic reactions, and can be split into contact sensitisers, spices and fruit concentrates. Those which can cause contact allergy such as dermatitis include the cinnamon family which includes Balsam of Peru. Balsam of Peru is a cinnamon-containing flavouring compound that can be found in toothpaste, hard sweets, marmalade, ice cream, cinnamon, clove or vanilla (see also Chapter 2). Other flavouring products which could be involved in contact dermatitis include clove oil, anise, fennel oil, d-limonene, menthol, peppermint oil and spearmint oil[77]. Spices and fruit concentrates can both cause reactions which have the potential to be IgE-mediated (see also Chapter 7). In addition to spices, there are other food additives which are derived from plant foods such as guar gum (E412), carageenan (E407) and tragacanth (E413). The literature contains case reports of reactions to all of these foods.

10.1.3 Diagnosis

History

It can be difficult from the history to pinpoint whether an additive is likely to be the cause of any reaction. Many people may suspect a food additive, especially when there is no obvious cause for their allergy. It is clear from the literature that a very small percentage of those who suspect they have an allergic reaction to additives actually do so, but this does not mean that it should be ruled out entirely, as case reports have shown good evidence for remission of symptoms by removal of a food additive. Wilson and Bahna suggest that although adverse reactions to additives are rare, they are likely to be under-diagnosed due to a low index of suspicion on the part of the physician[78]. Sometimes reported reactions to particular foods may be misleading. For example, reported reactions to wine, a beverage commonly thought to be implicated in sodium metabisulphite hypersensitivity, need careful investigation to rule out other triggers such as vasoactive amines, grape allergy and hypersensitivity to other added ingredients.

It has been proposed that adverse reactions to food additives should be suspected when symptoms after foods and drinks happen but not every time the food in question is consumed[29]. Food-additive hypersensitivity can also be suspected in those who report symptoms to multiple unrelated foods, or to a certain foods when commercially prepared but not when homemade[78]. Although an IgE-mediated reaction is usually not involved, it is not always the case that a reaction to a food additive can be characterised by delayed reactions. For example, sodium metabisulphite hypersensitivity can cause symptoms within 30 minutes of ingestion, and occasionally bronchospasm will be immediate.

Tests

Tests for specific IgE estimation are not usually helpful, as the reactions are not normally IgE-mediated, although where a naturally derived food colouring or flavouring is suspected, then tests to specific IgE antibodies may be helpful if available. Some studies have reported positive skin prick tests for sodium metabisulphite and tartrazine, but these have not always been validated by positive DBPCFCs and are usually not reliable and not available commercially. Patch testing is useful for contact dermatitis where parabens, spices or Balsam of Peru are suspected[25]. However, for most suspected food-additive allergy following ingestion, the best method will be a complete elimination of the offending additive from the diet for 3 weeks followed by reintroduction of the additive, with symptoms scored throughout the period if possible by recording skin, nasal or respiratory symptoms on an agreed scale, or using objective measures such as monitoring of peak flow. However, not all additives will be found in the same quantities in all foods; one study took eight subjects with sulphite sensitivity previously confirmed by capsule challenge, and exposed them to a variety of sulphited foods, finding that 50% failed to respond to any exposures[79]. However, those who derive benefit from the exclusion and report worsening of symptoms on reintroduction of the additive should have an oral food challenge. The normal method in most studies is the additive given in a standard or incrementally increasing dose, sometime over several days, but this may be difficult as such additives are not commercially available and cannot always be purchased in small quantities. It also needs to be borne in mind that some additives may not respond in the same way in a capsule challenge. For example, this method may bypass sodium metabisulphite reactions due to inhalation, and also some additives may act as haptens and therefore require the presence of protein in order to cause a reaction. Di Lorenzo and others have reported that DBPCFCs with single allergens were less often positive than DBPCFCs containing mixed additives in the same patients[10].

10.1.4 Management

Management of a hypersensitivity to any additive requires the avoidance of all foods containing the relevant additive. All of the additives have an identifiable E number, but it is also helpful to know which foods are more likely to contain them.

Some people may be able to tolerate small amounts of additives. For example, people sensitive to sodium metabisulphite may be able to eat some sulphited foods, but unable to tolerate foods containing the sulphite above a certain threshold level. There should not be any nutritional consequences as a result of removal of food additives from the diet, although the diets of children may be lower in energy as a consequence due to a lower consumption of sweets, fizzy drinks and snack foods.

10.2 Pharmacologic food reactions

10.2.1 Salicylates

Prevalence

Salicylate is a signalling molecule in plants with a spectrum of activities including anti-inflammatory actions[80]. Willow and meadowsweet were used in ancient times to treat fevers and pain, and it is suggested that this is due to their high salicylic acid content[81]. Aspirin is a synthetic derivative of salicylic acid called acetylsalicylic acid which is rapidly hydrolysed to salicylate in the gut following oral administration[82]. Aspirin acts by preventing the conversion of arachidonic acid to cyclic prostenoids by inhibiting the enzyme cyclooxygenase (COX)[83]. There are two isoforms of COX, COX-1 and COX-2, and aspirin is a potent inhibitor of COX-1, whereas non-acetylated salicylate such as salicylic acid inhibits COX-2[82,84]. Salicylic acid is found in many food plants, and there is wide range of published values for salicylates in foods[84-86]. Aspirin and other non-steroidal anti-inflammatory drugs (NSAIDS) are common causes of drug reactions, and the prevalence of aspirin hypersensitivity is thought to range from 0.6% to 2.5%, but this increases to 4.3–11% in asthmatics[87]. Aspirin-sensitive asthmatics may often have nasal polyposis, and aspirin triad disease was first reported in 1922, but characterised by Samter and Beers in 1967 as a non-immunologic systemic disease[88], and the condition is often known as Samter's triad.

It is unknown whether non-acetylated salicylate such as the naturally occurring salicylic acid in foods can also provoke response in aspirin-sensitive asthmatics or those with additional nasal polyposis. Studies have suggested that responses do occur, and also that it is dose-dependent, with an intake of 2.6 mg of salicylate reported to be the mean dose eliciting a 15% decrease in FEV1 in sensitive asthmatics[89]. It has been suggested that intolerance of NSAIDS was of clinical import for 2–7% of patients suffering from food allergy and inflammatory bowel disease, and that salicylate intolerance should always be considered in these cases[90]. However, other studies have shown that many aspirin-intolerant asthmatics can tolerate dietary salicylate in high amounts[91].

Foods involved

One of the main issues, apart from the efficacy of a dietary exclusion of salicylate, is the fact that the reported levels of salicylic acid in foods vary greatly. In 1985 Swain *et al.* published the salicylate content of 333 foods[85], and for many years this has remained the mainstay of advice on salicylate avoidance. However, studies in the last two decades have bought those values into question, with data from Venema *et al.* in 1995 showing marked differences in the amounts of salicylate in foods[86], being at much lower levels than those published by Swain. It was estimated by Swain *et al.* that the normal diet could provide 10–200 mg natural salicylates[85], whereas from Venema *et al.* it appears that a level of 0–5 mg is more likely[86]. The variation is thought to be due to differences in methodology, but it is possible that varietal differences, shelf-life and growing conditions could all affect salicylate content[92], with one study on soups demonstrating that organic vegetable soups contained more salicylic acid than non-organic ones[93]. The salicylic acid in spices has also been reassessed, having been found to be very high in Swain's data; Paterson and colleagues showed that total salicylic acids in spices were comparable to the levels in the Swain data, and that the salicylate content of blood and urine increased following consumption of the meal, indicating that this dietary source of salicylic acid was bioavailable[94].

As the data from Swain are now more than 20 years old, it is helpful that we have some more recent data published in 2007 by Scotter and colleagues, who analysed the free salicylic acid and acetylsalicylic acid content of 76 foods[84]. Their data for the salicylate contents of some foods were very different to those published by Swain *et al.*[85], especially for some fresh fruits and vegetables: bananas are salicylate-free according to Swain's data, but Scotter showed they contained 0.4 mg/kg of salicylic acid. Herbs, spices and loose tea were the most consistent food items tested, with all studies showing them to contain high levels of salicylic acid. Other foods which have been identified as being high in salicylate include oil of wintergreen, coffee, wine, bilberries, blackcurrants, grapes, peaches, strawberries, tomatoes, toothpastes and chewing gum (Table 10.2).

Diagnosis and management

There are no effective diagnostic tests for salicylate intolerance, and no studies showing the efficacy of dietary exclusion. The best method of choosing who would benefit from a salicylate exclusion is therefore an evaluation of the clinical history. The presence of aspirin sensitivity or Samter's triad is a good starting point, also looking for clues in the dietary history such as reported problems with black pepper, herbs or spices. Since salicylate occurs in many foods, and the quantities are a subject of controversy, it is probably more effective to trial an avoidance of only those foods known to be very high in salicylate. It needs to be remembered that the amount of salicylate in foods is much lower than in a typical dose of aspirin: for example, Scotter's data suggest that although curry powder contains 15.2 mg of salicylic acid per kg, the actual amount in a curry will only be in the region of 0.05 mg. Therefore a 4-week trial of the avoidance of high-salicylate foods should help to establish whether more stringent avoidance will be worth the subsequent dietary restrictions.

In the long term, people who are avoiding salicylate-containing foods may need dietary assessment to ensure that they are still maintaining an adequate intake of

Table 10.2 Foods high in salicylates.

Fruits	Green apples, apricot, blackberry, blackcurrant, blueberry, cherry, cranberry, currants, grapefruit, grapes, guava, lemon, loganberry, nectarine, orange, peach, plum, prunes, raisins raspberry, redcurrant, rhubarb, strawberry, sultanas, tangerine
Vegetables	Alfalfa sprouts, artichoke, aubergine, broad beans, carrot (raw), chicory, chilli peppers, courgette, cucumber, endive, gherkins, mushrooms, okra, olives, peas, peppers green, radishes, tomatoes, water chestnut
Nuts and snacks	Almonds, Peanuts, Flavoured crisps/snacks Muesli/cereal bars
Herbs, sauces and pickles	Cloves, Commercial sauces and gravies, cumin, tumeric, curry powder, ginger, thyme, large amounts of other herbs and spices, pickles, tomato paste, wine or cider vinegar, Worcester sauce, yeast extract
Sweets and spreads	Honey, jam, marmalade, liquorice, chewing gum, peppermints, other mint flavoured sweets
Beverages	Coloured fizzy drinks, fruit cordials, fruit squashes, fruit juices, peppermint tea, chamomile tea, leaf tea, champagne, liqueurs, port, rum, sherry, wine
Fats and oils	Coconut oil, creamed coconut, olive oil
Other sources of salicylate	Products flavoured with mint or menthol, such as toothpaste and mouthwash, also cough sweets containing menthol or oil of wintergreen

Adapted from the leaflet *Salicylate Information* by Catherine O'Donnell. Based on data from Scotter *et al.*[84] and Swain *et al.*[85]. Reproduced with permission from the author.

fresh fruits and vegetables. The intake of high-salicylate foods has been extensively investigated to assess its beneficial effects on cancer and heart disease. It is therefore very important to establish the efficacy of the diet and make sure any long-term exclusions are being balanced by the inclusion of other foods with the same health benefits.

10.2.2 Vasoactive or Biogenic amines

Prevalence

Vasoactive amines are the commonest cause of pharmacologic food reactions, and unlike food allergic reactions can affect a wide and diverse group of individuals, with the quantity of food necessary to elicit a reaction varying between individuals[95]. The vasoactive amines include norepinephrine, tryptamine, dopamine, histamine, phenylethylamine, serotonin and tyramine, and all except the first two can be present in food in amounts with the potential to cause an effect in sensitive individuals[96]. A review of the literature in 2003 concluded that 'The current scientific literature shows no relation between the oral ingestion of biogenic amines and food intolerance reactions. There is therefore no scientific basis for dietary recommendations concerning biogenic amines in such patients'[97]. Others have concluded that reactions to histamine and other vasoactive amines are only going to affect a small percentage of people with the inability to break down histamine, and it is food allergy which should be of greater concern[98]. However, a review by Maintz in 2007 concluded that the incidence of histamine-intolerance has been underestimated and further studies are needed[99].

Foods involved

Histamine

Histamine is a diamine, and probably the best-known vasoactive amine responsible for pharmacologic reactions to food. Reactions involving histamine are probably those most frequently confused with food allergy. They appear to be dose-dependent, with the ingestion of anything from 36 to 250 mg of histamine eliciting reactions[96], although reactions to amounts as low as 2.5 mg have been reported[100]. Dietary histamine is usually rapidly detoxified by diamine oxidase, but in people with reduced diamine oxidase activity histamine cannot be degraded and the excess may cause symptoms similar to those elicited by an IgE-mediated food allergic reaction involving histamine release from mast cells[99]. These symptoms are on a spectrum ranging from headache, rhinoconjunctivitis, flushing and pruritis through to urticaria, asthma, arrhythmia, hypotension and abdominal cramping. The most severe symptoms tend to be related to histamine poisoning from the consumption of fish containing excessive histamine due to the bacterial decarboxylation of histidine: this is known as scombroid poisoning (see Chapter 6). In addition to those with low levels of diamine oxidase, it has been proposed that histamine may also play a role in chronic idiopathic urticaria, with one study showing that an oligoantigenic and histamine-free diet induced significant improvement of symptoms in ten patients[11].

The foods generally thought to contain more histamine include three specific types of cheese (Parmesan, blue, Roquefort), red wine (Chianti and Burgundy), spinach, aubergines, yeast extract and scombroid fish such as tuna, mackerel[95]. There have been several studies examining wine, as this is particularly associated with flushing, headache and nasal congestion. Although histamine has been suggested as being causative of these reactions, studies have been inconclusive or have shown no correlation between the histamine content of wine and wine intolerance[101,102]. There are other foods which do not contain histamine but may trigger the degranulation of mast cells. These histamine-releasing foods include egg white, chocolate, strawberries, ethanol, tomatoes and citrus fruits[103].

Monoamines

There are a number of other vasoactive amines which have been reported to cause symptoms in sensitive individuals and these are the monoamines, in particular tyramine and phenylethylamine. Monoamines are metabolised by monoamine oxidase (MAO), and people susceptible to monoamines include those with rare genetic variations of the MAO subtype, or those taking MAO inhibitor (MAOI) drugs[95]. Dietary tyramine may affect those who are taking MAOI drugs or who have migraine headaches, although the results of studies looking at migraine and

Table 10.3 Foods high in vasoactive amines.

Vegetables	Pumpkin, broad beans, aubergine, spinach, tomato and tomato products, sauerkraut
Fruit	Avocado, citrus fruits, ripe bananas, tinned figs, pineapple, strawberries
Cheese	Any ripened, hard or mature cheese especially Roquefort cheese, parmesan and very strong cheddar cheese,
Fish	Tuna, sardine, anchovy, mackerel, salmon, caviar, herring, prawn, shrimp, crab, lobster, cockles, mussels, scallops, processed fish products, pickled and dried fish
Meat and egg	All cured meat and pork including salami, pepperoni, cured ham such as Parma ham, game, bacon, pork chops etc, egg white such as meringues
Alcohol	Red wine (including vinegar), white wine, beer, cider, spirits
Other	Chocolate, cocoa, yeast extract, egg white, miso, tempeh and cola drinks

tyramine have not shown a consistent link (for more about migraine, see Chapter 2). Tyramine is usually found in fermented foods such as cheese (Camembert and Cheddar), yeast extract, red wine (especially Chianti), chicken liver, fermented beans such as soya and miso soup, and pickled rollmop herring. Phenylethylamine, found in cheese, wine and chocolate, is thought to induce headache in susceptible individuals. One study suggested that 3 mg of phenylethylamine provoked headache in people who suffered from chocolate-induced headaches[104], although a criticism of this study was that patients would have to consume a great deal of chocolate in order to ingest 3 mg of phenylethylamine[25]. Other monoamines include dopamine, which has a similar effect to tyramine, and is present in broad beans, and serotonin, the dietary form of which does not appear to produce any clinical symptoms.

Diagnosis and management

The only way to diagnose hypersensitivity to dietary vasoactive amines is to undertake a thorough dietary history and trial an exclusion of foods high in vasoactive amines, to include symptom scoring of objective symptoms before and during the trialled exclusion. Patients who report benefits should be asked to reintroduce the foods and reassess symptoms. Table 10.3 lists examples of foods which are high in vasoactive amines.

10.2.3 Caffeine and chocolate

Caffeine belongs to a group of substances known as dietary methylxanthines, which also includes theophylline and theobromine. The latter two are not normally the cause of adverse reactions to the foods they are contained in, as only cocoa and chocolate contain any appreciable amount of theobromine, and theophylline is only present in tiny amounts in food[95]. Caffeine is a natural stimulant found in the seeds

Table 10.4 The amount of caffeine in different beverages and foods[105,106].

Food	Portion size	Caffeine content (mg)
Ground roasted coffee	140 ml	85
Instant coffee	140 ml	60
Decaffeinated coffee	140 ml	3
Leaf or bag tea	140 ml	30
Instant tea	140 ml	20
Cola drink	170 ml	18
Caffeine drink	1 serving	0–141
Other soft drinks, including various cola drinks	1 serving	0–48
Cocoa/hot chocolate	140 ml	4
Chocolate milk	170 ml	4
Chocolate bar	100 g	5–21

of the coffee, tea and cocoa plants, which increases arterial tension, stimulates the central nervous system, promotes urine formation and increases the activity of the heart and lungs. The amount in beverages and chocolate varies (Table 10.4), and it has been estimated that the average consumption is 4 mg per kg bodyweight per day[105,106]. This is a much higher estimate than that produced by a more recent study, which showed average caffeine consumption to be 193 mg per day, i.e. 1.2 mg caffeine/kg/day[107]. This study also showed that as age increased, caffeine consumption increased: adults aged 35–64 years were among the highest consumers of caffeine, with major sources of caffeine being coffee (71%) for adults and soft drinks (16%) for children and teens.

Caffeine can cause anxiety symptoms in normal individuals, especially in vulnerable patients, such as those with pre-existing anxiety disorders[108]. Caffeine can reduce cerebral blood flow[109], and consumption has been linked to disordered sleep[110]. It has also been suggested that pregnant women who had high intakes of caffeine were more likely to have low-birth-weight babies, although reducing caffeine intake had no effect on birth weight or length of gestation[111]. There have been several case reports of allergic reactions to caffeine, including one patient who had anaphylaxis to coffee as a child and had symptoms of urticaria and pruritis on consumption of large volumes of cola drink[112]. Cola drinks have also been reported to cause urticaria in someone who did not drink tea or coffee but tolerated chocolate and had a positive DBPCFC with caffeine[113].

Chocolate is manufactured from the seeds of the cacao nut (*Theobroma cacao* in the Sterculiaceae family) and contains theobromine, which like caffeine is also a methylxanthine. Although not related to other tree nuts botanically, there is a similarity between the seed storage proteins of cacao and walnut[114]. Chocolate has been cited as a common cause of self-reported allergy in surveys both in the USA[115] and in Russia and neighbouring countries[4]. Although there have been case reports of chocolate allergy[116,117], and it has also been linked to migraine (see Chapter 2), an allergy to chocolate is uncommon[118]. This is because the seeds are extensively processed, which means the proteins in chocolate are present in non-allergic complexes[29,119]. However, Chapman *et al.* suggest that an increasing trend towards the consumption of gourmet chocolate, containing pieces of roasted or raw cacao nut, could see an increase in reported reactions[29]. Chocolate extract may not reflect the allergens present in processed chocolate, because this extract may be manufactured from raw cacao seeds[29]; therefore the best method of ascertaining the likelihood of a chocolate allergy is to take a detailed diet history and perform open and blinded oral food challenges. It is also important to consider the many other ingredients added to chocolate which could be the real culprit.

10.2.4 Alcohol

Prevalence

Alcohol has many well-known pharmacological properties, but can also cause sensitivity reactions through alcohol-induced peripheral vasodilation, which manifests as flushing, tachycardia, hypotension and nausea and vomiting. About 50% of people of Asian ethnicity are unable to tolerate alcohol, because of diminished or inhibited aldehyde dehydrogenase enzymatic activity[120]. There are individuals who have a hypersensitivity to alcohol, but there are only a handful of case reports in the literature[121]. One study challenged patients who had reported symptoms to alcoholic drinks with pure ethanol, and 50% of them had reactions, but these were thought unlikely to be IgE-mediated as skin prick tests were negative[122]. The rest of these patients may have been hypersensitive to the components in alcoholic drinks rather than to the alcohol itself. Vally suggests that asthmatics often report that alcoholic drinks trigger their symptoms, and has undertaken studies which show that wine is an especially common reported trigger, possibly due to its sulphite content[123,124]. However, the relationship between alcoholic drinks and allergic symptoms may be more complex; alcohol intake is associated with increased total serum IgE levels[125]. Further work by this group has shown that levels of sensitivity to cross-reactive carbohydrate determinants were greatly increased in heavy drinkers, and were associated with positive IgE to pollens and hymenoptera venom[126]. Another study showed that in 3,317 subjects there was a statistically significant association between alcohol consumption and aeroallergen sensitisation, but only in those who consumed 15–20 alcoholic drinks a week after adjustment[127]. In a cohort of 5,870 women, alcohol consumption was associated with an increased risk of developing perennial allergic rhinitis[128]. A questionnaire survey of over 4,000 people in Denmark showed that 13.9% had experienced alcohol-induced hypersensitivity symptoms, and these were significantly more prevalent in those with asthma and allergic rhinitis[129].

Foods involved

Ehlers and colleagues have shown that reactions to ethanol might not be as uncommon as previously supposed, and it is important to evaluate ethanol alone before considering other factors[122]. Nonetheless, many people who report reactions to alcoholic drinks may in fact be reacting to other components in alcoholic drinks. These include histamine and other biogenic amines, sodium metabisulphite and sodium benzoate, additives used to 'fine' or clarify wine or beer, and non-specific lipid transfer protein (nsLTP) allergens in grapes, barley and wheat (see Chapter 7). Wine and beer are the two commonest alcoholic beverages reported to cause reactions, with no reactions to cider, vodka, gin, whisky or brandy reported in the literature. Severe reactions to beer have been reported, including urticaria and anaphylaxis both to traditional barley-based beer and to wheat beer[130-133]. In some patients this hypersensitivity is associated with a concomitant allergy to corn, and in the case of barley an nsLTP may be responsible for the reactions. Sodium metabisulphite can also be present in lager, and may also need to be considered as a possible cause of symptoms in the absence of positive specific IgE antibodies to the relevant cereal.

Wine is the main alcoholic drink eliciting reactions. Apart from the biogenic amines, the main agent thought to be responsible is sodium metabisulphite, a common preservative added to wine (see above). However, studies on wine-induced asthma have not been conclusive. Vally and colleagues studied low- and high-sulphite wines in patients with a history of wine-induced asthma, and found that only 2 out of 16 reacted to a high-sulphite wine[134]. Another study carried out by the same group in 2001 showed that only 4 out of 24 patients sensitive to wine reacted to a very high-sulphite wine, but did not respond to moderate or low levels of sulphites in wine[135]. A study from the same authors in 2007 showed conclusively that changes in bronchial hyper-responsiveness, in the absence of reductions in FEV1, were observed in some asthmatic patients following a challenge with high-sulphite wine, but these changes were not consistent with a single aetiology[136]. Various food derivatives are added to wine to fine or clarify the end product. Isinglass is one such additive, and although derived from fish it is not considered to be an allergen. One study looked at whether such additives could trigger an allergic response in a predisposed individual, and concluded that wines fined with egg white, isinglass (from fish), or non-grape-derived tannins present an extremely low risk of anaphylaxis to people who are fish-, egg- or peanut-allergic[137]. Wine can also cause an IgE-mediated reaction due to the presence of nsLTPs in the grapes, with several case reports of anaphylaxis to wine having been published[138,139] (see also Chapter 7). It has been suggested that there are many other factors which may contribute to the reactions, including the temperature and acidity of the wine, the rate it is consumed and even other stimuli such as laughing and talking[101].

Diagnosis and management

For reported reactions to alcohol, history is useful in ascertaining whether the reaction occurs when any alcohol is consumed. If so, then a challenge with incremental doses of ethanol is advisable. Ehlers recommended DBPCFC with a cumulative amount of 30 ml of ethanol[122]. If this is negative, or if the reaction is to a specific alcoholic drink, then further tests will be helpful, including specific IgE estimation to grapes in the case of wine, and to barley and/or wheat in the case of reported reactions to beer. Skin prick tests with grapes using prick-to-prick testing (PPT) may also be helpful for wine-induced reactions. For asthmatic patients, it is also worth excluding sodium metabisulphite or salicylate intolerance. Therefore, if the patient has asthma and the symptoms involve wine, lager or cider but also other foods such as dried fruit, frozen potatoes and fruit cordials, then it is possible that sodium metabisulphite is the culprit. In this case careful exclusion of foods containing sodium metabisulphite should be attempted, followed by oral challenge if available. If symptoms involve wine, but also dried herbs and spices, tea and some fruits and vegetables such as oranges and tomatoes, and the patient is also aspirin-sensitive, then an exclusion of high-salicylate foods may be useful. Benzoates are also added to beer, so if beer is eliciting symptoms but other foods such as prunes, raspberries and cranberries also cause symptoms, then it is also worth considering the exclusion of this food additive.

If diagnosis is achieved, management can be difficult due to the social effects of alcohol abstinence, but there are no nutritional consequences emanating from alcohol avoidance.

10.3 Food-dependent exercise-induced anaphylaxis

10.3.1 Prevalence

Food-dependent exercise-induced anaphylaxis (FDEIA) is a variant of exercise-induced anaphylaxis (EIA), which has been defined as 'the onset of allergic symptoms during, or immediately after, exercise[140]. FDEIA is characterised by a chronological sequence in which the eating of a certain food followed by exercise induces symptoms, but where the food is consumed or exercise taken independently of each other, there are no symptoms. The first case report of FDEIA appeared in 1979[141], since when there have been numerous case reports and reviews published. In 2001, Romano and colleagues reported on their clinical and laboratory findings of 54 subjects with FDEIA[142]. They studied all patients reporting at least one EIA episode which had occurred two hours after a meal, questioned patients about their food intake in the preceding 24 hours and performed skin prick and serum levels of specific food antibodies, with results showing that 48 of the 54 patients (89%) suspected a particular food in at least one episode. It is not known how common FDEIA is, although a study of anaphylaxis in Korea by Yang and colleagues showed that 13% of the 138 reported cases were thought to be caused by FDEIA, but only 2.9% were attributed to EIA[143]. Both Yang and Romano's studies showed that over 80% of cases of anaphylaxis involving exercise were food-related.

10.3.2 Foods involved

A summary statement from a practice guideline[29] states that there are two types of FDEIA: one subset of patients who develop anaphylaxis to any type of food when consumed in temporal proximity to exercise, and another subset who only experience symptoms after they have ingested a specific food in conjunction with exercise. A wide variety of foods have been implicated, with many case reports referring to individual and multiple foods[144,145]. Many of these suggest that wheat is the commonest cause of the condition[146]. A review by Beaudouin in 2006 suggested that wheat and crustaceans were the two commonest foods, but others can also be implicated[140]. Romano and colleagues in Italy showed that tomatoes were the commonest food to cause symptoms, affecting nearly a third of the cohort of 48 patients[142]. Wheat, peanuts, maize and soya beans all affected more than 10%, and many patients were affected by more than one food. Tomatoes are not the only fruit or vegetable to cause symptoms. Kidd and colleagues reported three cases of celery involved in FDEIA[147]. Data from the USA appear to show that wheat is less important as a precipitant of FDEIA there than it is in Japan or Europe. Shadick and colleagues showed that shellfish affected nearly 16% of all cases, with alcohol, tomato, cheese, celery and strawberries eliciting more reactions than wheat[148]. Although wheat appears to be the commonest food linked with FDEIA, so many different foods have been implicated that it is important not to rule out FDEIA if the reaction has involved exercise and a food other than the common triggers such as tomatoes, wheat or celery.

However, food may not be the only factor, and some have shown that aspirin can elicit symptoms in FDEIA patients in the absence of exercise[149]. Other factors which may be important include the menstrual cycle, the amount of food ingested and ambient temperature and humidity[29]. Comorbid pollen or house-dust-mite sensitisation may be an important factor in some cases, especially where the main trigger food is a cross-reacting food such as tomatoes in the case of grass-pollen allergy and crustaceans or molluscs in the case of house-dust-mite sensitisation[142,150]. Jogging is the most common exercise to provoke the reaction, but other activities such as dancing, cycling and even walking have all be implicated[148]. FDEIA has been associated with mast cell degranulation and elevated plasma histamine levels, and it has been suggested that exercise facilitates allergen absorption from the gastrointestinal tract into the bloodstream[149]. Matsuo and colleagues suggest that in the case of wheat-dependent exercise-induced anaphylaxis, gliadin absorption into the blood circulation is facilitated by exercise and also by aspirin intake, but they speculate this mechanism is not limited only to reactions involving wheat[149].

10.3.3 Diagnosis

As with all other types of food hypersensitivity, taking a good history is the cornerstone of diagnosis. As several different foods and/or augmentation factors may be involved, it is important to go through the precise history of each reaction and get a detailed history of the exact foods consumed, the proximity of ingestion to exercise, and whether aspirin and/or alcohol were consumed. All types of exercise should be considered, even if it is fairly low-level such as walking, shopping or sweeping up. O'Connor *et al.* suggest that the best clue comes from the presence of intermittent reactions, superimposed on the baseline of consistent uneventful exercise[151].

Whenever a food is suspected, then it is useful to undertake tests to assess whether there is any specific IgE antibody to the suspected food present. Although the symptoms are at the severe end of the spectrum, practice guidance suggests that it is acceptable to use both skin prick testing and serum specific IgE estimation in the diagnosis of FDEIA[29]. For foods such as milk, crustaceans and nuts, tests with standardised reagents will be sufficient. For fruits and vegetables, prick-to-prick testing (PPT) may be better in order to ensure high sensitivity[152]. Romano *et al.* showed that, for all foods, PPT revealed positivities not disclosed by SPT[142]. For wheat, however, neither reagents nor PPT have shown good positive or negative predictive values, and they are often a poor way of assessing the presence of IgE antibodies (see Chapter 9). Therefore much of the work on the individual allergens responsible for these reactions has concentrated on wheat. Palosuo and colleagues identified that the major allergen involved is the omega-5 gliadin[153], which is also involved in wheat allergy in children. Omega-5 gliadin measurement using recombinant allergens has been shown to be an effective way of diagnosing wheat-dependent exercise-induced anaphylaxis[154].

The final diagnostic test is exercise challenge with and without prior consumption of the suspect food[29]. However, a negative challenge does not rule out FDEIA, and augmentation factors such as alcohol, aspirin and the amount of food consumed may all affect the outcome of challenge. Chong *et al.* suggest that it is beneficial to challenge with the composite meal reported to cause symptoms if the single food does not provoke a response[152]. Pre-treatment of the patient with aspirin is recommended by some for those patients where food alone does not elicit a response[149,152]. The interval between the oral food challenge and the exercise is important; in Romano's study the reported time elapsed between the meal and exercise ranged from 30 to 120 minutes, and some patients in the challenge did not react after a 2-hour gap between ingestion and exercise challenge[142]. However, there are some patients where the time lag can be up to 12 hours after the ingestion of food, and so accurate history may help determine this[151].

10.3.4   Management

The main management consists of advising patients to avoid exercising in proximity to specific food consumption[29]. Patients may also be advised to exercise on an empty stomach, such as first thing in the morning[143]. The length of time between eating and exercise is controversial, with some recommending 1–6 hours[152] and others recommend waiting for at least 4 hours before exercising[142]; best-practice guidelines suggest that a waiting period of 4–6 hours is prudent[29]. Wearing medical identification jewellery and carrying adrenaline is also recommended. Those who have life-threatening anaphylaxis should be advised to avoid or modify their exercise routines, and to take account of the fact that warm humid conditions and the taking of aspirin will enhance their chances of experiencing an attack. Finally, it is advised that everyone with FDEIA should have with them an exercise 'buddy', to ensure that should they require emergency aid there is someone there to give it. There are no data to support the effectiveness of premedication with steroids, cromoglycate or antihistamines[29].

Although there are only 8–10 foods which commonly cause food hypersensitivity, it is important to remember that there is a very wide range of other foods and food

Table 10.5 Food hypersensitivity triggered by composite meals or unrelated foods.

Food(s) reported to cause reactions	Connected foods with reported tolerance	Potential triggers	Additional information
Pizza	Bread, pasta, tomatoes, cheese	Soya, celery, mustard, milk	
Indian curry	Bread, rice, vegetables, meat and seafood	Mustard; herbs or spices such as coriander, cumin, fenugreek, tumeric; pistachio, almond or cashew nuts; lentils, chickpeas or salicylates. Some curries have almond paste added which is ground peanuts with almond essence	If reacts to all curries whether restaurant, takeaway, ready meal or homemade, then likely to be a spice. If also aspirin-sensitive, consider salicylates. If only reacts to curries containing fresh raw herbs such as coriander then it could be OAS.
Thai or Malaysian food	Chilli and other spicy food, Atlantic prawns, rice, bread	Peanuts, tiger prawns, sesame oil, fish sauce, lemongrass, lime, coconut, buckwheat noodles, cashew nuts	Do not rule out prawns or sesame if eats them normally, as whole sesame may not get a reaction. Can also get single-species allergy to individual shellfish.
Chinese food	Rice, noodles, chicken, seafood, vegetables	MSG, black beans, soya, gelatine, ginger, cashew nuts, peanuts, loosely cooked egg in spring rolls, egg fried rice	
Dessert or cake (unspecified)	Wheat, sugar, margarine and butter, milk and eggs	Gelatine, carrageen, soya, cinnamon, cloves, coconut, arrowroot, orange or lemon oil, nuts, especially almonds (check for marzipan) and hazelnuts or nut oil, annatto (custard powder), lupin	

Corn, malted foods, certain fruits and vegetables	Wheat, other fruits and vegetables	Lipid transfer proteins, which are found in wide variety of foods	If only fruits and vegetables, check pollen allergies as may have OAS. If not allergic to pollen then either do a skin prick test with peach reagent or if available a Pru p 3 specific IgE test, as this is a marker for LTP allergy.
Certain gluten-free products, or onion rings, apple fritters or pastry products, especially if eaten in EU country	Can tolerate other pastry and GF products without a problem, also OK with wheat	Lupin	Those with a wheat allergy may have de-glutenised wheat thinking that it is wheat-free because it is labelled gluten-free.
Alcoholic drink (unknown which one, as had mixed drinks)	Wheat, grapes	Barley (malt), alcohol, sodium metabisulphite, benzoates, colouring or flavouring added to shots, juniper berries, vasoactive amines Sesame in aqua libra	To clarify whether it is an additive, ask about other foods. For sulphites, ask about similar reactions to dried fruit, burgers, sausages or commercially prepared lime or lemon juice. For benzoates, ask about reactions to orange drinks, jam and fruit-based desserts.
Dried herbs, black pepper, tomatoes, tea, peppermint, blackcurrants	Can tolerate other fruits and vegetables, meat and fish	Salicylates	Check for aspirin sensitivity.

ingredients which could be implicated in reactions. This is particularly true where a patient reports symptoms to a composite meal, where the culprit food may not be obvious. Table 10.5 illustrates the types of food triggers most likely to cause reactions to composite meals.

References

1. Pereira B, Venter C, Grundy J *et al.* Prevalence of sensitization to food allergens, reported adverse reaction to foods, food avoidance, and food hypersensitivity among teenagers. *J Allergy Clin Immunol* 2005; **116**: 884–92.
2. Schäfer T, Böhler E, Ruhdorfer S *et al.* Epidemiology of food allergy/food intolerance in adults: associations with other manifestations of atopy. *Allergy* 2001; **56**: 1172–9.
3. Jansen JJ, Kardinaal AF, Huijbers G *et al.* prevalence of food allergy and intolerance in the adult Dutch populations. *J Allergy Clin Immunol* 1994; **93**: 446–56.
4. Eriksson NE, Möller C, Werner S *et al.* Self-reported food hypersensitivity in Sweden, Denmark, Estonia, Lithuania and Russia. *J Investig Allergol Clin Immunol* 2004; **14**: 70–9.
5. Falcão H, Lunet N, Lopes C, Barros H. Food hypersensitivity in Portuguese adults. *Eur J Clin Nutr* 2004; **58**: 1621–5.
6. Woods RK, Thien F, Raven J, Walters EH, Abramson M. Prevalence of food allergies in young adults and their relationship to asthma, nasal allergies, and eczema. *Ann Allergy Asthma Immunol* 2002; **88**: 183–9.
7. Young E, Patel S, Stoneham M, Rona R, Wilkinson JD. The prevalence of reaction to food additives in a survey population. *J R Coll Physicians Lond* 1987; **21**: 241–7.
8. Osterballe M, Hansen TK, Mortz CG, Bindslev-Jensen C. The clinical relevance of sensitization to pollen-related fruits and vegetables in unselected pollen-sensitized adults. *Allergy* 2005; **60**: 218–25.
9. Zuberbier T, Edenharter G, Worm M *et al.* Prevalence of adverse reactions to food in Germany: a population study. *Allergy* 2004; **59**: 338–45.
10. Di Lorenzo G, Pacor ML, Mansueto P *et al.* Food-additive-induced urticaria: a survey of 838 patients with recurrent chronic idiopathic urticaria. *Int Arch Allergy Immunol* 2005; **138**: 235–42.
11. Guida B, De Martino C, De Martino S *et al.* Histamine plasma levels and elimination diet in chronic idiopathic urticaria. *Eur J Clin Nutr* 2000; **54**: 155–8.
12. Weber RW, Hoffman M, Raine DA, Nelson HS. Incidence of bronchoconstriction due to aspirin, azo dyes, non-azo dyes, and preservatives in a population of perennial asthmatics. *J Allergy Clin Immunol* 1979; **64**: 32–7.
13. Simon RA. Update on sulfite sensitivity. *Allergy* 1998; **53** (Suppl 46): 72–4.
14. Papazian R. Sulfites: safe for most, dangerous for some. *FDA Consumer* December 1996.
15. Timberlake CM, Toun AK, Hudson BJ. Perception of asthma attacks in Melanesian adults by sodium metabisulphite. *Papua New Guinea Med J* 1992; **35**: 186–90.
16. Bush RK, Taylor SL, Holden K, Nordlee JA, Busse WW. The prevalence of sensitivity to sulfiting agents in asthmatics. *Am J Med* 1986; **81**: 816–20.
17. Buckley CE III, Saltzman HA, Seiker HO. The prevalence and degree of sensitivity to ingested sulfites. *J Allergy Clin Immunol* 1985; **75**: 144.
18. Bateman B, Warner JO, Hutchinson E *et al.* The effects of a double blind, placebo controlled, artificial food colourings and benzoate preservative challenge on hyperactivity in a general population sample of preschool children. *Arch Dis Child* 2004; **89**: 506–11.
19. Ross MP, Ferguson M, Street D *et al.* Analysis of food-allergic and anaphylactic events in the National Electronic Injury Surveillance System. *J Allergy Clin Immunol* 2008; **121**: 166–71.
20. Colver AF, Nevantaus H, Macdougall CF, Cant AJ. Severe food-allergic reactions in children across the UK and Ireland 1998–2000. *Acta Paediatr* 2005; **94**: 689–695.
21. European Union. Council Directive of 21 December 1988 on the approximation of the laws of the Member States concerning food additives authorized for use in foodstuffs intended for human consumption (89/107/EEC). *Official Journal of the European Union* 1989; **L40**: 27.

22. Sumner SS, Eifert JD. Risks and benefits of food additives. In: Branen AL, Davidson PM, Salminen S, Thorngate JH, eds. *Food Additives*, 2nd edn. New York, NY: Marcel Dekker, 2002: 27–42.
23. Salminen S, Tahvonen R. Food additive intake assessment. In: Branen AL, Davidson PM, Salminen S, Thorngate JH, eds. *Food Additives*, 2nd edn. New York, NY: Marcel Dekker, 2002: 11–26.
24. Food Standards Agency. Current EU approved additives and their E numbers. www.food. gov.uk/safereating/chemsafe/additivesbranch/enumberlist. Accessed September 2008.
25. Hannuksela M, Haahtela T. Food additives and hypersensitivity. In: Branen AL, Davidson PM, Salminen S, Thorngate JH, eds. *Food Additives*, 2nd edn. New York, NY: Marcel Dekker, 2002: 43–86.
26. Chafee FH, Settipane GA. Asthma caused by FD&C approved dyes. *J Allergy* 1967; **40**: 65–72.
27. DeFranco AL, Locksley RM, Robertson M. *Immunity: the Immune Response in Infectious and Inflammatory Disease*. London: New Science Press, 2007.
28. Simon R. Adverse reactions to food and drug additives. *Immunol Allergy Clin North Am* 1996: **16**: 137–76.
29. Chapman JA, Bernstein IL, Lee RE *et al.* Food allergy: a practice parameter. *Ann Allergy Asthma Immunol* 2006; **96**: S1–68.
30. Stevenson DD, Simon RA, Lumry WR *et al.* Adverse reactions to tartrazine. *J Allergy Clin Immunol* 1986; **78**: 182–91.
31. Chung K, Baker JR, Baldwin JL, Chou A. Identification of carmine allergens among three carmine allergy patients. *Allergy* 2001; **56**: 73–7.
32. Wüthrich B, Kägi W, Stücker W. Anaphylactic reactions to ingested carmine (E120). *Allergy* 1997; **52**: 1133–7.
33. Nish WA, Whisman BA, Goetz DW, Ramirez DA. Anaphylaxis to annatto dye: a case report. *Ann Allergy* 1991; **66**: 129–31.
34. Bosso JV, Simon RA. Urticaria, angiooedema and anaphylaxis provoked by food and drug additives. In: Metcalfe DD, Sampson HJ, Simon RA, eds. *Food Allergy: Adverse Reactions to Foods and Food Additives*, 3rd edn. Oxford: Blackwell, 2003: 310–23.
35. Lucas CD, Hallagan JB, Taylor SL. The role of natural color additives in food allergy. *Adv Food Nutr Res* 2001; **43**: 195–216.
36. Surendranath Lal MB, Srinivas CR. Allergic contact dermatitis to turmeric in kumkum. *Indian J Dermatol* 2006; **51**: 200–1.
37. Arup Fischer L, Agner T. Curcumin allergy in relation to yellow chlorhexidine solution used for skin disinfection prior to surgery. *Contact Dermatitis* 2004; **51**: 39–40.
38. Lee JH, Kim JW, Ko Y *et al.* Curcumin, a constituent of curry, suppresses IgE-mediated allergic response and mast cell activation at the level of Syk. *J Allergy Clin Immunol* 2008; **121**: 1225–31.
39. Wüthrich B, Schmid-Grendelmeyer P, Lundberg M. Anaphylaxis to saffron. *Allergy* 1997; **52**: 476–7.
40. Juhlin L, Michaelsson G, Zetterstrom O. Urticaria and asthma induced by food and drug additives in patients with aspirin sensitivity. *J Allergy Clin Immunol* 1972; **50**: 92–102.
41. Nettis E, Colanardi MC, Ferrannini A, Tursi A. Suspected tartrazine-induced acute urticaria/angioedema is only rarely reproducible by oral rechallenge. *Clin Exp Allergy* 2003; **33**: 1725–9.
42. Worm M, Ehlers I, Sterry W, Zuberbier T. Clinical relevance of food additives in adult patients with atopic dermatitis. *Clin Exp Allergy* 2000; **30**: 407–14.
43. Worm M, Vieth W, Ehlers I, Sterry W, Zuberbier T. Increased leukotriene production by food additives in patients with atopic dermatitis and proven food intolerance. *Clin Exp Allergy* 2001; **31**: 265–73.
44. Park HW, Park Chang H, Park SH *et al.* Dermatologic adverse reactions to 7 common food additives in patients with allergic diseases: a double-blind, placebo-controlled study. *J Allergy Clin Immunol* 2008; **121**: 1059–61.
45. Stevenson DD. Tartrazine, azo dyes and non-azo dyes. In: Metcalfe DD, Sampson HJ, Simon RA, eds. *Food Allergy: Adverse Reactions to Foods and Food Additives*, 3rd edn. Oxford: Blackwell, 2003: 351–9.

46. Feingold BF. Hyperkinesis and learning disabilities linked to artificial food flavors and colours. *Am J Nurs* 1975; **75**: 797–803.
47. McCann D, Barrett A, Cooper A *et al*. Food additives and hyperactive behaviour in 3-year-old and 8/9-year-old children in the community: a randomised, double-blinded, placebo-controlled trial. *Lancet* 2007; **370**: 1560–7.
48. Farenholz JM, Simon RA. Adverse reactions to benzoates and parabens. In: Metcalfe DD, Sampson HJ, Simon RA, eds. *Food Allergy: Adverse Reactions to Foods and Food Additives*, 3rd edn. Oxford: Blackwell, 2003: 369–76.
49. Ortolani C, Pastorello E, Luraghi MT *et al*. Diagnosis of intolerance to food additives. *Ann Allergy* 1984; **53**: 587–91.
50. Nettis E, Colanardi MC, Ferrannini A, Tursi A. Sodium benzoate-induced repeated episodes of acute urticaria/angio-oedema: randomized controlled trial. *Br J Dermatol* 2004: **151**: 898–902.
51. Asero R. Sodium benzoate-induced pruritus. *Allergy* 2006; **61**: 1240–1.
52. Asero R. Food additives intolerance: does it present as perennial rhinitis? *Curr Opin Allergy Clin Immunol* 2004; **4**: 25–9.
53. Pacor ML, Di Lorenzo G, Martinelli N *et al*. Monosodium benzoate hypersensitivity in subjects with persistent rhinitis. *Allergy* 2004; **59**: 192–7.
54. Karovicova J, Simko P. Preservatives in food. In: Nollet LML, ed. *Handbook of Food Analysis*. New York, NY: Marcel Dekker, 1996: 1745–7.
55. Martin LB, Nordlee JA, Taylor SL. Sulfite residues in restaurant salads. *J Food Protection* 1986; **49**: 126–9.
56. European Union. European Parliament and Council Directive No 95/2/EC of 20 February 1995 on food additives other than colours and sweeteners. *Official Journal of the European Union* 1995; **L61**.
57. Leclercq C, Molinaro MG, Piccinelli R *et al*. Dietary intake exposure to sulphites in Italy – analytical determination of sulphite-containing foods and their combination into standard meals for adults and children. *Food Add Contamin* 2000; **17**: 979–89.
58. European Union. Directive 2003/89/EC of the European Parliament and of the Council of 10 November 2003 amending Directive 2000/13/EC as regards indication of the ingredients present in foodstuffs. *Official Journal of the European Union* 2003; **L308**: 15–18.
59. Boushey HA. Bronchial hyperreactivity to sulphur dioxide: physiologic and political implications. *J Allergy Clin Immunol* 1982; **69**: 335.
60. Taylor SL, Bush RK, Nordlee JA. Sulfites. In: Metcalfe DD, Sampson HJ, Simon RA, eds. *Food Allergy: Adverse Reactions to Foods and Food Additives*, 3rd edn. Oxford: Blackwell, 2003: 324–41.
61. Asero R. Multiple intolerance to food additives. *J Allergy Clin Immunol* 2002; **110**: 531–2.
62. Moneret Vautrin DA, Einhorn C, Tisserand J. Le role du nitrite de sodium dans les urticares histaminiques d'origine alminetaire. *Ann Nutr Aliment* 1980; **34**: 1125–32.
63. Hawkins CA, Katelaris CH. Nitrate anaphylaxis. *Ann Allergy Asthma Immunol* 2000; **85**: 74–6.
64. Asero R. Nitrate intolerance. *Allergy* 2000; **55**: 678–9.
65. Berkes EA, Woessner KM, Monosodium glutamate. In: Metcalfe DD, Sampson HJ, Simon RA, eds. *Food Allergy: Adverse Reactions to Foods and Food Additives*, 3rd edn. Oxford: Blackwell, 2003: 342–50.
66. Food and Drug Administration. Monosodium glutamate. *FDA Med Bull* 1996; Jan: 3–4.
67. Kwok RHM. Chinese restaurant syndrome. *N Engl J Med* 1968; **178**: 796.
68. Settipane GA. The restaurant syndromes. *N Engl Reg Allergy Proc* 1987; **8**: 39–46.
69. Yang WH, Drouin MA, Herbert M, Mao Y, Karsh J. The monosodium glutamate symptom complex: assessment in a double-blind, placebo-controlled, randomized study. *J Allergy Clin Immunol* 1997; **99**: 757–62.
70. Geha RS, Beiser A, Ren C *et al*. Multicenter, double-blind, placebo-controlled, multiple-challenge evaluation of reported reactions to monosodium glutamate. *J Allergy Clin Immunol* 2000; **106**: 973–80.
71. Allen DH, Delohery J, Baker G. Monosodium L-glutamate-induced asthma. *J Allergy Clin Immunol* 1987; **80**: 530–7.

72. Woods RK, Weiner JM, Thien F, Abramson M, Walters EH. The effects of monosodium glutamate in adults with asthma who perceive themselves to be monosodium glutamate-intolerant. *J Allergy Clin Immunol* 1998; **101**: 762–71.
73. Woessner KM, Simon RA, Stevenson DD. Monosodium glutamate sensitivity in asthma. *J Allergy Clin Immunol* 1999; **104**: 305–10.
74. Stevenson DD. Monosodium glutamate and asthma. *J Nutr* 2000; **130**: 1067S–73S.
75. Simon RA. Additive-induced urticaria: experience with monosodium glutamate (MSG). *J Nutr* 2000; **130**: 1063S–6S.
76. Weber RW. Adverse reactions to butylated hydroxytoluene and butylated hydroxyanisole (BHT and BHA). In: Metcalfe DD, Sampson HJ, Simon RA, eds. *Food Allergy: Adverse Reactions to Foods and Food Additives*, 3rd edn. Oxford: Blackwell, 2003: 360–8.
77. Taylor SL, Dormendy ES. The role of flavouring substances in food allergy and intolerance. *Adv Food Nutr Res* 1998; **42**: 1–44.
78. Wilson BG, Bahna SL. Adverse reactions to food additives. *Ann Allergy Asthma Immunol* 2005; **95**: 499–507.
79. Taylor SL, Bush RK, Selner JC *et al*. Sensitivity to sulfited foods among sulfite-sensitive subjects with asthma. *J Allergy Clin Immunol* 1988; **81**: 1159–67.
80. Wu KK. Salicylates and their spectrum of activity. *Anti-Inflamm Anti-Allergy Agents Med Chem* 2007; **6**: 278–92.
81. Jeffreys D. *Aspirin: the Story of a Wonder Drug*. London: Bloomsbury, 2004.
82. Hare LG, Woodside JV, Young IS. Dietary salicylates. *J Clin Pathol* 2003; **56**: 649–50.
83. Amann R, Peskar BA. Anti-inflammatory effects of aspirin and sodium salicylate. *Eur J Pharmacol* 2002; **447**: 1–9.
84. Scotter MJ, Roberts DPT, Wilson LA *et al*. Free salicylic acid and acetyl salicylic acid content of foods using gas chromatography-mass spectrometry. *Food Chem* 2007; **105**: 273–9.
85. Swain AR, Dutton SP, Truswell AS. Salicylates in foods. *J Am Diet Assoc* 1985; **85**: 950–60.
86. Venema DP, Hollman PCH, Janssen KPLTM, Katan MB. Determination of acetylsalicylic acid and salicylic acid in foods, using HPLC with fluorescence detection. *J Agric Food Chem* 1996; **44**: 1762–7.
87. Nizankowska-Mogilnicka E, Bochenek, Mastalerz L *et al*. EAACI/GA2LEN guideline: aspirin provocation tests for diagnosis of aspirin hypersensitivity. *Allergy* 2007; **62**: 1111–18.
88. Samter M, Beers RF. Concerning the nature of intolerance to aspirin. *J Allergy* 1967; **40**: 281–93.
89. Corder EH, Buckley CE. Aspirin, salicylate, sulfite and tartrazine-induced broncho-constriction: safe doses and case definition in epidemiological studies. *J Clin Epidemiol* 1995; **48**: 1269–75.
90. Raithel M, Baenkler HW, Naegel A *et al*. Significance of salicylate intolerance in diseases of the lower gastrointestinal tract. *J Physiol Pharmacol* 2005; **56**: 89–102.
91. Dahlén B, Boréus LO, Anderson P, Andersson R, Zetterström O. Plasma acetylsalicylic acid and salicylic acid levels during aspirin provocation in aspirin-sensitive subjects. *Allergy* 1994; **49**: 43–9.
92. Paterson J, Baxter G, Lawrence J, Duthie G. Is there a role for dietary salicylates in health? *Proc Nutr Soc* 2006; **65**: 93–6.
93. Baxter GJ, Graham AB, Lawrence JR, Wiles D, Paterson JR. Salicylic acid in soups prepared from organically and non-organically grown vegetables. *Eur J Nutr* 2001; **40**: 289–92.
94. Paterson JR, Srivastava R, Baxter GJ, Graham AB, Lawrence JR. Salicylic acid content of spices and its implications. *J Agric Food Chem* 2006; **54**: 2891–6.
95. Fritz SB, Baldwin JL. Pharmacologic food reactions. In: Metcalfe DD, Sampson HJ, Simon RA, eds. *Food Allergy: Adverse Reactions to Foods and Food Additives*, 3rd edn. Oxford: Blackwell, 2003: 395–407.
96. Malone MH, Metcalfe DD. Histamine in foods: its possible role in non-allergic adverse reactions to ingestants. *N Engl Reg Allergy Proc* 1986; **7**: 241–5.
97. Jansen SC, van Dusseldorp M, Bottema KC, Dubois AEJ. Intolerance to dietary biogenic amines: a review. *Ann Allergy Asthma Immunol* 2003; **91**: 233–40.
98. Fogel WA, Lewinski A, Jochem J. Histamine in food: is there anything to worry about? *Biochem Soc Trans* 2007; **35**: 349–52.

99. Maintz L, Novak N. Histamine and histamine intolerance. *Am J Clin Nutr* 2007; **85**: 1185–96.
100. Morrow KJ, Margolies GR, Rowland BS, Roberts LJ. Evidence that histamine is the causative toxin of scombroid fish poisoning. *N Eng J Med* 1991; **324**: 716–20.
101. Vally H. Allergic and asthmatic reactions to alcoholic drinks: a significant problem in the community. *Clin Exp Allergy* 2008; **38**: 1–3.
102. Kanny G, Gerbaux V, Olszewski A *et al.* No correlation between wine intolerance and histamine content of wine. *J Allergy Clin Immunol* 2001; **107**: 375–8.
103. American Academy of Allergy and Immunology Committee on Adverse Reactions to Foods. *Adverse Reactions to Foods.* NIH Publication 84-2442. Bethesda, MD: National Institutes of Health, 1984.
104. Moneret-Vautrin DA. False food allergies: non-specific reactions to foodstuffs. In: Lessof MH, ed. *Clinical Reactions to Food.* Wiley. Chichester: Wiley, 1983: 135–53.
105. Barone JJ, Roberts HR. Caffeine consumption. *Food Chem Toxicol* 1996; **34**: 119–29.
106. McCusker RR, Goldberger BA, Cone EJ. Caffeine content of energy drinks, carbonated sodas, and other beverages. *J Analyt Toxicol* 2006; **30**: 112–14.
107. Frary CD, Johnson RK, Wang MQ. Food sources and intakes of caffeine in the diets of persons in the United States. *J Am Diet Assoc* 2005; **105**: 110–13.
108. Broderick P, Benjamin AB. Caffeine and psychiatric symptoms: a review. *J Okla State Med Assoc* 2004; **97**: 538–42.
109. Mathew RJ, Wilson WH. Behavioral and cerebrovascular effects of caffeine in patients with anxiety disorders. *Acta Psychiatr Scand* 1990; **82**: 17–22.
110. Pollak CP, Bright D. Caffeine consumption and weekly sleep patterns in US seventh-, eighth-, and ninth-graders. *Pediatrics* 2003; **111**: 42–6.
111. Bech BH, Obel C, Henriksen TB, Olsen J. Effect of reducing caffeine intake on birth weight and length of gestation: randomised controlled trial. *BMJ* 2007; **334**: 409.
112. Infante S, Baeza ML, De Barrio M *et al.* Anaphylaxis due to caffeine. *Allergy* 2003; **58**: 681–2.
113. Fernandez-Nieto M, Sastre J, Quirce S. Urticaria caused by cola drink. *Allergy* 2002; **57**: 967.
114. Teuber SS, Jarvis KC, Dandekar AM, Peterson WR, Ansari AA. Identification and cloning of a complementary DNA encoding a vicilin-like proprotein Jug r 2 from English walnut (*Juglans regia*), a major food allergen. *J Allergy Clin Immunol* 1999; **104**: 1311–20.
115. Altman DR, Chiaramonte LT. Public perception of food allergy. *Environ Toxicol Pharmacol* 1997; **4**: 95–9.
116. Businco L, Falconieri P, Bellioni-Businco B, Bahna S. Severe food-induced vasculitis in two children. *Pediatr Allergy Immunol* 2002; **13**: 68–71.
117. Aziz O, Dioszeghy C. Allergic hemiglossitis as a unique case of food allergy: a case report. *J Med Case Reports* 2008; **2**: 71.
118. Bock SA, Sampson HA, Atkins FM *et al.* Double-blind, placebo-controlled food challenge (DBPCFC) as an office procedure: a manual. *J Allergy Clin Immunol* 1988; **82**: 986–97.
119. Zak DL, Keeney PG. Changes in cocoa proteins during ripening of fruit, fermentation and further processing of cocoa beans. *J Agric Food Chem* 1976; **24**: 483–6.
120. Agarwal DP, Harada S, Goedde HW. Racial differences in biological sensitivity to ethanol: the role of alcohol dehydrogenase and aldehyde dehydrogenase isozymes. *Alcohol Clin Exp Res* 1981; **5**: 12–16.
121. Kanny G, Mouton C, Morisset M, Moneret-Vautrin AD. Food allergy to alcohol. *Allergy* 2003; **58**: 535.
122. Ehlers I, Hipler UC, Zuberbier T, Worm M. Ethanol as a cause of hypersensitivity reactions to alcoholic beverages. *Clin Exp Allergy* 2002; **32**: 1231–5.
123. Vally H, Thompson PJ. Allergic and asthmatic reactions to alcoholic drinks. *Addict Biol* 2003; **8**: 3–11.
124. Vally H, de Klerk N, Thompson PJ. Alcoholic drinks: important triggers for asthma. *J Allergy Clin Immunol* 2000; **105**: 462–7.
125. Gonzalez-Quintela A, Vidal C, Gude F. Alcohol, IgE and allergy. *Addict Biol* 2004; **9**: 195–204.

126. Gonzalez-Quintela A, Garrido M, Gude F *et al.* Sensitisation to cross-reactive carbohydrate determinants in relation to alcohol consumption. *Clin Exp Allergy* 2008; **38**: 152–60.
127. Linneberg A, Berg ND, Gonzalez-Quintela A, Vidal C, Elberling J. Prevalence of self-reported hypersensitivity symptoms following intake of alcoholic drinks. *Clin Exp Allergy* 2008; **38**: 145–51.
128. Bendtsen P, Grønbaek M, Kjaer SK *et al.* Alcohol consumption and the risk of self-reported perennial and seasonal allergic rhinitis in young adult women in a population-based cohort study. *Clin Exp Allergy* 2008; **38**: 1179–85.
129. Linneberg A, Hertzum I, Husemoen LLN, Johansen N, Jargensen T. Association between alcohol consumption and aeroallergen sensitisation in Danish adults. *Clin Exp Allergy* 2006; **36**: 714–21.
130. Curioni A, Santucci B, Cristaudo A *et al.* Urticaria from beer: an immediate hypersensitivity reaction due to a 10-kDa protein derived from barley. *Clin Exp Allergy* 1999; **29**: 407–13.
131. Figueredo E, Quirce S, del Amo A *et al.* Beer-induced anaphylaxis: identification of allergens. *Allergy* 1999; **54**: 630–4.
132. Asero R, Mistrello G, Roncarolo D, Amato S, van Ree R. A case of allergy to beer showing cross-reactivity between lipid transfer proteins. *Ann Allergy Asthma Immunol* 2001; **87**: 65–7.
133. Herzinger T, Kick G, Ludolph-Hauser D, Przybilla B. Anaphylaxis to wheat beer. *Ann Allergy Asthma Immunol* 2004; **92**: 673–5.
134. Vally H, Carr A, El-Saleh J, Thompson P. Wine-induced asthma: a placebo-controlled assessment of its pathogenisis. *J Allergy Clin Immunol* 1999; **1**: 41–6.
135. Vally H, Thompson PJ. Role of sulfite additives in wine induced asthma: single dose and cumulative dose studies. *Thorax* 2001; **56**: 763–9.
136. Vally H, Thompson PJ, Misso NLA. Changes in bronchial hyper-responsiveness following high- and low-sulphite wine challenges in wine-sensitive asthmatic patients. *Clin Exp Allergy* 2007; **37**: 1062–6.
137. Rolland JM, Apostolou E, Deckert K *et al.* Potential food allergens in wine: double-blind, placebo-controlled trial and basophil activation analysis. *Nutrition* 2006; **22**: 882–8.
138. Kalogeromitros DC, Makris MP, Gregoriou SG *et al.* Grape anaphylaxis: a study of 11 adult onset cases. *Allergy Asthma Proc* 2005; **26**: 53–8.
139. Schad SG, Trcka J, Vieths S *et al.* Wine anaphylaxis in a German patient: IgE-mediated allergy against a lipid transfer protein of grapes. *Int Arch Allergy Immunol* 2005; **136**: 159–64.
140. Beaudouin E, Renaudin JM, Morisset M *et al.* Food-dependent, exercise-induced anaphylaxis: update and current data. *Allerg Immunol Paris* 2006; **38**: 45–51.
141. Maulitz RM, Pratts DS, Schocket AL. Exercise-induced anaphylactic reaction to shellfish. *J Allergy Clin Immunol* 1979; **63**: 433–4.
142. Romano A, Di Fonso M, Guiffreda F *et al.* Food-dependent exercise-induced anaphylaxis: clinical and laboratory findings in 54 subjects. *Int Arch Allergy Immunol* 2001; **125**: 264–72.
143. Yang MK, Lee SH, Kim TW *et al.* Epidemiologic and clinical features of anaphylaxis in Korea. *Ann Allergy Asthma Immunol* 2008; **100**: 31–6.
144. Morimoto K, Hara T, Hide M. Food-dependent exercise-induced anaphylaxis due to ingestion of apple. *J Dermatol* 2005; **32**: 62–3.
145. Caffarelli C, Cataldi R, Giordano S, Cavagni G. Anaphylaxis induced by exercise and related to multiple food intake. *Allergy Asthma Proc* 1997; **18**: 245–8.
146. Dohi M, Suko M, Sugiyama H *et al.* Food-dependent, exercise-induced anaphylaxis: a study on 11 Japanese cases. *J Allergy Clin Immunol* 1991; **87**: 34–40.
147. Kidd JM 3rd, Cohen SH, Sosman AJ, Fink JN. Food-dependent exercise-induced anaphylaxis. *J Allergy Clin Immunol* 1983; **71**: 407–11.
148. Shadick NA, Laing MH, Partridge AJ *et al.* The natural history of food-dependent exercise-induced anaphylaxis: survey results from 10-year follow-up study. *J Allergy Clin Immunol* 1999; **104**: 123–7.
149. Matsuo H, Morimoto K, Akaki T. Exercise and aspirin increase levels of circulating gliadin peptides in patients with wheat-dependent exercise-induced anaphylaxis. *Clin Exp Allergy* 2005; **35**: 461–6.

150. Peroni DG, Piacentini GL, Bodni A, Boner AL. Snail anaphylaxis during house dust mite immunotherapy. *Pediatr Allergy Immunol* 2000; **11**: 260–1.
151. O'Connor ME, Schocket AL. Exercise- and pressure-induced syndromes. In: Metcalfe DD, Sampson HJ, Simon RA, eds. *Food Allergy: Adverse Reactions to Foods and Food Additives*, 3rd edn. Oxford: Blackwell, 2003: 262–9.
152. Chong SU, Worm M, Zuberbier T. Role of adverse reactions to foods in urticaria and exercise-induced anaphylaxis. *Int Arch Allergy Immunol* 2002; **129**: 19–26.
153. Palosuo K, Alenius H, Varjonen E *et al*. A novel wheat gliadin as a cause of exercise-induced anaphylaxis. *J Allergy Clin Immunol* 1999; **103**: 912–17.
154. Matsuo H, Dahlström J, Tanaka A *et al*. Sensitivity and specificity of recombinant omega-5 gliadin-specific IgE measurement for the diagnosis of wheat-dependent exercise-induced anaphylaxis. *Allergy* 2008; **63**: 233–6.

Part 3
Other Aspects of Management, Allergy Prevention and Nutritional Considerations

11 Nutritional Consequences of Avoidance, and Practical Approaches to Nutritional Management

Ruth Kershaw

11.1 Introduction

It is vital to take into consideration the nutritional consequences of an avoidance diet in both the diagnosis and management of food hypersensitivity. This chapter briefly considers the assessment of dietary adequacy and reviews a range of factors that need to be considered when implementing an avoidance diet. Each of the common food allergens are discussed, with consideration given to the nutritional consequences of the removal of these foods from the diet. Practical strategies to ensure ongoing dietary adequacy are also considered. This review is concluded by considering other common nutritional issues encountered when implementing food-avoidance diets.

11.2 Assessment of dietary adequacy

In both children and adults, the assessment of nutritional status is vital both prior to and during any nutritional intervention. This is specifically the case when foods are being removed from the diet.

Prior to implementing a food-avoidance diet, it is useful to assess the individual's nutritional status for a number of reasons. This assessment can provide a baseline from which to assess ongoing nutritional status while following a food-avoidance diet. Also, if it is found that a person's nutritional status is suboptimal, it may be appropriate to review whether an aggressive food-avoidance regimen is appropriate, weighing up the nutritional implications of the diet against the severity and extent of the symptoms. For example, in a child with faltering growth whose parents suspect that foods may be exacerbating disruptive behaviour, it may be appropriate to address the reasons for faltering growth prior to considering eliminating further foods from the diet. However, if an individual reports a history of severe reactions to a food then this food and its derivatives must be eliminated from the diet regardless of the individual's current nutritional status.

If it is found that a person's nutritional status is suboptimal, this will impact on the dietary advice that is provided when a food-avoidance diet is initiated. For example, in an adult who suspects that cow's milk products may be exacerbating their abdominal symptoms and who is therefore commencing a 4-week trial of a cow's-milk exclusion, it may not be necessary to consider calcium supplementation initially if calcium intake has been adequate up to that point. However, if there are already concerns about calcium status, immediate calcium supplementation may be essential to ensure nutritional status is not compromised further.

It is also vital that a person's nutritional status is reviewed regularly while they are following a food-avoidance diet. There have been a number of case reports in the literature of severe signs and associated symptoms of nutritional deficiency as a result of nutritionally inadequate elimination diets. This is the case for both perceived and diagnosed food hypersensitivity[1–15]. These reports suggest adverse consequences of inadequately supervised food-avoidance diets, ranging from faltering growth affecting both weight and height, to iron deficiency anaemia, inadequate bone mineralisation, rickets and kwashiorkor (a severe form of protein-energy malnutrition). For example, Lui et al. reported the cases of 12 children diagnosed with kwashiorkor in tertiary referral centres in the United States[1]. His group concluded that 50% of these cases were due to the individuals following a protein-deficient diet because of a perceived intolerance to milk. This body of evidence highlights the importance of all food-avoidance diets being supervised by an appropriate specialist healthcare professional with nutritional knowledge such as a registered dietitian[16,17]. The regular assessment of nutritional status during a period of food avoidance will also inform the decision as to whether to continue an elimination diet or consider food challenges in an attempt to broaden the scope of a person's diet.

Assessment of dietary adequacy has been covered in great depth in a number of textbooks[18,19]. In an adult population, review of sequential weight, body mass index (BMI) or other anthropometric measurements can prove a simple marker to assess nutritional adequacy. The simplest way of monitoring infants and children for nutritional deficiencies is to assess growth velocity using approved growth curves[20]. Unfortunately, nutritional deficiencies can occur without inappropriate changes in growth velocity or BMI. Consequently, if there is any suspicion of nutritional deficiency, further assessment of nutritional adequacy by an experienced health professional is essential.

There are a number of methods which may be used to assess dietary adequacy, including dietary recall, a quantitative food diary for a given number of days, weighed food intakes (again taken over a number of days), or a food frequency questionnaire[20,21]. The information obtained from these methods, taking into consideration their accepted limitations, can be used to assess current intake in comparison to known nutritional requirements, in order to ascertain potential nutritional deficiencies. A number of biochemical markers of nutritional intake and nutritional status of both macro- and micronutrients also exist. In certain cases, these markers may also be used to assess recent intake, body stores or a combination of these. However, as with all methods of nutritional assessment, it is necessary to consider the assessment of biochemical markers in the light of a number of confounding factors such as homeostatic mechanisms and the distribution of nutrients between body compartments[18].

11.3   Factors affecting nutritional status

When implementing a food-avoidance diet, it is necessary to consider a number of factors.

11.3.1   Number of foods being eliminated

It is likely that as the number of foods to be avoided increases, the impact on the nutritional adequacy of the resulting diet will also increase[17]. If items from a single food group need to be avoided it is likely that, with appropriate dietary counselling, alternative foods can be used to ensure that no nutritional deficiencies occur. However, the larger the number of food groups to be avoided, the more limited are the available macro- and micronutrient alternatives, with a consequent adverse affect on dietary adequacy. As the number of foods to be excluded increases, the resultant diet has the potential to become monotonous. In children, this may cause food refusal due to the boredom of having a limited variety of permitted foods, with a further adverse impact on dietary adequacy. Specialist advice will help to ensure that an elimination diet remains as varied as possible, in an attempt to prevent food fatigue and its associated consequences.

11.3.2   Range of products containing food allergen

The nutritional impact of a food-avoidance diet is likely to increase if the food allergen is found in a large number of foods. For example, an allergy to a food that is not commonly used in food manufacturing will both make it simpler to avoid that food and also mean that the range of foods to be avoided is limited. However, if the suspected or known food allergen is found in a large number of manufactured foods (e.g. cow's milk, egg, soya, wheat, nuts), the range of 'allowed' foods will be limited and consequently the risk of nutritional deficiencies occurring will be greater. As food manufacturers become increasingly 'allergy aware', a large number of manufactured products bear 'may contain' warnings (for example when a chocolate bar that does not have nuts listed as an ingredient is produced in a factory where nuts are processed for use in other products). For the most sensitive patients, who need also to avoid products which bear these types of warning, their food choices are limited further, and this may have a resultant impact on their nutritional status[9].

11.3.3   Length of the elimination period

As discussed previously, the nutritional impact of a short-term exclusion diet in a patient whose nutritional status is optimal is likely to be minimal, and therefore detailed dietary assessment and support may not be required to asses the nutritional adequacy of the diet, although specialist advice may be required to support the client in the practicalities of food avoidance. However, if the exclusion diet is likely to last for a longer period (and in some cases for life), the impact on a patient's nutritional status will be significant, as their nutritional stores will soon be depleted and need to be replenished. Appropriate support is therefore vital.

11.3.4   Other dietary restrictions

It is recognised that people do not include certain foods in their diet for a range of reasons. These may include cultural or religious expectations, ethical beliefs, food preferences or food availability. When implementing an elimination diet, it is vital to take these factors into consideration both when assessing the risk of possible nutritional deficiencies and when providing advice on how to ensure an ongoing balanced diet. For example, the nutritional consequences of removing nuts from the diet are likely to be much lower in a patient who is happy to eat a range of other protein-rich foods such as meat, fish, animal-derived dairy products, eggs and legumes. However, if the patient has chosen to follow a vegan diet, the nutritional impact of commencing a nut-free diet is likely to be more significant and would warrant specialist support to ensure that the patient's diet remains adequate.

It is also necessary to consider food preferences when providing advice to ensure a nutritionally adequate elimination diet. There is no benefit in recommending alternative foods that will lead to nutritional adequacy, if these foods are disliked or refused. The dietary advice needs to be expertly tailored to meet the needs of each individual patient and provide support as new foods are integrated into the diet. Regular follow-up is also required, to ensure that the patient is able to implement effectively the advice that has been provided.

11.3.5   Changing nutritional requirements

It is important to recognise that an individual's nutritional requirements for both macro- and micronutrients change with age, weight and medical condition. This means that, even if a food-avoidance diet is deemed adequate at one point in time, patients may be at risk of developing nutritional deficiencies if their nutritional requirements increase but their diet does not alter to meet these increased needs. This is specifically relevant when providing support for children, whose nutritional needs for optimal growth and development change rapidly.

Table 11.1 demonstrates that there is a vast difference between a person's calcium requirement at different ages and stages of life. A cow's-milk-free diet which has been assessed to ensure that it meets the calcium requirement of an 18-month-old may not meet the calcium requirement of a 5-year-old, further highlighting the importance of regular review to ensure ongoing dietary adequacy[20].

11.4   Ensuring optimal nutritional status while following a food-avoidance diet

To ensure a nutritionally adequate food-avoidance diet while taking into consideration the above factors, it can be helpful to consider the following three basic questions (adapted from Geissler & Powers[18]):

Table 11.1   Changing calcium requirements from birth to adulthood[22].

Age	Calcium requirement (mg/day) Reference nutrient intake (RNI)	
0–12 months	525	
1–3 years	350	
4–6 years	450	
7–10 years	550	
11–18 years	Male – 1000	Female – 800
19+ years	700	
Lactation	Additional 550	
Coeliac disease and	Adults – 1000	
inflammatory bowel disease[23]	Postmenopausal women and men > 55 years old – 1200	

- Which nutrients are going to be reduced in the prescribed food-avoidance diet?
- Are other components of the current diet adequate to fulfil the resulting nutritional deficits?
- Are further dietary manipulations required, for example the use of food substitutes or nutritional supplements, in order to ensure the diet remains nutritionally adequate?

When aiming to achieve dietary adequacy while eliminating foods from the diet, it is helpful to use guidelines which have been endorsed by organisations such as the Food Standards Agency or the British Dietetic Association, describing what constitutes a balanced diet. Doing this helps to identify alternative foods to ensure that the avoidance diet remains balanced. For example, the UK government has published recommendations for the types and proportions of foods which ensure a healthy and well-balanced diet at www.eatwell.gov.uk[24].

11.5   The nutritional consequences of avoiding a number of common food allergens

11.5.1   Cow's milk

Cow's milk is the most complete of all foods, containing nearly all the constituents of nutritional importance to humans, apart from iron[25]. Following breast milk, cow's-milk-based infant formulas are the second most appropriate sole source of nutrition for healthy infants under 6 months of age, if mothers choose not to breast-feed or if a supplement to breast milk is needed[26]. Cow's milk is a particularly good source of high-quality protein, easily assimilated calcium and riboflavin[25]. Cow's milk also provides significant levels of vitamin B_{12}, magnesium and phosphate. Whole milk is also a good source of vitamin A and energy from fat[27]. Consequently, the nutritional impact of removing cow's milk from the diet has the potential to be significant.

There have been numerous reports concerning the nutritional consequences of both supervised and unsupervised elimination of cow's milk from the diet. Isolauri *et al.* studied 100 children with a mean age of 7 months presenting with atopic dermatitis and challenge-proven cow's-milk allergy[28]. This group found that despite achieving symptom control, indices of both length and weight-for-length were decreased in patients following a cow's-milk-free diet compared to healthy controls.

There have also been a number of published reports concerning the impact on calcium status of eliminating cow's milk. It is known that approximately 80% of peak bone mass should be achieved from birth to adolescence, and the role of calcium in this process is well recognised[4]. Inadequate levels of calcium in childhood can result in stunted growth and rickets. In adults, calcium deficiency can result in osteomalacia[25]. Over 20 years ago, David *et al.* analysed the nutrient intake over a five-day period of 23 children whose atopic dermatitis was being treated with a multiple avoidance diet and showed significantly low calcium intakes in 57% of these children[7]. McGowan and Gibney looked at a group of 38 adults with self-reported milk allergy and found significantly lower intakes of calcium ($p < 0.002$) than in age-, sex- and occupation-matched controls[12]. Black *et al.* reported on a group of children following a cow's-milk-free diet who had lower total-body bone mineral content ($p < 0.01$) than controls who drank cow's milk[8]. Fox *et al.* described a case of a toddler with atopic dermatitis and reported immediate onset of symptoms following his first exposure to cow's-milk formula[13]. He had been commenced on a cow's-milk-free diet and was slow to progress with the introduction of solids due to parental anxiety. He presented with delayed motor development and clinical and biochemical markers of rickets, with raised levels of alkaline phosphatase and parathyroid hormone, and low serum calcium, phosphate and vitamin D.

This body of evidence highlights the importance of appropriate medical and dietetic support for all patients presenting with suspected cow's-milk-protein allergy (CMPA).

For infants, it is essential that an alternative, non-allergy-provoking formula which meets current infant formula guidelines[29] is identified as an alternative to cow's milk. Table 11.2 shows the nutritional composition of a selection of infant formulas designed to meet the nutritional requirements of infants (under 1 year of age) with suspected or diagnosed cow's-milk allergy, compared with the nutritional composition of other cow's-milk substitutes suitable for older children and adults. This comparison shows the varied nutritional profile of cow's-milk substitutes suitable for older children and adults. For example, soya milk and rice milk are significantly lower in calories compared to suitable infant formulas and will therefore not promote appropriate growth in infants and young children. It is important that a specialist healthcare practitioner such as a registered dietitian is consulted in order to identify the most appropriate cow's-milk substitute.

Despite the availability of infant formulas designed specifically to meet the needs of an infant with suspected or diagnosed CMPA, it is still vital to assess the nutritional adequacy of the resulting diet. This is particularly the case when the intake of formula declines appropriately as weaning progresses, but where the weaning diet is limited. Figure 11.1 provides a worked example of calculating an infant's calcium

Table 11.2 Nutritional profile of a range of cow's-milk substitutes: (a) infant formulas designed to meet the nutritional requirements of infants with suspected or diagnosed cow's-milk allergy; (b) other cow's-milk substitutes suitable for older children and adults.

Product	Energy (per 100 ml)	Protein (per 100 ml)	Calcium (per 100 ml)	Age group for which product suitable
Nutramigen® AA	68 kcal 100 ml	1.89 g 100 ml	64 mg 100 ml	From birth
Nutramigen® 1 (Mead Johnson)	68 kcal	1.9 g	64 mg	From birth
Pepti® (Cow and Gate)	66 kcal	1.6 g	52 mg	From birth
Neocate® (SHS)	71 kcal	1.95 g	49 mg	From birth
Nutramigen® 2 (Mead Johnson)	72 kcal	2.3 g	90 mg	From 6 months
Infant soya formula	66 kcal	1.8 g	65 mg	From 6 months[30]
Organic soya milk	41 kcal	3.3 g	12 mg	From 2 years*
Calcium-enriched soya milk	42 kcal	3.3 g	120 mg	From 2 years*
Unfortified rice milk	47 kcal	0.1 g	nil	From 2 years*
Calcium-enriched rice milk	47 kcal	1.1 g	120 mg	From 2 years*

* In special circumstances, following the detailed assessment of a child's diet, these milks may be recommended to younger children if other milks have been refused.

Figure 11.1 Worked example of calculating an infant's calcium.

Calcium requirement for a 9-month-old infant – 525 mg calcium per day
Current diet free from cow's milk
Cow's-milk substitute – Neocate (SHS)
Average daily intake of Neocate – 600 ml, providing 294 mg calcium
Calcium-rich foods included in weaning diet:
   Broccoli, calcium-fortified bread
Average daily calcium intake from solids – 70 mg
Total daily calcium intake – approximately 365 mg/day
Additional calcium required to meet requirements – 160 mg/day

needs when on a cow's-milk-free diet. In this example, it would be appropriate to consider introducing other, non-dairy, calcium-rich foods. However, if this is not possible, a calcium supplement may be required to ensure that the infant is meeting his or her calcium requirement consistently. Vitamin and mineral supplementation is discussed later in this chapter.

If the infant continues to be breast-fed, and there is suspicion that he or she is reacting to traces of allergenic proteins in the mother's breast milk, a maternal dietary restriction may be recommended[31]. In this instance it is vital to consider how to maintain the nutritional status of the lactating mother. This is especially important as, during lactation, a woman's nutritional requirements for energy, protein, vitamins and minerals are elevated. Although it is known that the calcium content of breast milk is not affected by the mother's nutritional status, it is known that her own calcium stores will be depleted if she is not meeting her increased requirements[22]. It is therefore essential that mothers are counselled on appropriate methods of ensuring that their own diet remains adequate in macro- and micronutrients even when dietary restrictions are implemented. If it is impractical to manage this through diet alone, it may be necessary to consider a suitable micronutrient supplement.

Once a child is older than 1 year, it may be appropriate for an infant formula to be continued, in view of the lower energy content of other cow's-milk substitutes. If the child is also following a very restricted diet, he or she may benefit from the additional micronutrients in infant formulas compared with cow's-milk substitutes. When choosing a cow's-milk substitute for older children (> 2 years) and adults, since other calcium-rich foods are unlikely to be included in the diet regularly enough to ensure a consistently adequate calcium intake, it is helpful to ensure that the cow's-milk substitute used is fortified with calcium, ideally to a level similar to that of cow's milk (approximately 120 mg/100 ml). It is a common misconception that products marketed as being 'milks' naturally contain calcium, when in fact this is not always the case (Table 11.2). Patients require educating on which products will be suitable. It is also important to consider the protein and energy content of the cow's-milk substitute. If a substitute with a poor energy and protein level is chosen, then the nutritional adequacy of the diet will need further assessment to ensure that nutritional requirements continue to be met.

It is inevitable that the taste of cow's-milk alternatives will not always be accepted, particularly in large quantities, especially in older children and adults who have been used to cow's milk in the past. It may be appropriate to consider flavouring the cow's-milk substitute with fruit or a proprietary milkshake flavouring or liquid suitable for the individual's exclusion diet[32]. There are also a number of alternatives to commonly consumed cow's-milk-based products, such as soya-based yogurts and cheese, or custard or rice pudding made with a cow's-milk alternative such as soya milk or rice milk. These products not only add variety to the diet but can also help ensure dietary adequacy. As with cow's-milk substitutes, it is helpful to choose products fortified with calcium.

In some cases it may not be possible to provide appropriate quantities of cow's-milk substitutes to ensure an adequate calcium intake. If this is the case it is helpful to ascertain whether non-dairy calcium sources can be incorporated into the diet to meet an individual's calcium requirement. Table 11.3 provides a list of calcium-rich, non-dairy foods and their calcium content per 100 g and per average portion. When assessing whether the use of these foods will ensure the individual's calcium requirement is met, it is necessary to consider whether sufficient quantities of these foods can be included in the diet on a regular basis. If dietary assessment reveals that an individual with CMPA is not meeting his or her calcium requirement, despite trying to implement a diet containing other calcium-rich foods (as shown in the example at Figure 11.1 above), a calcium supplement may be necessary.

Although cow's milk provides a significant proportion of dietary protein and calcium, it is important to consider the other micronutrients which will be lacking in the diet if cow's milk is excluded. This can be done by assessing the diet using weighed food-intake records, followed by either manual or computer-aided assessment of the micronutrient content of the diet. If this analysis suggests deficiency, it

Table 11.3   Calcium content of a range of foods[25,33].

Food source	Calcium content (per 100g)	Calcium content per average portion[34]
Eggs (boiled)	57 mg	34.2 mg (60 g)
Beef – stewing steak (stewed)	15 mg	21 mg (140 g)
Cod fillet (baked)	22 mg	26.4 mg (120 g)
Sardines – canned in oil (fish only)	550 mg	275 mg (50 g)
Baked beans	53 mg	71.6 mg (135 g)
Courgettes (boiled)	19 mg	17.1 mg (90 g)
Cabbage (boiled)	33 mg	31.4 mg (95 g)
Okra (boiled)	120 mg	6 mg (5 g – 1 medium)
Onions (fried)	47 mg	18.8 mg (40 g)
Watercress	170 mg	34 mg (20 g)
Sultanas	64 mg	19.2 mg (30 g)
Peanuts (dried roasted)	52 mg	26 mg (50 g)
Bread – white	110 mg	39.6 mg (36 g)
Bread – wholemeal	54 mg	19.4 mg (36 g)
Rice – white (boiled)	18 mg	32.4 mg (180 g)

may be helpful to look at ways of incorporating other dietary sources of the nutrient into the diet (Table 11.4), or to consider vitamin or mineral supplementation.

11.5.2   Egg

Eggs are a good source of protein, vitamin A, vitamin B_{12}, vitamin D, vitamin E, riboflavin, pantothenic acid, selenium, biotin (only after avidin has been denatured during the cooking process) and iodine[25]. However, the nutritional consequences of avoiding egg in an individual following an otherwise varied, balanced diet are likely to be minimal, as all of the above nutrients can be provided from other sources. Egg avoidance may, however, have a greater nutritional impact upon an individual who is following a vegetarian diet and is relying on eggs as a principal source of protein. In this instance, the diet can remain nutritionally adequate through the inclusion of suitable alternative protein sources such as nuts, beans and pulses.

11.5.3   Legumes, nuts and seeds

Legumes such as peas, beans (including soya) and lentils are a good source of protein, fibre and a range of vitamins and minerals[36]. Nuts (including peanuts) are rich in fat and therefore a good source of energy when eaten in larger quantities. Like legumes, they are also an excellent source of protein and fibre and are also a good source of a range of B vitamins and vitamin E. Seeds (such as pumpkin and sesame) have a similar nutritional profile to nuts[25].

As with egg, the nutritional consequences of excluding certain foods from this group will be minimal if the rest of the diet is varied and contains a range of other

Table 11.4　Food sources of vitamins, minerals and trace elements[35].

Vitamin/mineral	Sources
Water-soluble vitamins	
Biotin	Egg yolk, liver, kidney, muscle and organ meats, certain vegetables
Folic acid (in the form of folates)	Liver, yeast extract, green leafy vegetables, legumes, certain fruits, fortified breakfast cereals and margarines
Niacin (nicotinic acid & nicotinamide)	Beef, pork, wheat flour, maize flour, eggs, cow's milk
Pantothenic acid	Chicken, beef, potatoes, oat cereals, tomato products, liver, kidney, yeast, egg yolk, broccoli, whole grains
Riboflavin	Milk, eggs, enriched cereals and grain, ice cream, liver, some lean meats, green vegetables
Thiamin (vitamin B_1)	Unrefined grain products, white and brown flour, meat products, vegetables, dairy products, legumes, fruits and eggs
Vitamin B_6 (pyridoxine)	Chicken, fish, liver, kidney, pork, eggs, milk, wheat germ, brewer's yeast, brown rice, soybeans, oats, whole-wheat grains, peanuts and walnuts
Vitamin B_{12}	Meat (particularly liver) and fish
Vitamin C	Citrus and soft fruits, leafy green vegetables, kidney and liver
Fat soluble-vitamins	
Vitamin A (retinol)	Dairy products, fortified margarine, liver, fish oils
β-Carotene	Yellow and green leafy vegetables, yellow fruits, EC160a
Vitamin D	Fatty fish, fish oils, liver, milk, eggs Fortified margarines, processed/powdered milk, breakfast cereals and chocolate bars
Vitamin E	Plant oils (e.g. soybean oil, corn oil, olive oil), meat, poultry, dairy products
Vitamin K	Green leafy vegetables, vegetable oils, dairy products, meat, eggs
Trace elements	
Boron	Nuts, fruit, green vegetables
Chromium	Processed meats, wholegrain products, pulses, spices
Cobalt	Fish, nuts, green leafy vegetables, fresh cereals
Copper	Nuts, shellfish, offal
Germanium	Beans, tomato juice, oysters, tuna, garlic
Iodine	Marine fish, shellfish, sea salt, cereals and grains, cow's milk
Manganese	Green vegetables, nuts, bread and other cereals, tea
Molybdenum	Legumes, leafy vegetables, cauliflower, nuts, canned vegetables, cereals
Nickel	Pulses, oats, nuts

Table 11.4 *(cont'd)*

Vitamin/mineral	Sources
Selenium	Fish, offal, brazil nuts, eggs, cereals
Tin	Fruit products, canned vegetables, E512
Vanadium	Spinach, parsley, nuts, oils, wholegrains, meats, seafood, dairy products
Zinc	Meat, cereal products
Minerals Calcium	Milk, cheese, other dairy products, green leafy vegetables (except spinach), fortified soybean products, breads and other baked goods made with calcium fortified flour, almonds, brazil nuts, hazel nuts
Iron	Liver, meat, beans, nuts, dried fruit, poultry, fish, whole grains or enriched cereals, fortified flour, soybean flour, green leafy vegetables
Magnesium	Leafy vegetables, grains, nuts, dairy products, meats
Phosphorus	Red meats, fish, dairy products, poultry, bread and other cereals
Potassium	Milk, fruit, vegetables, fish, shellfish, beef, chicken, turkey, liver, salt substitutes
Silicon	Grains (e.g. oats, barley, rice), beer
Sodium chloride	Table salt, cereals and cereal products (particularly bread), meat and meat products, crisps and savoury snacks

protein sources. However, if an individual is following a vegetarian or vegan diet, it will be necessary to ensure that alternative energy and protein options are provided. It should also be noted that soya is found unexpectedly in a large range of manufactured products (for example breads, baked goods, sweets, drinks, breakfast cereals, ice cream, margarine, pasta and processed meats)[24]. Therefore, for those individuals (who tend to be the minority) who are particularly sensitive to soya and need to avoid these traces of soya, the nutritional impact on their diet will be more significant due to the wide range of foods that will need to be excluded. Specialist support will ensure that nutritional deficiencies are prevented.

If an individual needs to avoid both cow's milk and soya, the nutritional consequences will also be more significant. As discussed previously, calcium-fortified soya-protein-based products are a common alternative for people who need to follow a cow's-milk-free diet. Therefore, if both cow's-milk protein and soya protein need to be excluded, the options for ensuring an adequate calcium intake, in addition to energy and protein, will be limited and a calcium supplement may need to be recommended.

Soya beans contain significant levels of isoflavines, a compound belonging to the phyto-oestrogen family. Phyto-oestrogens are naturally occurring plant compounds that have been found to have both weak oestrogenic and anti-oestrogenic actions[18]. There is currently growing interest as to the potentially beneficial or adverse effects of these compounds in a range of population groups[37]. Alternative sources of isoflavines include other pulses and cereals, such as sorghum and millet. Lignans, also part of the phyto-oestrogen family, are found in wholegrain products, seeds, grains and other fibre-rich foods[37].

11.5.4 Seafood

Fish and shellfish are valuable sources of high-quality protein. Fatty fish (such as herring, mackerel and salmon, as well as fish livers) contains high levels of the fat-soluble vitamins A and D. Fish muscle contains a variety of minerals including iodine, and fish where the bones are commonly eaten (for example sardines or tinned salmon) are a good source of calcium, phosphorus and fluoride[25]. Fatty fish also contain high levels of long-chain n-3 polyunsaturated fatty acids[36], which have been shown to have a number of beneficial effects, including helping to protect against cardiovascular disease[18]. It is also known that these fats are important in the development of an infant's central nervous system[38]. A number of groups have also investigated the long-chain polyunsaturated fatty acid requirements for the brain and retina development of preterm and term infants. However, a recent Cochrane review focusing on preterm infants concluded that when the results of randomised controlled studies were pooled, no clear long-term benefit was seen in the groups receiving formula supplemented with long-chain polyunsaturated fatty acid. The Cochrane review considering the evidence for the routine supplementation of term infant formulas with long-chain polyunsaturated fatty acids concluded that the current evidence showed no proven benefit regarding vision, cognition or physical growth[39,40]. There is also current interest in the possible link between prenatal omega-3 polyunsaturated fatty acid status and the development of allergic disease[41].

The UK government has recognised that, due to the potential health benefits, the population as a whole should increase their consumption of oily fish, and have recommended that everyone should eat at least two portions (a portion being 140 g) of fish a week, including one portion of oily fish[24]. However, due to the low levels of pollutants which may be found in oily fish, maximum levels have also been recommended, as follows[24]:

- two portions per week for girls, women who are planning to have a baby and women who are pregnant or breastfeeding;
- four portions per week for boys, men and women who do not fall into the above categories.

It has also been recommended that women who are trying for a baby or who are pregnant, as well as children, should avoid shark, swordfish (classified as an oily fish) and marlin due to the levels of mercury in these fish, which can affect the development of children's developing nervous systems[24].

It should be noted that a recent government inquiry considering the links between diet and behaviour has recommended, in view of the ongoing research in this area, that the Scientific Advisory Committee on Nutrition (SACN) should further define the optimum intake of omega-3 polyunsaturated fatty acids at different life stages, including pregnancy and childhood[42].

For people who need to avoid seafood in their diet, alternative sources of omega-3 fatty acids include certain vegetable oils, such as linseed, flaxseed, walnut, rapeseed and algae. However, the fatty acids found in these products are not the same as those found in fish, and they may not have the same benefits[24]. Fish-oil supplements may not be suitable for people with a fish allergy due to the risk of them containing or being contaminated with the allergenic fish protein. In this instance, the potential risks for a fish-allergic individual of having a severe allergic reaction outweigh the potential benefits of the n-3 polyunsaturated fatty acids found in oily fish. However, non-fish sources of omega-3 fatty acids could be recommended. It is worth asking the manufacturer of a particular fish oil supplement if there are any traces of fish protein left.

11.5.5 Cereals

Cereal grains are a major component of the human diet. In Britain, it is estimated that wheat, wheat-based products and other cereals (for example rice, oatmeal and breakfast cereals) contribute approximately 30% of the total energy, 25% of the protein and nearly 50% of the carbohydrate in the average diet[18]. In addition to being a good energy source, cereals also significantly contribute to our intake of a range of other nutrients, either due to their high natural content or through fortification; however, the variety and content of nutrients vary from one cereal to another.

Cereals also contribute significantly to our intake of both insoluble and soluble fibre (non-starch polysaccharides). Wholegrain bread, brown rice and wholegrain breakfast cereals are all rich in insoluble fibre, which is thought to increase faecal weight and therefore to be important in the treatment of constipation and diverticular disease. Oats, barley and rye contain higher amounts of soluble fibre (which may be particularly helpful in the control of plasma glucose levels and cholesterol levels)[18,19].

Wheat is considered the most significant source of cereals in the United Kingdom, while rice is of greater significance in Far Eastern countries and maize is a common staple in much of Africa and Central America[18]. These differences highlight the importance of taking into consideration an individual's cultural background when assessing the impact of a food-avoidance diet. Although it is impossible to generalise, the impact of eliminating wheat from the diet is likely to be greater in population groups who rely on wheat as their main source of carbohydrate. As the number of grains to be avoided increases, the options for alternative products will also diminish.

When providing support to an individual who needs to avoid one or more cereals in the diet, it is vital that alternative products are identified in order to ensure that the resulting diet remains varied and balanced. A range of alternatives to common wheat-based products are available to purchase in both supermarkets and more specialist health-food shops. A number of staple wheat-free products are also available on prescription. These products are primarily prescribable for patients with coeliac disease, but general practitioners can also prescribe it for other wheat related diagnoses (see also Chapter 9). These products include breads, pastas and biscuits based on alternative grains such as rice, maize or buckwheat. These products may not be fortified with vitamins and minerals to the same degree as their wheat-based equivalents, and do not always function in the same way when being prepared for eating. They may also have a unique taste. It is therefore important that patients using these products are encouraged to follow the preparation instructions on the packet and are provided with strategies to improve the palatability of the products – such as disguising the taste of wheat-free pasta with a suitable sauce, eating bread immediately after it has been 'refreshed', and using spreads and jams to moisten the products.

For individuals who need to eliminate one or more cereals from their diet, it is important that alternative fibre sources are also provided. Current government recommendations are that adult diets should contain an average of 18 g of fibre per day (individual range 12–24 g/day of non-starch polysaccharides)[22]. Certain wheat-free breads, mixes and pastas are available in fibre-containing varieties. There is also a range of non-cereal foods that are good sources of both insoluble and soluble fibre (Table 11.5).

Table 11.5   Fibre (non-starch polysaccharide) content of selected foods (edible portion)[33].

Food	Fibre content (total non-starch polysaccharides) (g/100 g)	Fibre content (total non-starch polysaccharides) (g/average portion)[34]
Meat	0	0
Baked beans	3.7	5 (135 g)
Beans, red kidney, boiled	6.7	4.7 (70 g)
Beans, runner, boiled	1.9	1.7 (90 g)
Cabbage, boiled	1.8	1.7 (95 g)
Carrots, boiled	2.5	1.5 (60 g)
New potatoes, boiled, with skins	1.5	2.6 (175 g)
Yam, boiled	1.4	1.8 (130 g)
Apples with skin, raw	1.8	1.8 (100 g)
Raisins	2.0	0.6 (30 g)
Nuts, mixed	6.0	3.0 (50 g)
Bread, white	1.9	0.7 (36 g)
Bread, brown	3.5	1.3 (36 g)
Bread, wholemeal	5.0	1.8 (36 g)
Flour, white, plain	3.1	–
Flour, wholemeal	9.0	–
All Bran	24.5	9.8 (40 g)
Oatmeal, raw	7.1	3.6 (50 g)
Weetabix	9.7	3.9 (40 g)
Rice Krispies	0.7	0.2 (30 g)
Rice, white, boiled	0.1	0.2 (180 g)
Rice, brown, boiled	0.8	1.4 (180 g)
Spaghetti, white, boiled	1.2	2.6 (220 g)
Spaghetti, wholemeal, boiled	3.5	7.7 (220 g)

11.5.6 Fruit and vegetables

The nutritional consequences of eliminating fruit and vegetables from the diet may, initially, appear minimal. However, this family of foods is an extremely rich source of a range of vitamins, minerals and trace elements. Leafy vegetables, despite being low in energy, are a significant source of carotenoids, vitamin C, folates and, to a lesser extent, B vitamins. Green vegetables are an important source of non-haem iron. Potassium and magnesium are also present in significant levels, in addition to trace elements absorbed from the soil. Fruits, including citrus fruit, berries, currants, tomatoes, apples and melons, are significant sources of vitamin C. Green and yellow fruits are also an important source of carotenoids. The majority of fruits and vegetables are also a valuable source of non-starch polysaccharides, although the concentrations of both the soluble and insoluble forms differ between varieties. It is thought that fruit and vegetables provide approximately one-third of the total intake of dietary fibre in the UK diet[18].

As a result of their nutritional value, the government recommends that a variety of fruits and vegetables should make up a third of our daily intake of food. In order to promote an increased intake of fruit and vegetables, it is recommended that five portions of foods from this group are eaten daily[24]. For individuals who need to avoid certain fruits and vegetables, it is important that they are provided with strategies to ensure that they continue to meet the target of five portions per day regularly. This could mean encouraging someone to try new fruits or vegetables that are unlikely to provoke an allergic reaction and may require education on how these products can be easily incorporated into the diet. If a large range of fruits and vegetables need to be excluded from the diet then it may be necessary to consider recommending a multivitamin supplement.

11.6 Vitamin and mineral supplements

Despite being aware of the nutritional deficits caused by a food-avoidance diet, it may not be possible to ensure dietary adequacy is maintained by simply using food substitutes. This can be the case for a number of reasons:

- the number of foods to be avoided means that the range of alternatives is too limited to ensure nutritional adequacy;
- an individual's food preferences mean that food substitutes are not accepted;
- the use of food substitutes becomes monotonous, and compliance with dietary advice to ensure nutritional adequacy is not achieved;
- poor availability or high cost of food substitute.

In the above instances, it may be appropriate to consider using micronutrient supplements to ensure consistent dietary adequacy.

Micronutrient supplements should only be recommended following a thorough assessment of an individual's current nutritional intake. In infants under 6 months of age, the 24-hour recall method may be sufficient to assess dietary adequacy.

However, in all other individuals it is important to analyse dietary adequacy using a food diary kept for three days or more[17]. If it is considered necessary to commence dietary supplements, a number of factors need to be taken into consideration:

11.6.1   Composition

Detailed analysis of an individual's current intake will identify whether a single nutrient needs to be supplemented or whether the diet requires supplementation with a range of nutrients. This assessment will ascertain the composition of the micronutrient supplement that needs to be recommended. Single-nutrient supplements are available, as are supplements containing a range of micronutrients.

When considering which supplement to recommend it is also essential to ensure that the supplement is free from the foods that are being excluded from the diet. This can be achieved by reviewing the ingredients list of a product, or by liaising with the drug information team at the local hospital, a community pharmacist or the manufacturer of the micronutrient supplement. Individuals who need to avoid food additives or other naturally occurring food compounds may find it particularly difficult to identify suitable products, and will need support in order to ensure appropriate supplements are recommended.

11.6.2   Dose

Assessment of an individual's current diet in conjunction with an awareness of their micronutrient requirements will allow estimation of the dose of supplementary micronutrients required. This information can then be equated to a dose of a single micronutrient (e.g. calcium or iron) or used to review the suitability of a supplement containing a range of micronutrients. Although a product may be marketed as containing a specific micronutrient, the dose that the product contains may not be therapeutically significant. This highlights the importance of checking the doses of micronutrients in a product instead of assuming from the marketing information that a supplement is a rich source of a micronutrient.

11.6.3   Presentation

Vitamin, mineral and trace-element supplements come in a range of presentations, for example as liquids, chewable tablets, effervescent tablets or tablets designed to be swallowed whole. Flavoured supplements are also available in many of these presentations. The preferred or most appropriate presentation for an individual will help facilitate compliance with the recommended supplement regime. As mentioned previously, it is also possible to source individual micronutrient supplements (for example calcium or iron) or supplements containing a range of micronutrients (for example calcium and vitamin D or a multivitamin supplement). As an example, Table 11.6 provides a list of calcium supplements that are available on prescription

Table 11.6   Prescribable calcium supplements[43].

Name of product	Contents	Presentation	Nutritional profile
Calcium gluconate	Calcium gluconate 600 mg	Tablets	Calcium 53.4 mg Sodium 4.46 mmol
Calcium gluconate	Calcium gluconate 1 g	Effervescent tablets	Calcium 89 mg Sodium 4.46 mmol
Calcium lactate	Calcium lactate 300 mg	Tablets	Calcium 39 mg
Adcal®	Calcium carbonate 1.5 g	Chewable tablets	Calcium 600 mg
Cacit®	Calcium carbonate 1.25 g	Effervescent tablets	Calcium 500 mg
Calcichew®	Calcium carbonate 1.25 g	Tablets	Calcium 500 mg
Calcichew Forte®	Calcium carbonate 2.5 g	Tablets	Calcium 1000 mg
Calcium-500	Calcium carbonate 1.25 g	Tablets	Calcium 500 mg
Calcium Sandoz®	Calcium glubionate 1.09 g, calcium lactobionate 727 mg	Syrup	Calcium 108.3 mg/5 ml
Sandocal-400®	Calcium lactate gluconate 930 mg, calcium carbonate 700 mg, anhydrous citric acid 1.189 g	Effervescent tablets	Calcium 400 mg
Sandocal-1000®	Calcium lactate gluconate 2.263 g, calcium carbonate 1.75 g, anhydrous citric acid 2.973 g	Effervescent tablets	Calcium 1000 mg

for both adults and children where only calcium supplementation is indicated, and highlights the range of presentations and doses that are available.

11.6.4   Availability

A number of micronutrient supplements are available on prescription. The British National Formulary (updated regularly in book format and available online) is an essential resource detailing all prescribable vitamin and mineral supplements[43]. A range of micronutrient supplements are also available over the counter in chemists, supermarkets, specialist health-food shops or online. If a non-prescription product is going to be recommended, it is important that the family or individual has easy access to the product to ensure compliance and therefore ongoing dietary adequacy.

11.6.5   Cost

If an over-the-counter micronutrient supplement is recommended, it is also important to consider the cost of the supplement. The cost of micronutrient supplements varies greatly, and in order to ensure long-term compliance with a product it is important to ensure that the long-term cost is not prohibitive.

11.6.6   Length of supplementation

In some instances, the micronutrient supplementation may be required for the length of the exclusion. However, there are a number of instances when this may not be the case. As mentioned earlier in this chapter, an individual's nutritional requirements change with age. In the case of calcium, the requirement for a 0–1 year old is 525 mg calcium/day, compared to 350 mg calcium/day for a 1–3 year old[22]. In this instance, supplementation may be required in infancy but could be stopped when the child is 1 year old if the diet is adequate to meet the reduced calcium requirements. Micronutrient supplementation may also be able to be stopped if assessment suggests adequate levels (for example of ferritin levels), or if assessment of dietary adequacy indicates that the diet has become adequate to meet nutritional requirements. All these scenarios highlight the importance of regular dietetic review for all individuals on an exclusion diet, to ensure that the diet continues to meet an individual's nutritional needs.

11.7   Other common nutritional issues encountered when implementing food-avoidance diets

11.7.1   Faltering growth/weight loss

There are a number of reports of faltering growth in the paediatric population following a food-avoidance diet. Following a retrospective case review to examine the link between perceived food allergy and failure to thrive, Roesler *et al.* concluded that parental beliefs about food allergy can lead to dietary restrictions severe enough to cause failure to thrive[6]. Christie *et al.* reported that children with two or more food allergies were shorter, based on height-for-age percentiles, than the children with only one food allergy[9], a finding similar to that of Isolauri's group[28].

If, prior to commencing a food-avoidance diet, an individual is assessed as not growing or maintaining weight appropriately, and the symptoms are mild, it may be deemed appropriate to address the growth failure prior to implementing further dietary restrictions. However, if delaying the implementation of a food-avoidance diet is not possible, or if growth failure is observed as a consequence of a nutritionally inappropriate food-avoidance diet, it will be essential to identify methods of promoting appropriate growth in conjunction with necessary dietary restrictions. Specialist advice with regard to increasing the energy density of a food-avoidance diet using allowed food sources will be required. However, in some instances, prescribable nutritional supplements may be required.

In children with a cow's-milk-allergy and faltering growth, evidence suggests that an amino-acid-based formula is the most appropriate formula choice[44]. There are also a number of energy-dense, cow's-milk-free supplements that are suitable for

Table 11.7   Energy-dense, cow's-milk-free, prescribable supplements[43].

Product name	Indications	Energy content (kcal/100 ml)	Protein content (g/100 ml)
Neocate Active (SHS)	Amino-acid-based Suitable from 1 year Flavoured and unflavoured varieties Designed to provide dietary supplementation for children with cow's milk allergy	100 (21% standard concentration)	2.8
Neocate Advance (SHS)	Amino-acid-based Suitable over 1 year Flavoured and unflavoured varieties Suitable as a sole source of nutrition under careful medical supervision	100 (25% standard concentration)	2.5
Elemental 028 (SHS)	Amino-acid-based Suitable over 1 year Flavoured and unflavoured varieties Suitable as a sole source of nutrition under careful medical supervision	78 (20% standard concentration)	2
Elemental 028 Extra (SHS)	Amino-acid-based Suitable over 1 year Flavoured and unflavoured varieties Suitable as a sole source of nutrition under careful medical supervision	89 (20% standard concentration)	2.5
ProvideExtra (Fresenius Kabi)	Based on soya and pea proteins To be used with caution in children under 5 years Flavoured, fat-free supplement	125	3.75

older children (of various ages from 1 year and upwards) or adults with faltering growth or weight loss (Table 11.7).

Individual carbohydrate and fat supplements are also available, and may be of use in individuals who are unable to incorporate the above supplements into their diet. However, these products should only be used following a specialist nutritional review.

There are also a number of cow's-milk-free enteral feeds (based on alternative proteins such as soya or free amino acids) which may be used as a suitable enteral feed for individuals with cow's-milk allergy.

11.7.2 Iron deficiency

Iron deficiency most commonly occurs when the diet cannot provide adequate levels of iron to meet an individual's requirement[18]. Iron deprivation can affect a number of essential body systems including cardiovascular, respiratory, brain and muscle function. In children, iron deficiency may also impact on mental and motor development[19]. Despite the important roles of iron, the National Diet and Nutrition Survey of young people aged 4–18 years showed that 50% of the older girls had an iron intake below the lower RNI (reference nutrient intake)[45].

There are a number of published reports of iron deficiency associated with food hypersensitivity. In a retrospective review of the causes of iron deficiency in childhood and adolescence, Ferrara *et al.* concluded that in younger children (7.5 months – 2 years) the most important cause of iron deficiency was blood loss associated with the gastrointestinal symptoms of cow's-milk intolerance[2]. There have also been case reports of iron-deficiency anaemia as a result of unsupervised dietary restrictions[13].

In infants with a diagnosed cow's-milk-allergy, it is vital that a suitable alternative is identified that meets the guidelines for infant formulas and is fortified with iron. In older children and adults, it is important to assess the contribution that the food or foods to be avoided make to the overall iron content of the diet, and to provide suitable alternatives. If iron deficiency is suspected, medical assessment and support is vital to ensure that it is corrected appropriately.

11.8 Conclusion

When providing support to an individual embarking on a food-avoidance diet, it is vital to consider the impact of the diet on the person's nutritional status, alongside providing support with regard to eliminating the required foods. It is also essential to review the impact of a food-avoidance diet regularly, to ensure that optimal nutritional status is maintained. The impact of inappropriate and unsupervised food-avoidance diets can be immense. A multidisciplinary approach to the treatment of individuals with suspected or diagnosed food hypersensitivity is, therefore, essential. Specialist healthcare practitioners such as registered dietitians can provide vital support to allow individuals to enjoy a varied, nutritionally balanced food-avoidance diet.

References

1. Lui T, Howard RM, Mancini AJ *et al.* Kwashiorkor in the United States: Fad Diets, Perceived and True Milk Allergy and Nutritional Ignorance. *Arch Dermatol* 2001; **137**: 630–6.
2. Ferrara M, Coppola L, Coppola A, Capozzi L. Iron deficiency in childhood and adolescence: retrospective review. *Hematology* 2006; **11**: 183–6.
3. Katz KA, Mahlberg MH, Honig PJ, Yan AC. Rice nightmare: kwashiorkor in 2 Philadelphia-area infants fed Rice Dream beverage. *J Am Acad Dermatol* 2005; **52**: S69–72.
4. Infante D, Tormo R. Risk of inadequate bone mineralization in diseases involving long-term suppression of dairy products. *J Pediatr Gastroenterol Nutr* 2000; **30**: 310–13.

5. Carvalho NF, Kenney RD, Carrington PH, Hall DE. Severe nutritional deficiencies in toddlers resulting from health food milk alternatives. *Pediatrics* 2001; **107**: E46.
6. Roesler TA, Barry PC, Bock SA. Factitious food allergy and failure to thrive. *Arch Pediatr Adolesc Med* 1994; **148**: 1150–5.
7. David TJ, Waddington E, Stanton RH. Nutritional hazards of elimination diets in children with atopic eczema. *Arch Dis Child* 1984; **59**: 323–5.
8. Black RE, Williams SM, Jones IE, Goulding A. Children who avoid drinking cow milk have low dietary calcium intakes and poor bone health. *Am J Clin Nutr* 2002; **76**: 675–80.
9. Christie L, Hine J, Parker JG, Burks W. Food allergies in children affect nutrient intake and growth. *J Am Diet Assoc* 2002; **102**: 1648–51.
10. Price CE, Rona RJ, Chinn S. Height of primary school children and parents' perceptions of food intolerance. *Br Med J* 1988; **296**: 1696–9.
11. Stallings VA, Oddleifson NW, Negrini BY, Zemel BS, Wellens R. Bone mineral content and dietary calcium intake in children prescribed a low-lactose diet. *J Pediatr Gastroenterol Nutr* 1994; **18**: 440–5.
12. McGowan M, Gibney MJ. Calcium intakes in individuals on diets for the management of cows' milk allergy: a case control study. *Eur J Clin Nutr* 1993; **47**: 609–16.
13. Fox AR, Du Toit G, Lang A, Lack G. Food allergy as a risk factor for nutritional rickets. *Pediatr Allergy Immunol* 2004; **15**: 566–9.
14. MacDonald A, Forsyth A. Nutritional deficiencies and the skin. *Clin Exp Dermatol* 2005; **30**: 388–90.
15. Barth GA, Weigl L, Boeing H, Disch R, Borelli S. Food intake in patients with atopic dermatitis. *Eur J Dermatol* 2001; **11**: 199–202.
16. Niggemann B, Heine RG. Who should manage infants and young children with food induced symptoms? *Arch Dis Child* 2006; **91**: 379–82.
17. Grimshaw KEC. Dietary management of food allergy in children. *Proc Nutr Soc* 2006; **65**: 412–17.
18. Geissler C, Powers H. *Human Nutrition*, 11th edn. Edinburgh: Elsevier Churchill Livingstone, 2005.
19. Thomas B, Bishop J. *Manual of Dietetic Practice*, 4th edn. Oxford: Blackwell, 2007.
20. Mofidi S. Nutritional management of pediatric food hypersensitivity. *Pediatrics* 2003; **111**: 1645–53.
21. Shaw V, Lawson M. *Clinical Paediatric Dietetics*, 3rd edn. Oxford: Blackwell, 2007.
22. COMA. *Dietary Reference Values for Food Energy and Nutrients for the United Kingdom*. Report of the Panel on Dietary Reference Values of the Committee on Medical Aspects of Food Policy. London: HMSO, 1991.
23. British Society of Gastroenterology. *Guidelines for Osteoporosis in Inflammatory Bowel Disease and Coeliac Disease*. London: BSG, 2007. www.bsg.org.uk.
24. Food Standards Agency. Eat well, be well. www.eatwell.gov.uk.
25. Ministry of Agriculture, Fisheries and Food. *Manual of Nutrition*, 10th edn. London: Stationery Office, 1995.
26. Department of Health. *Infant Feeding Recommendation*. London: DoH, 2004.
27. Dairy Council. Nutrients in milk. www.milk.co.uk.
28. Isolauri E, Siitas Y, Salo M, Isosomppi R, Kaila M. Elimination diet in cow's milk allergy: Risk for impaired growth in young children. *J Pediatr* 1988; **132**: 1004–9.
29. Infant Formula and Follow-on Formula (England) Regulations 2007 (S.I. 2007/3521) (as amended by The Infant Formula and Follow-on Formula (England) (Amendment) Regulations 2008 (S.I. 2008/2445)). This implements EC Directive 2006/141/EC. Similar regulations apply for Scotland, Wales and Northern Ireland.
30. British Dietetic Association Paediatric Group. *Paediatric Group Position Statement: Use of Infant Formulas based on Soy Protein for Infants*. London: BDA, 2008. www.bda.uk.com.
31. Vandenplas Y, Brueton M, Dupont C *et al.* Guidelines for the diagnosis and management of cow's milk protein allergy in infants. *Arch Dis Child* 2007; **92**: 902–8.
32. MacDonald S. Managing GI disorders in children one year and older. Cited in *Complete Nutrition* 2008; **8** (1): 23–5.

33. Food Standards Agency. *McCance and Widdowson's The Composition of Foods*, 6th summary edn. Cambridge: Royal Society of Chemistry, 2002.
34. Ministry of Agriculture, Fisheries and Food. *Food Portion Sizes*, 2nd edn. London: Stationery Office, 1993.
35. Food Standards Agency Expert Group on Vitamins and Minerals. *Safe Upper Levels of Vitamins and Minerals*. London: FSA, 2003.
36. Garrow JS, James WPT, Ralph A. *Human Nutrition and Dietetics*, 10th edn. Edinburgh: Churchill Livingstone, 2000.
37. Committee on Toxicity. *Phytoestrogens and Health*. London: Food Standards Agency, 2003.
38. Committee on Toxicity and Scientific Advisory Committee on Nutrition. *Advice on Fish Consumption: Benefits and Risks*. London: Stationery Office, 2004.
39. Simmer K, Schulzke SM, Patole S. Longchain polyunsaturated fatty acid supplementation in preterm infants. *Cochrane Database Syst Rev* 2008; (1): CD000375.
40. Simmer K, Patole SK, Rao SC. Longchain polyunsaturated fatty acid supplementation in infants born at term. *Cochrane Database Syst Rev* 2008; (1): CD000376.
41. Prescott SL, Dunstan JA. Prenatal fatty acid status and immune development: the pathways and the evidence. *Lipids* 2007; **42**: 801–10.
42. Food and Health Forum. *The Links Between Diet and Behaviour: the Influences of Nutrition on Mental Health*. Report of an inquiry held by the Associate Parliamentary Food and Health Forum, 2007.
43. British National Formulary. *BNF 56*, September 2008. London: Pharmaceutical Press, 2008. www.bnf.org.
44. Isolauri E, Sutas Y, Makinen-Kiljunen S *et al*. Efficacy and safety of hydrolyzed cow milk and amino acid-derived formula in infants with cow milk allergy. *J Pediatr* 1995; **127**: 550–7.
45. National Diet and Nutrition Survey: young people aged 4 to 18 years. Volume 1: Report of the diet and nutrition survey. London: Stationery Office, 2000.

12 Lifestyle Issues

Tanya Wright

12.1 Introduction

Living on a restricted diet usually requires changes to lifestyle to accommodate dietary needs and prevent reactions. This can impact on many areas of the sufferers' and their families' lives and severely affect quality of life[1-3]. The level of the restriction imposed and the severity of the reaction to accidental food consumption are the dictating factors that impose these limitations and changes. This chapter will cover issues that either directly or indirectly affect the lifestyle of the sufferer and the family, and it aims to provide information that will significantly reduce the impact of this. Sufferers of severe allergies who are at risk of a potentially fatal reaction may be given most press and have to deal with the most compromising lifestyle issues, but sufferers of other types of food hypersensitivity also have a plethora of issues to navigate – including, not least, the sceptical attitudes of other people. This group of FHS sufferers also need support and understanding.

12.2 The burden of anaphylaxis and food allergy

A diagnosis of food allergy, potential anaphylaxis and the prescription and carriage of adrenaline is a burden that has an impact on the whole family[4,5] (see Chapter 14). The impact has been found to be much worse in peanut-allergic children compared with children who have other chronic diseases[6]. In social, educational and home settings such a diagnosis has been confirmed to have a negative impact on quality of life[7-9], for both the sufferer and their family. Furthermore, dietary and lifestyle parameters are imposed which can be compounded further by cultural, ethical and personal preferences. Effective care for individuals at risk of anaphylaxis requires a comprehensive management approach[10] involving the child at risk, the family and carers, including medical, social and educational personnel. Together they can help with the effective management of this life-threatening condition, thus minimising the impact on their lifestyle.

12.3 The importance of reintroduction of foods

Reintroduction of foods, once an allergy has been outgrown, will lead to a better and more achievable nutritional quality in the diet. There is little evidence in the literature regarding the reintroduction of foods. In one study Eigenmann *et al.* found that one-quarter of patients who had had a negative food challenge continued to avoid the food[11]. Those with a previously confirmed peanut allergy were less likely to reintroduce the food than those allergic to other foods, and girls were found to reintroduce the challenge food significantly less frequently than boys. Fear of persistence of allergies was a reason cited for not reintroducing the food and failing to cease dietary restrictions.

This has a negative effect on quality of life, social life, psychological wellbeing and nutrition. Growth faltering in children is more likely with milk or wheat avoidance, but it can occur with any food, depending on the dietary habits of the individual. Non-allergy-related restrictions can compound this further. These include food avoidance for religious, cultural and ethical reasons, as well as food taste and texture preferences. Once an allergy has resolved, many of these restrictions can cease. Allergy rescue medications no longer have to be carried, food labels no longer have to be read, and those preparing foods no longer require constant scrutiny. Life should be more relaxed and enjoyable.

12.4   Cross-contamination

Cross-contamination is the inadvertent transfer of food allergens or particles from one food to another. This contamination can occur during manufacturing of foods, when foods are prepared, or from touching or drinking from a vessel someone else has used after eating. When foods are sold loose, such as in a bakery or delicatessen, or served together, such as at a buffet, the risks of cross-contamination are extremely high. This will usually only be an issue for those with a severe IgE-mediated food allergy, where minuscule amounts are enough to trigger a severe reaction.

In 2006 the Food Standards Agency produced a report aimed at food manufacturers and caterers on adapting practices that will reduce cross-contamination[12]. The food advisor for the anaphylaxis campaign has also produce guidance on the website www.allergytraining.com. In 2008, the FSA produced posters and leaflets to help caterers by providing a practical guide to reduce the risks of cross-contamination and the provision of suitable meals for those with 'food allergies'.

Personal contact is another consideration for these sufferers who must be wary of others who have eaten the foods they are allergic to. Kissing on the lips presents the highest risk, as particles of foods containing allergens may be transferred and ingested. Even a trace of allergen could be sufficient to trigger a life-threatening allergic reaction in the severely allergic population. This can be a real problem for a teenager, who may not like to broach the subject of what his or her partner has been eating if they are not well acquainted. Furthermore, teenagers are the group who are least likely to be carrying their medication for a variety of reasons, putting them at further risk. The Anaphylaxis Campaign runs workshops to help teenagers and young adults deal effectively with this and other pertinent age-related issues.

12.5   Items on prescription

Managing the diet of patients on restricted diets can have financial implications. One factor is the elevated cost of most replacement foods. The cumulative effect of this can impact on many areas of the sufferer's and the family's lives. The cost may inhibit special foods being purchased, which may have not only nutritional effects but also social and psychological implications. This has been recognised, and the following foods have been approved by the Advisory Committee on Borderline Substances (ACBS) so they may be prescribed to those requiring them:

- whole-egg and egg-white replacers;
- gluten-free foods for coeliacs;
- specialised formula milks;
- nutritional supplements.

12.6   Recipe information

Managing any diet is not just about obtaining adequate nutrition. Diets should also be varied and tasty irrespective of any restrictions which may be imposed due to food hypersensitivity. In addition, factors that restrict food choice also require consideration. These include food and texture dislikes, unacceptable foods due to cultural or religious reasons and self-imposed restrictions such as those imposed by veganism and vegetarianism. It may be a challenge, but with the correct planning, information, knowledge and support providing a nutritious, varied and tasty diet despite these restrictions in addition to a food allergy is almost always possible.

Most everyday recipes can be easily adapted and replacement products can be used. To help with this there are specialised recipe books, support groups, special diet cookery classes and recipes available for specific products. Specialist healthcare professionals such as allergy dietitians should also always have tried and tested recipes to give to patients.

For infants and children using specialised formula milks, the manufacturers will usually have recipes available on request that have been tested using their formulas. Likewise the companies making gluten- and wheat-free flours have recipes available using their products. This is usual for any special diet product. Generally the higher-profile the product the greater the level of their recipe resources. In most cases these are available on their websites or by telephone on request and are usually free of charge (see Section 12.15, below).

12.7   Product information

Awareness of products available to enhance the nutrition, taste and quality of restricted diets is one of the most important features of successfully managing them. Both clinicians and patients should endeavour to keep abreast of available products. Availability of products can be an issue but increasingly they are available in super-markets, health-food stores, chemists (gluten- and wheat-free foods and egg replacers) and online.

Another option is for patients to make their own products. Any vegan cookery book will have a recipe to make soya milk and on the use of foods such as pureed

Table 12.1 Replacements for common food ingredients.

Food avoided	Replacement product for this diet
Cow's milk	Soya-based dairy-free milk, soft cheese, hard cheese, yoghurt, cream, custard, ice cream, chocolate
Soya and cow's milk	Rice- or oat-based milk, cream, desserts, ice cream. Other milk such as quinoa, almond, chufa and potato milks are also available
Wheat	Flours based on rice, corn, potato, soya, millet, rye, barley, oat; bread, cakes, pasta, pizza, bakery items, pies etc
Gluten	Deglutenised wheat-based flours, bread, cakes, pasta, pizza, bakery items, pies etc
Fish and shellfish	Any vegetarian or vegan product including nutritional supplements

apple to replace the properties of eggs in a recipe free from them. There are whole books available on making dairy-free cheeses and egg-free cakes

Unacceptability in terms of taste, texture, cooking properties, variety, cultural and cost are often reasons given by those not using these products. Encouragement to try new products usually leads to satisfaction. Table 12.1 shows some of those available.

12.8   Awareness products

To reduce the chance of a child being given a food he or she should be avoiding, the use of identification on the person can be helpful. Suitable items include T-shirts, badges, stickers, lunch boxes and key rings with logos. For older children and adults with severe reactions, awareness jewellery with a universally identifiable logo can be life-saving in an emergency situation. These are particularly helpful if the sufferer has a reaction when alone, or in a foreign country, where communication may be difficult. Examples of companies making these products area listed in Section 12.15, below.

12.9   Nurseries, childminders and carers

Leaving an infant or child with others when the diet is restricted often requires organisational skills to ensure the diet is safe but also varied, nutritious and tasty. When the child has a potentially life-threatening reaction to a food that would require emergency treatment if ingested this is a totally different matter: the child's food will need careful planning, cross-contamination is a risk, and the storage and management of the medications and their indications and use will need careful consideration. Some nurseries have a nut-free policy, but it is rare for other foods to be excluded.

For parents who are unwilling to place the child's wellbeing in the hands of others, it will mean changing their work arrangements or giving up altogether so they can care for their otherwise healthy child. This can have many knock-on effects, financially, socially and psychologically.

Choices made by the parents can also curb the child's lifestyle in a number of ways. Some parents will home educate and refuse participation in social activities away from them, whilst others live in fear, and they can pass these negative emotions on to their child. With the correct management of the diet, with information, knowledge, advice and support, a normal life is achievable, and many parents succeed in providing this for their child. The alternative may be exclusion of the child, anxiety for the parent and carer, and stress for everyone.

Helpful information for childcare providers includes:

- a list of the exact foods the child can and cannot eat;
- suitable savoury and sweet recipes;
- information about replacement products and where to buy them;
- advice for the childcare provider about 'fitting in' and 'not feeling different';
- indications and use of any prescribed medications;

The parents should ask about the policies of the childcare facility in relation to:

- food swapping and cross-contamination issues;
- foods banned from the facility and what this means in practical terms;
- un-policed foods bought in from home by parents of other children being cared for at the same time (though it should be noted that in recent years health-and-safety concerns have meant that parents are not permitted to provide food for a child whilst in most formal childcare settings).

A particularly useful information resource for carers of children with severe IgE-mediated food allergy is the Allergy in Schools website, run by the Anaphylaxis Campaign at www.allergyinschools.org.uk. This site includes advice and information for parents, teachers, preschool childcare providers and caterers providing food for these children. It can be used alongside the Department of Health publication *Managing Medicines in Schools and Early Year Settings* (www.teachernet.gov.uk/wholeschool/healthandsafety/medical).

12.10   Managing food allergy at school

The Allergy in Schools website is an essential tool for schools managing children who have severe IgE-mediated food allergy. There are also children who are on restricted diets who have reactions that are not life-threatening but still need careful management, such as coeliacs who require a strict gluten-free diet, lactose-intolerants who require a low-lactose diet, and any other type of food hypersensitivity which needs appropriate and individual management. If these diets are not precise then the result is the predictable onset of symptoms, but long-term the effects commonly include time off school leading to low self-esteem, poor learning, fear of eating and poor social interaction.

Separate allergy tables, feeling different and bullying are among the other re-ported problems associated with being on a restricted diet, and they can have both a direct and an indirect impact on the child and his or her family.

For those who must have prescribed medications available at all times careful planning is essential, and regular discussions with the school should be scheduled. Issues to be discussed include where to keep the medication, who is to give it, the indications and usage, what happens on days or activities away from the school. Keeping the medications up to date and how to store them is another consideration. Older children may wish to carry their medications, but this is rarely allowed due to health-and-safety regulations. It has been known for parents to request their child to be 'statemented' to keep them safe: this is where a learning support assistant is designated to watch the child at every moment in school to ensure that risks of inadvertent exposure to a food are minimised. If this is to be considered it should not be undertaken lightly, as the long-term effects may be far-reaching. Equally it may be entirely appropriate, so a thorough multidisciplinary approach to the final decision is essential.

Training of school personnel in the indications and usage of prescribed medica-tions can be done by the paediatric community nurse or the school nurse. The most important aspect is to ensure that the training is done and that available competent staff are accessible whenever the child is around. The school nurse, the head teacher, the class teacher and the parent are usually all involved in agreeing a suitable man-agement plan, based on the Department of Health's *Managing Medicines in Schools and Early Year Settings*.

For other types of food hypersensitivity it may be helpful to join a support group related to the condition, such as those run by Coeliac UK, to gain a useful insight into managing the diet and lifestyle of a school-aged child.

12.11 Managing food allergy at home

Managing food allergy at home is a really great opportunity for sufferers and their families to try new products, to adapt recipes and to try new recipes. This will give confidence and hope that the new diet can be managed successfully. The infor-mation can then be passed onto others who wish to cater for the sufferer. Feeling positive about a new regime can make a great difference to how the sufferer and his or her family view the diet and management of the condition, and can make a significant difference in the short and long term. This should not be underestimated.

How a food allergy is managed at home will depend on the severity of the reaction suffered and what quantity of the food is required to trigger a reaction. For severe allergies it may be appropriate and easier to ban the food from the house altogether. If the allergic food is a staple such as milk, egg or wheat this could be difficult to manage. In this case the next best option is to have separate cooking vessels, chop-ping boards and utensils, and also to prepare the foods separately. For those with the luxury of two sinks, keeping preparation and washing-up separate is another way of managing cross-contamination risks. For the less severe hypersensitivities such extremes are unnecessary, but care with reading labels remains essential.

The sufferer should feel safe and relaxed eating in his or her own home. For children, sibling rivalry may be an issue, and other children may feel jealous because of the sibling's special diet. In their eyes, their sibling is always the focus of attention, and it seems that everyone talks about nothing but the allergic child, cooking special dishes and looking for special foods to buy. The power of this should not be underestimated – especially if the allergic child also has eczema with daily wet-wraps which require much time and attention. In this instance parents may require a reminder about the feelings of other children in the household.

12.12   Managing food allergy at work

The best way to manage food allergy at work is to be well prepared and organised. Good planning will omit the need for sufferers to be hungry because there is nothing suitable to eat. For those who travel as part of their job this will be more difficult, but it is achievable. See Sections 12.13 and 12.14 (below) for further advice when work takes the sufferer away from home.

For those with milk allergy it is worth being aware that vending-machine drinks often have cross-contamination issues, and ingredients are also unknown. It is not unusual for a white coffee to contain milk, wheat and soy.

Another issue at work concerns the food that colleagues supply for special occasions. It is worth having a few treats in a cupboard so that the sufferer does not feel left out, and is not tempted to take the risk of eating a food whose ingredients are unknown.

12.13   Eating out

Most reactions to foods occur when eating away from home[13]. This is generally because ingredients are often unknown, mistakes are made and cross-contamination is common. Another important factor, which may account for the majority of very severe reactions occurring in teenagers, is that this group can be self-conscious and reticent about asking probing questions about ingredients and the way foods are prepared. Risk taking is common amongst this age group, and in some cases reluctance to carry prescribed medications or wear identification jewellery can amplify the problem[14].

Some reactions occur because the sufferer is poorly informed about the food that is to be avoided. In this case advice and support should be sought from a specialist healthcare professional, such as a registered dietitian specialising in managing food allergy. A referral through the general practitioner is the usual route.

To reduce the risks involved in eating out, the following can be helpful:

- If possible a quiet time of day and day of the week should be chosen to eat out, until the caterer learns about the sufferer's needs. Visiting by appointment prior to eating is the best way for needs to be explained for the caterer's full attention.
- Clear communication of the allergy sufferer's needs is vital, and this may mean choosing an English-speaking restaurant.

- Menu choices should be simple, steering away from soups, sauces and dressings where ingredients are easily hidden and where there are so many that the caterer could easily forget the exact ingredients.
- It should be remembered that EU food-allergen labelling laws apply only to manufactured prepacked foods. Other foods are not legally bound to label ingredients.
- For those with a severe IgE-mediated allergy special considerations such as cross-contamination must be discussed with the chef to minimise risks. It may be helpful to direct the caterer to some of the suitable advice available on the Internet (see Section 12.15, below).
- Organisation and forward planning are essential. The caterer should be advised in advance when possible (or at least on arrival) of the dietary restriction, with details of the food(s) to be avoided and the potential severity of the reaction.
- The ingredients of the chosen dish should be discussed and the ingredients label studied if available. In most cases this can be done prior to the sitting.
- In some cases it will be possible for the order to be prepared earlier and placed under wrap and then just heated up as required. This reduces the risk of cross-contamination, and of staff being so busy they make errors.
- For sufferers who may be having a reaction, they should tell those with them and take any prescribed medications without delay. For those with a potentially life-threatening reaction an ambulance should be called immediately. A chef card is frequently used in the USA (see www.foodallergy.org).

12.14   Going on holiday

Holidays should be fun and relaxing. By planning ahead and being organised, managing a restricted diet should not compromise this. Going on holiday could be in the sufferer's home country or when going abroad, so the arrangements should be adjusted accordingly. Self-catering is usually the safest option, especially if the reactions are severe or there are multiple restrictions.

As always, there are two aspects to managing a restricted diet. First there is the issue of managing the food preparation, and deciding whether to prepare it oneself or take the risks associated with eating foods someone else has prepared. Second, there may be language and cultural barriers: if the sufferer is abroad the caterer may speak little English or may have a poor understanding of the potential reaction.

When flying, taking favourite foods may be feasible only on a short-haul flight, so choosing a holiday destination near a well-stocked international supermarket may be a consideration for those deciding to self-cater.

In terms of managing a severe reaction whilst abroad, there are many steps that can be taken:

- prescribed medications should be carried at all times;
- ID should be worn in the language of the country visited;
- translation cards should be made up that are specific to the individual;

- aeroplane food should be avoided, as ingredients are usually unknown and mistakes in the provision of ordered special-diet meals are common;
- staples and favourite foods should be taken on holiday if possible, to aid enjoyment and reduce risk taking or feeling left out;
- it is important to be aware that product ingredients are not always the same despite the product looking the same;
- it should be highlighted that outside the EU food labelling laws are different.

12.15 Support and resources

There is a huge number of resources available to aid the management of restricted diets, and sharing those that are pertinent to the individual patient's requirements is essential.

Eating out in the UK and abroad

When eating out, both in the UK and abroad, the following sites will aid safe food choice, and help with the identification of suitable foods, making eating a safer and more pleasurable experience.

- www.allergyfreepassport.com – guide to eating out safely
- www.allergyaction.org – for names of most common allergens in many different European languages
- www.specialdietsconsulting.co.uk – information on special diets for individuals, catering organisations and restaurants; includes detailed product information, recipes and resources
- www.leaveitout.co.uk – a directory for people with special dietary needs who wish to eat out; includes detailed information about the diagnosis and management of food allergy and other hypersensitivity reactions

Translation cards

Translation cards will aid communication and reduce the risk of inadvertent exposure to potentially harmful foods. They also help when reading labels and when calling an ambulance in the event that it is required.

- www.kidsaware.co.uk
- www.yellowcross.co.uk

Identification

Identification jewellery is recommended for any patient with an unpredictable potentially acute medical emergency. Anaphylaxis is one such condition. If someone is found collapsed and they are alone and have no ID a diagnosis of anaphylaxis is not necessarily made immediately. Heart attacks, stroke, overdose and diabetic coma are just some of the other possible conclusions a passer-by could come to. With anaphylaxis, time is of the essence when administering the medication, so wearing ID could make the difference.

- www.medicalert.org.uk – identification jewellery
- www.sostalisman.com – identification jewellery and watches
- www.yellowcross.co.uk – mail-order range of bags and travelling containers for medicines, translation cards for travelling
- www.kidsaware.co.uk – awareness clothing and accessories for children with severe allergies, awareness bibs, babygrows and teddies for babies with allergies, key rings, stickers, T-shirts
- www.icegems.co.uk – selection of awareness jewellery
- www.iceideas.co.uk – selection of awareness jewellery aimed at children

Carry bags for food and medication

Being on a restricted diet sometimes means taking your own food when eating away from home and carrying medication at all times. The following sites help do this in an organised and refined manner:

- www.yellowcross.co.uk
- www.kidsaware.co.uk

Nut-free products

Rather than risking having foods that 'may contain traces of nuts' it is sensible to use the foods that are made in a nut-free factory (see also Chapter 8). For those patients who choose to continue to eat 'may contain traces' foods, it could be suggested they use nut-free products when away from emergency healthcare, such as when they are on an aeroplane, on a ferry or walking in isolated areas.

- www.bakinboys.co.uk – flapjacks, cupcakes etc
- www.itsnutfree.com – cakes, biscuits, flapjacks etc
- www.kinnerton.com – sweets, chocolates, seasonal goods

Anaphylaxis resources

Anaphylaxis is much easier to manage when informed. The following sites provide essential resources, enabling the sufferer to be in control of the condition, rather than it controlling the sufferer and the family.

- www.anaphylaxis.org.uk – the Anaphylaxis Campaign: advice, resources, information, helpline, support groups, product alerts, newsletter
- www.allergyinschools.org.uk – information from the Anaphylaxis Campaign for nurseries, preschools and schools
- www.cateringforallergy.org

- www.epipen.co.uk – all about the EpiPen, including videoclip of its use
- www.teachernet.gov.uk/wholeschool/healthandsafety/medical – Department of Health publication *Managing Medicines in Schools and Early Year Settings* (2005)

Special diet food suppliers

Food on a restricted diet can be just as varied, tasty and nutritious as an unrestricted diet using the following sites.

- www.goodnessdirect.co.uk – extensive website for special diet foods, including nutritional breakdown, dietary suitability, mail order
- www.dietaryneedsdirect.co.uk – online and mail-order shopping for special diet products
- www.ok-foods.co.uk – wheat-, gluten- and dairy-free biscuits, cake and snacks
- www.plamilfoods.co.uk – vegan chocolate bars and drops, carob, mayonnaise, chocolate spreads
- www.viva.org.uk – dairy-free (and vegan) foods
- www.wheatanddairyfree.com – wheat- and dairy-free foods
- www.juvela.co.uk – gluten-free foods
- www.intolerablefood.com – gluten- and dairy-free foods

Recipes

Having savoury and sweet tried and tested recipes will enhance the taste, variety and nutrition of the diet

- www.foodyoucaneat.com – extensive recipes sent in by the website users
- www.specialdietsconsulting.co.uk – recipe information, product information etc
- www.foodsmatter.com – recipes and product information
- www.allergycooks.co.uk – recipes free from wheat dairy and egg
- www.glutenfreecatering.com – dairy-, egg-, wheat- and gluten-free recipes, product information etc

Allergy alert services

Allergy alert services allow sufferers to learn immediately about recipe mistakes in manufactured foods.

- www.alert4allergy.org
- www.anaphylaxis.org.uk – the Anaphylaxis Campaign

IBS resources

Resources to help with the management of irritable bowel syndrome and other gastrointestinal-related symptoms.

- www.theguttrust.org – IBS Network
- www.corecharity.org.uk – Core (the Digestive Disorders Foundation)
- www.ibsgroup.org – internet-based self-help group:

Other useful sites

- www.asthma.org.uk – Asthma UK
- www.eczema.org – National Eczema Society
- www.skinhealth.co.uk – information site written by dermatologists on skin conditions
- www.ctpa.org.uk – Cosmetic, Toiletry and Perfume Association
- www.food.gov.uk – Food Standards Agency (FSA)
- www.eatwell.gov.uk – part of the FSA, offering advice on dietary matters for all ages and stages; includes information on many food allergies and intolerances as well as information for consumers on eating out, buying food and current food labelling laws
- www.vegansociety.com – Vegan Society
- www.lasg.co.uk – Latex Allergy Support Group
- www.nhsdirect.nhs.uk – NHS Direct: government health information website
- www.bda.uk.com – British Dietetic Association: includes useful factsheets on food allergy and intolerance, autistic spectrum and allergy testing amongst others
- www.nos.org.uk – National Osteoporosis Society
- www.allergicchild.com – useful American website for food-allergics: includes information on American food labelling laws and books on food allergy for children

Resources for health professionals

- www.infantandtoddlerforum.org – up-to-date resources including factsheets, study days, resources. on infant and toddler feeding and food hypersensitivity
- www.actagainstallergy.co.uk – educational initiative designed to increase the awareness of childhood food allergy
- foodallergens.ifr.ac.uk – a searchable database with detailed information on allergenic foods

References

1. Teufel M, Biedermann T, Rapps N *et al*. Psychological burden of food allergy. *World J Gastroenterol* 2007; **13**: 3456–65.
2. Marklund B, Ahlstedt S, Nordstrom G. Food hypersensitivity and quality of life. *Curr Opin Allergy Clin Immunol* 2007; **7**: 279–87.
3. Östblom E, Egmar AC, Gardulf A, Lilja G, Wickman M. The impact of food hypersensitivity reported in 9-year-old children by their parents on health-related quality of life. *Allergy* 2008; **63**: 211–18.

4. Primeau MN, Kagan R, Joseph L *et al*. The psychological burden of peanut allergy as perceived by adults with peanut allergy and the parents of peanut-allergic children. *Clin Exp Allergy* 2000; **30**: 1135–43.

5. Cohen BL, Noone S, Muñoz-Furlong A, Sicherer SH. Development of a questionnaire to measure quality of life in families with a child with food allergy. *J Allergy Clin Immunol* 2004; **114**: 1159–63.

6. Avery NJ, King RM, Knight S, Hourihane JO. Assessment of quality of life in children with peanut allergy. *Pediatr Allergy Immunol* 2003; **14**: 378–82.

7. Sicherer SH, Noone SA, Muñoz-Furlong A. The impact of childhood food allergy on quality of life. *Ann Allergy Asthma Immunol* 2001; **87**: 461–4.

8. Bollinger ME. Dahlquist LM, Mudd K *et al*. The impact of food allergy on the daily activities of children and their families. *Ann Allergy Asthma Immunol* 2006; **96**: 415–21.

9. LeBovidge JS, Stone KD, Twarog FJ *et al*. Development of a preliminary questionnaire to assess parental response to children's food allergies. *Ann Allergy Asthma Immunol* 2006; **96**: 472–7.

10. Sicherer SH, Simons FE. Self-injectable epinephrine for first-aid management of anaphylaxis. *Pediatrics* 2007; **119**: 638–46.

11. Eigenmann PA, Caubet JC, Zamora SA. Continuing food-avoidance diets after negative food challenges. *Pediatr Allergy Immunol* 2006; **17**: 601–5.

12. Food Standards Agency. *Guidance on Allergen Management and Consumer Information: Best Practice Guidance on Managing Food Allergens with Particular Reference to Avoiding Cross-Contamination and Using Appropriate Advisory Labelling (e.g. 'May Contain' Labelling)*. London: FSA, 2006.

13. Pumphrey RSH. Lessons for management of anaphylaxis from a study of fatal reactions. *Clin Exp Allergy* 2000; **30**: 1144–50.

14. Sampson MA, Muñoz-Furlong A, Sicherer SH. Risk-taking and coping strategies of adolescents and young adults with food allergy. *J Allergy Clin Immunol* 2006; **117**: 1440–5.

13 Allergy Prevention and the Effect of Nutrition on the Immune System

Carina Venter

13.1 Introduction

Allergic diseases such as asthma, rhinitis and eczema are increasing in both the developed and the developing world[1,2]. In the UK, 39% of children and 30% of adults are diagnosed with asthma, eczema or hay fever at some point in their lives[3]. It is estimated that about 1.3–3.4% of adults suffer from food allergy[4–8] and around 0.5–8%[8–14] of children. Data from the Isle of Wight indicate that the prevalence of food hypersensitivity may not be increasing[11]. Nevertheless, there remain two important reasons for preventing sensitisation to food allergens early in life. For those children who develop allergies to foods (in particular milk and egg[15]) it could have a huge impact on their quality of life[16–18]. Most importantly, food allergy is not an isolated phenomenon but often the beginning of an atopic career: those children with food allergy are very likely to develop eczema, asthma and hay fever/allergic rhinitis later in life[19].

Most nutritional recommendations are based on populations, and until we are able to screen for specific genes, this will most probably be the case for some time. However, based on family history[20,21], we are to some extent able to identify those at highest risk of developing allergic diseases, and most of the nutritional recommendations regarding allergy prevention are directed to this group. The risk of a child developing allergies is as follows[20]:

- both parents with identical allergy: 72%;
- both parents with non-identical allergy: 43%;
- one parent with allergy: 20%;
- one sibling with allergy: 32%;
- neither parent allergic: 12%.

The European Academy of Allergy and Clinical Immunology (EAACI) defines a high-risk infant as one with at least one first-degree relative (mother, father or sibling) with documented allergic disease such as asthma, eczema, hay fever or food allergies[22]. This definition was also adopted by the American Academy of Pediatrics (AAP). This method of screening is not entirely satisfactory, however, as a significant number of children with no history of allergy will develop allergic disease. It is also important to realise that it does not mean that the child will develop the same types of allergies as the parents or the siblings.

In future, however, developments in genotyping, and in the fields of nutrigenetics and nutrigenomics, may enable us to provide allergy-preventive recommendations on an individual level.

This chapter deals with primary prevention of allergic disease and the involvement of the immune system, i.e. preventing infants from becoming sensitised to allergens[23]. Allergic sensitisation is a failure to develop tolerance to allergens, an active immunological response induced by tolerogenic food proteins. The chapter therefore does not include any advice for infants already sensitised to foods or aeroallergens (secondary prevention) or those who are already clinically allergic and need pharmacotherapy (tertiary prevention).

A large number of studies, including both observational and intervention studies, have been conducted in order to look at preventive measures for allergic disease. Presently, two major strategies for allergy prevention in high-risk children are being pursued:

1   Avoidance of potential allergens early in life, i.e. from conception. The principle behind allergen avoidance strategies is the hypothesis that reducing allergen levels may reduce the risk of sensitisation, hence a reduced risk of becoming clinically allergic. It is known that allergens pass from the placenta to the fetus and via breast milk to the infant[24]. However, intervention studies have not been able to show such a clear pattern of events, i.e. that reduced exposure to allergens equals reduced levels of clinical allergy.
2   Induction of tolerance early in life using certain prebiotics, probiotics, long-chain fatty acids, vitamin supplementation and hypoallergenic infant formulas.

13.2   Introduction to the immune system

The fetal immune system starts to develop very early on in pregnancy and is influenced by maternal factors. Birth and feeding/weaning during the first year of life are critical control points in the development of appropriate responses to pathogens and harmless dietary and commensal antigens. The development of the fetal immune system and further development during the first few years of life are crucial in promoting a fully functional, healthy immune system.

The immune system comprises cells and tissues, which play an important role in recognising and destroying pathogens (invaders) such as viruses, bacteria and parasites. It also prevents the body from destroying its own cells or tissues.

The human immune system is divided into the *innate* and the *adaptive* immune systems[25,26].

13.2.1   Innate immune system

The innate system is the most basic part of the immune system, and it is almost fully functional from birth[25,26]. It is non-specific and will therefore react similarly to all foreign material. This immune system does not develop a memory, and will react to any pathogen as if it is exposed to it for the first time (Figure 13.1).

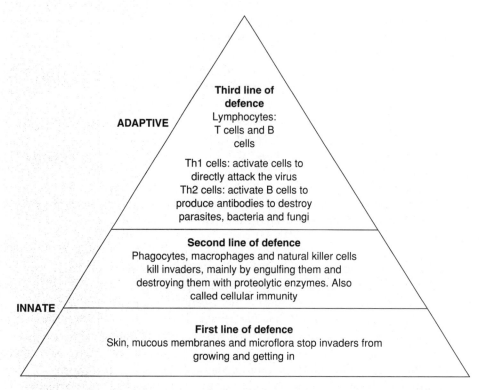

The **innate system** basically stays in 'infancy' and does not develop any further, but needs to be nourished through good nutrition and stimulated by invaders to be able to fulfil its function.

The **adaptive system** is like the 'eternal student' who will continue to develop throughout life (but mostly in the first six years). In order to keep up this process of lifelong 'learning and development', this immune system also needs to be nourished and stimulated, as each exposure will increase the potency of the next reaction.

Figure 13.1   The innate and adaptive immune system.

- The first line of defence is provided by non-specific physical barriers such as the skin, the mucous membranes of the mouth, nose, respiratory, gastrointestinal and genitourinary tract and the natural microflora (gut bacteria).
- The second line of defence is provided by cells such as phagocytes (eosinophils and neutrophils), macrophages and natural killer cells, which kill invaders mainly by engulfing them and destroying them with the help of specialised proteins and proteolytic enzymes. This is also called cellular immunity.

13.2.2   Adaptive immune system

The adaptive immune system provides the third line of defence. It is immature at birth and takes about 2–6 years to fully develop. The components of the adaptive immune system are more sophisticated, having the ability to learn, to adapt, and to remember. The adaptive immune system is therefore able to distinguish different

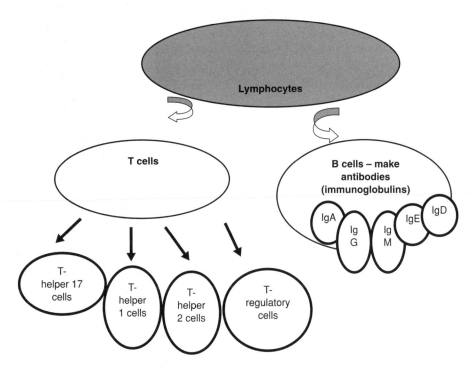

Figure 13.2   Cells of the adaptive immune system.

viruses, bacteria, parasites and food proteins from one another. For each of these there will be a specific immune reaction based on the memory developed, and the reaction may be more severe at each encounter[25,26]. Lymphocytes are the cells involved in the adaptive immune system, and they can be divided into two major groups[25,26]: T cells are further divided into 4 types: T-helper 1 cells, T-helper 17 cells, Thelper 2 cells and T-regulatory cells. The T-regulatory cells are divided into T-regulatory 1 and T-regulatory 3 cells which are made by the thymus, and B cells, made by bone marrow. T cells play a primary role directing the immune response[25,26] (Figures 13.2 and 13.3). Once B cells are activated, they produce immunoglobulins, which enable them to destroy pathogens (Table 13.1).

Table 13.1   Immunoglobulins and their roles in the human body.

Immunoglobulin	Role
IgA	Found in mucous secretions and prevents infection in gut and respiratory tract
IgE	Destroys parasites and is involved in allergic reactions
IgG	Important in passing immunity from mother to fetus Plays an important role in developing tolerance to antigens (food proteins)
IgM	Plays an important role in the first days of infections

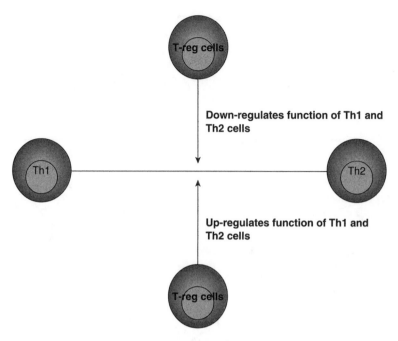

Figure 13.3   The role of T-regulatory cells in allergy.

13.3   Supporting the immune system through nutrition

13.3.1   During pregnancy

There is a fine balance of immune cell activity and production of immune cells between the pregnant woman, the placenta and the fetus, to encourage normal fetal growth and immunological responsiveness[27,28].

Birth and feeding/weaning during the first year of life are critical control points in preventing infants from becoming sensitised (producing IgE) to foods or launching an attack on harmless bacteria. Pregnancy involves a subtle alteration (favours Th2 cells) of the maternal immune system that promotes tolerance of the fetus and prevents its rejection. The maternal immune system affects the fetus's immune system as the fetus can swallow IgEs and cytokines produced by the mother and IgG is transferred across the placenta[27]. Maternal immunity may therefore have long-term, perhaps even lifelong, consequences for her infant.

Development of the fetal immune system starts very early in pregnancy. Stem cells are present in the human yolk sac at 21 days of gestation, with the first lymphocytes seen in the thymus at the end of the ninth week of gestation[22,27–29]. The amniotic fluid is sterile to protect the fetus, so in order to get a functional immune system in place, maternal–fetal interactions are needed. Two factors therefore determine development of the infant's immune system. The first is the maternal immune system, whereby immunoglobulin G passes from the mother to the fetus and the fetus swallows immunoglobulin E from the mother. The second determining factor is the maternal diet.

Maternal diet

The maternal diet affects the general development of the fetus's immune system, and the pregnant woman should therefore consume a healthy balanced diet consisting of all the immune-supporting vitamins and minerals. In general it has been shown that vitamin and mineral deficiencies adversely affect immune system function. Lack of vitamin A[30], iron[31], zinc[32,33], selenium[34], and in particular vitamin D[35] has been shown to impair immune function and increase susceptibility to infection. This is probably due to the role of these nutrients in ensuring fully developed and functioning immune cell membranes. A healthy immune system relies on these healthy cell membranes to correctly identify pathogens, as well as dead and malfunctioning cells. The maternal diet could also affect the development of allergic disease in the infant. There are a number of papers dealing with allergy prevention during pregnancy, breast-feeding and the infant's first year of life. It is difficult to compare the data from these studies, however, due to different methodologies and outcome measures.

Observational studies during pregnancy

Studies looking at maternal intake during pregnancy and its influence on the development of allergic disease in the infant have focused mainly on fatty-acid intake, including fish consumption[36–40], antioxidant intake based on fruit, vegetable and supplement consumption[37,38,40–44], vitamin D and zinc intake[45], as well as seed[37] and peanut consumption[46,47].

These studies have shown that:

- Maternal fatty acid intake, particularly saturated fatty acids and omega-6 fatty acids, may play a role in increased prevalence of atopic disease in the infant.
- Fish intake of at least more than once per week may have an allergy-preventive effect.
- The role of total fruit and vegetable intake on the development of allergic disease is still controversial.
- Vitamin E, vitamin D and zinc intake may be preventive against the development of allergic disease, particularly wheeze, in the infant.
- Vitamin C intake may increase the risk for development of allergic disease, particularly wheeze and eczema.
- More information is needed regarding peanut intake during pregnancy. A 1998 report on peanut allergy by the Committee on Toxicity of Chemicals in Food, Consumer Products and the Environment (COT) stated that 'pregnant or breast feeding women who are themselves atopic, or where another first-degree relative of the child is atopic, may wish to avoid eating peanuts and peanut products during pregnancy and breast feeding'[48]. Researchers on the Isle of Wight have

found that this advice has been misunderstood and incorrectly implemented by both health professionals and pregnant women[49]. The COT report is currently under review.

Intervention studies during pregnancy

Dietary avoidance
A number of studies have looked at whether maternal food avoidance during pregnancy or supplementing the maternal diet with certain dietary factors had an effect on the prevalence of allergic disease[50-56]. The data obtained from these intervention studies, however, do not give indisputable evidence to support incorporating any of these measures into clinical practice.

Supplementation of the maternal diet with probiotics
The gut microbiota is the major source of microbial exposure, composed of 10 times the number of cells in the entire body (10^4 microorganisms). Microbes play an important role in postnatal maturation of the immune response, particularly through their role in regulating Th2 cells and Th1 cells. Differences in gut microbiota composition have been reported in infants who go on to develop allergic disease compared with those who do not[57], and it has been found that different bacteria may be associated with different types of allergic disease[58]. This has raised the question as to whether supplementation with probiotic microbes (Table 13.2) may have an effect in allergy prevention.

Five studies performed in high-risk families are cited in the literature looking at the effect of probiotic supplementation during pregnancy and the infant's first few months of life on the prevention of allergic disease. Four of these were conducted during pregnancy in the last 2–4 weeks[59-61] or last 4–6 weeks[62] and continued for

Table 13.2 Definitions used in immunology.

Prebiotics are non-digestible food ingredients that beneficially affect the host (you and me) by selectively stimulating the growth and activity of specific 'friendly' bacteria (also called probiotics) in the intestinal tract. In other words, prebiotics are foods not for us but for our 'good' bacteria, because they stimulate their growth in our digestive tracts.

Probiotics are a live microbial feed supplement which beneficially affects the host animal by improving its intestinal microbial balance.

Long-chain polyunsaturated fatty acids (LCPUFAs) play an important role in regulating the immune system. They are divided mainly into omega-3 and omega-6 fatty acids.

Passive immunity is immunity passed from mother to child via placenta or breast milk. Passive immunity is effective, but protection is generally limited and diminishes over time (usually a few weeks or months). For example, maternal antibodies are passed to the infant prior to birth; temporarily protect the baby for the first 4–6 months of life[12].

Active immunity refers to the activated immune system during infection or after immunisation.

6 months post partum utilising *Lactobacillus rhamnosus* GG, *Bifidobacterium breve* and *Proprionibacterium freudenreichii* plus a prebiotic mixture[59], *Lactobacillus rhamnosus* GG[60,62] or *Lactobacillus reuteri* for 12 months[61] of the infant's life. One study used *Lactobacillus acidophilus* during the first 6 months of the infant's life only[63]. The main benefit from these studies seems to be a reduction in eczema, found in some studies[59,60,64,65] but not all[61–63].

It is thought that the effects of probiotics are strain-specific, and that environmental factors such as maternal and infant diet or factors specific to the host such as genetic profile and susceptibility to colonisation may have an effect on the results seen[66]. However, Kopp *et al.* showed that different outcomes can be seen with the same strain as well[62].

Omega-3 fatty acids

Two reports from Australia of randomised-controlled trials suggest that dietary n-3 polyunsaturated fatty acid (PUFA) supplements during pregnancy[67] or in the early postnatal period[68] could have immunomodulatory properties and/or associated clinical effects on atopy and asthma in offspring.

Recommendations regarding the maternal diet

- Women should consume a variety of foods according to the five food groups: meat and alternatives, starchy food, fruit and vegetables, dairy foods and fat and sugars.
- Whole grains, leafy green and yellow vegetables, and fruit should be consumed daily to meet nutrient needs and provide enough fibre. Meat, poultry, seafood, legumes and nuts are important sources of protein, as are zinc, iron and magnesium.
- Iron, zinc, selenium, vitamin A and vitamin C are particularly important for maintaining a healthy immune system. Pregnant women should never be tempted, however, to take any mineral or vitamin supplementation without consulting a medical practitioner and dietitian. It is also important to note that vitamin A supplementation is contraindicated in pregnancy.
- Fish-oil supplementation should not be recommended at present unless the fatty-fish intake is insufficient (see www.food.gov.uk or for advice on fatty-fish consumption during pregnancy).
- The efficacy and safety of probiotics, and whether different organisms may have different effects on the immune system, need further clarification.
- There is no evidence to suggest maternal avoidance of any of the allergic foods[69,70].
- However, the current advice in the UK is that pregnant women from high-risk families may wish to avoid peanuts and foods containing peanut[48].

Method of delivery

The method of delivery can also affect the infant's immune system. As infants are born with a sterile gut, exposure to bacteria is very important to enhance gut colonisation, which strengthens the immune system (the hygiene hypothesis'[71]). Vaginally born infants obtain their gut flora mainly through the mother's vaginal tract, which is very similar to the mother's gut flora. Children born by Caesarean section, on the other hand, obtain their gut flora through skin contact and the environment. This results in a significant difference of bacterial microflora in the gut of those infants born by Caesarean versus those born by vaginal delivery[72] – an effect which may last into childhood. There is also some evidence to suggest that Caesarean-born infants are more likely to suffer from allergic disease[73]. Caesarean-born children may therefore have an amplified need for correcting and nurturing their gut flora in the first few years of life.

13.3.2   Method of feeding after birth

The gut is the biggest organ in the human body and houses as much as two-thirds of the immune system. In addition to its role in digestion (processing and absorbing ingested food), an important function of the gut is to provide a healthy immune system (by discharging waste products)[74,75]. The mucosal immune system therefore fulfils the primary function of defence against potential pathogens that may enter across vulnerable (especially in the first year of life) surface epithelia. However, a secondary function of the intestinal immune system is to discriminate between pathogen-associated and 'harmless' antigens, expressing active responses against the former and tolerance to the latter. Two critical time points for the infant are the period immediately after birth and at weaning.

The mucosal immune system encounters a large number of antigens (food proteins/commensal organisms) on a daily basis, and generally suppresses an immune response to these harmless substances even though it is fully capable of launching a quick protective response to pathogens. The mucosal barrier uses physical barriers and cells to prevent antigens from entering the circulation. The physical barriers include:

1   epithelial cells joined by tight junctions;
2   a thick mucous layer that covers these cells;
3   factors that help strengthen and restore the barrier;
4   luminal and brush border enzymes;
5   bile salts;
6   a range of different pH;
7   gut bacteria.

These factors all lead to destruction of pathogens and render antigens non-immunogenic, although 2% of food proteins will reach the circulation intact. Cells involved in providing gut immunity includes cells form both the innate (natural killer cells, macrophages, epithelial cells) and adaptive (lymphocytes, Peyer's patches, secretory IgA, cytokines) systems.

A number of these factors are either lacking or immature in the infantile gut, such as suboptimal enzyme production and insufficient production of secretory IgA[76].

This is primarily because infants are born with a sterile gut, which is immature in terms of handling large food proteins and foreign organisms causing infections. It is therefore important to provide the infant with the correct nutrition to enhance the colonisation and maturation of the gastrointestinal tract. This occurs in the first few months and continues up to 6 years of age[77]. Breast milk contains nutritional and immunomodulatory components that play an important role in this process. These factors include prebiotics[78], long-chain polyunsaturated fatty acids (LCPUFAs), immunoglobulins (Table 13.1)[74,79], nucleotides[79] and proteins[79].

The *prebiotics* (mainly oligosaccharides) and *LCPUFAs* in breast milk enhance colonisation of the gut with bifidobacteria. These bacteria suppress development of an allergy-prone immune system (Th2 system) and allergic inflammation. *Probiotics* also reduce the dietary allergen load by degrading and modifying these large food proteins, therefore possibly reducing food allergy[80]. It is well known that the gut microflora of breast-fed babies contains more *Lactobacillus* and *Bifidobacterium* than that of bottle-fed babies[78].

There is also evidence to suggest that apart from the effect on prevention of allergy, probiotics may positively affect the immune system, e.g. genitourinary tract infection and cancer[79,81]. Breast-fed babies have been shown to be less likely to suffer from diarrhoea and gastroenteritis, and seem to have more protection against infections, such as ear infections, than bottle-fed babies.

One of the most important aspects of breast milk is that secretory IgA is passed from the mother to the infant when feeding. The *nucleotides* in breast milk have multiple functions. They are the building blocks of RNA and DNA and play an important role in cell division[79]. The κ-*casein* and *lactoferrin* present in breast milk have also been shown to provide protection against bacteria, viruses and fungus as well as showing anti-inflammatory effects[79].

Breast milk is therefore considered to be the best source of nutrition for infants, not only because of the immunological components, but also because it contains just the right nutrients to support the infant's development. The nutritional uniqueness of breast milk lies in the fact that it 'adapts' during the feed and during the infant's first months of life. In early lactation, breast milk contains a high protein content, with a higher whey : casein ratio. This changes to a 50 : 50 whey : casein ratio later in lactation. The lactose and fat content of breast milk is lower earlier on, while the prebiotic and zinc content are much higher.

13.3.3   Breast-feeding and the development of allergic disease

The effect of breast-feeding on allergy prevention is still very controversial, due to a number of studies with contradicting results. One major problem is that we have to rely on observational studies rather than randomised controlled trials, as infants could never ethically be randomised into a breast-feeding and a formula-feeding group. Previous studies performed both in the general population[82–88] and among high-risk infants[89,90] indicate that breast-feeding may not protect against all types of allergic disease in all infants. There are a number of factors that could have led to the discrepancy in the data:

- All breast milk is not created equal. The lower omega-3 fatty acid levels of the serum and breast milk of atopic mothers versus non-atopic mothers may play a role in the development of asthma and eczema in the infant[91]. The reduced levels of soluble CD14 (allergy-preventive immune cells) and omega-3 fatty acids in breast milk could also favour the development of atopy in the infant[92].

- It has been suggested that perhaps those with the highest degree of atopic heredity will tend to be breast-feeding for the longest period. This implies that when we are looking at the effect of breast-feeding on allergy prevention, the breast-feeding group may naturally include more of those highest at risk, as they are the group that breast-feed for a longer period.

- It is also frequently mentioned that children are more likely to be breast-fed than formula-fed if they were born to parents of higher socioeconomic status. One could speculate that aeroallergen exposure may be lower or at least different in this group. Furthermore, children born into a higher socioeconomic class probably have better access to healthcare facilities, resulting in their being prescribed more antibiotics.

Eczema

Two systematic reviews reached the conclusion that exclusive breast-feeding (for at least 4 months) does seem to have a protective effect on the development of allergic diseases, particularly eczema, and that this effect is greater when there is a family history of atopic disease[93,94].

Asthma

The effect of exclusive breast-feeding on the prevention of asthma is less clear. It does not seem that breast-feeding in high-risk children will prevent the infants from developing asthma, but it can reduce wheezing in children under 4 years of age[95].

Food allergy

Until recently, only one study had examined the effect of exclusive breast-feeding (for 4 months) on food allergy, and found it had no effect[82]. A new study performed on the Isle of Wight, however, has shown that breast-feeding of any duration (either any breast-feeding or exclusive) does not seem to affect the prevalence of FHS[96]. A review paper concluded that firm conclusions about the role of breast-feeding in either preventing or delaying the onset of food allergies are not possible at this stage[95]. It is known that nutrients such as fatty acids[97] and proteins such as β-lactoglobulin[98] and ovalbumin[24] are present in breast milk, and that their levels are influenced both by maternal diet and by maternal bodily stores.

Observational studies during breast-feeding

Observational studies during breast-feeding found that fat intake could affect development of atopy. Saturated-fat intake is associated with an increased sensitisation to allergens[99] and the development of atopic dermatitis in the infant[100]. Seven studies are cited in the literature looking at breast-milk fatty-acid levels and allergic disease in the offspring, with five studies finding that breast milk fatty acid levels can affect development of allergic disease in infants[100–104], one finding an effect in the infant but not later in childhood (5 years)[105], and one study finding no effect[106]. In addition, antioxidant intake may also play a role: Hoppu *et al.* showed that low intake of vitamin C together with a high intake of saturated fats increased the risk of developing allergy[99]. Finally, based on one study, it did not seem that the prebiotic/oligosaccharide content of milk directly affected the development of allergic disease in the offspring[107].

Intervention studies during breast-feeding

Reviews by the EAACI[70] and the American Academy of Pediatrics Committee on Nutrition and American Academy of Pediatrics Section on Allergy and Immunology[95] conclude that there is no evidence for maternal dietary intervention during pregnancy or lactation in the prevention of allergic disease.

Recommendations regarding breast-feeding

Table 13.3 summarises the recommendations from three review papers regarding dietary allergy prevention and the role of breast-feeding and formula-feeding. These include a paper by the AAP[95], a joint statement of the European Society for

Table 13.3 Recommendations regarding allergy prevention in high-risk infants by AAP, ESPACI/ESPGHAN and EAACI.

	AAP (2007)[95]	ESPACI/ESPGHAN (1999)[108]	EAACI (2004, updated 2008)[70,109]
Who is at risk?	If one first-degree relative with documented allergic disease	If one affected parent or one affected sibling	If one first degree relative with documented allergic disease
Breast-feeding recommendations	Exclusive breastfeeding for at least 4 months	Exclusive breast-feeding to 4–6 months	Exclusive breast-feeding for 6 months but at least 4 months, combined with avoidance of solid foods and cow's milk.
Alternatives if breast-feeding not possible/sufficient	Extensively hydrolysed formula may be more effective in preventing allergic disease than partially hydrolysed formula, but the cost should be taken into account with any decision made.	Use formula with proven reduced allergenicity.	In case of a lack of breast milk, formulas with documented allergenicity should be used for at least 4 months.

Paediatric Allergology and Clinical Immunology (ESPACI) and the European Society for Paediatric Gastroenterology, Hepatology and Nutrition (ESPGHAN)[108] and a review by a committee of EAACI[70] with an update in 2008[109]. Recommendations for breast-feeding are as follows:

- Breast-feeding should always be the first choice for feeding infants, for a number of other reasons such as bonding, as well as because of the unique nutritional and immunomodulatory composition of breast milk[110,111].
- There is a need for dietetic counselling of mothers, as breast-feeding is recommended to be the sole source of nutrition for the first 6 months of life in infants.
- Nutritional factors in breast milk such as the fatty-acid content may play a role in allergy prevention, but more studies are needed.
- Exclusive breast-feeding for allergy prevention in high-risk children is recommended for the first 4–6 months of life.
- Maternal dietary avoidance during lactation for allergy prevention is not recommended at present.
- No recommendations regarding supplementation of breast milk with any nutrient so far exist, primarily due to a lack of evidence.

13.3.4   Use of infant formulas in the prevention of allergic disease

Some mothers are not able to breast-feed, or choose not to do so. In an attempt to avoid exposure to cow's-milk protein early in life, hydrolysed formulas (extensive or partial) have been investigated as a replacement for or supplement to breast milk.

Intervention studies in non-high-risk families

Only four intervention studies have been performed in unselected cohorts of children. Three of these found that early introduction of cow's-milk formulas does not lead to an increase in allergic disease[112–114]. However, two of these studies were performed in premature[112] or low-birthweight infants[114]. The only study using a reliable method of diagnosing FHS did find that early cow's-milk feeding increased cow's-milk allergy between 18 and 34 months[82].

Intervention studies in high-risk infants

No long-term studies have compared the effect of hydrolysed formulas to exclusive breast-feeding, and there is no evidence that the use of these formulas is any better than human milk in the prevention of atopic disease[95]. Hypoallergenic formulas could provide a possible alternative to cow's-milk formulas for mothers of high-risk infants who choose not to, or cannot, breast-feed. It is paramount that the results should be interpreted for each formula studied, rather than grouping results of partially hydrolysed formulas[115–120] and extensively hydrolysed formulas[116,120,121] together. It is known that the immunogenicity of these formulas will differ depending on the source of the protein (casein or whey), degree of hydrolysation (partial or extensive), site of hydrolysation, enzymes used and filtration methodology[109]. A formula for allergy prevention is therefore defined as a formula with documented reduced allergenicity[22,109].

Three studies in high-risk families did not compare the effect of a hydrolysed formula to cow's milk, but compared different hydrolysed formulas. Nentwich and colleagues found a significantly decreased sensitisation to cow's-milk proteins in the partially hydrolysed whey formula (pHF-w) compared to the extensively hydrolysed whey formula (eHF-w) group at 6 and 12 months[122]. Prevalence of eczema did not differ among the groups during the first 12 months. In addition, Halken and colleagues showed that pHF-w was less effective than extensively hydrolysed casein formula (eHF-c) in preventing cow's-milk allergy (4.7% vs. 0.6%) when the children were reviewed at 18 months of age[123]. This confirmed the results of an earlier study by Halken et al.[124].

In summary, it seems that some protein hydrolysates may reduce allergic manifestations during the high-risk infant's first few years of life, as either a replacement or a supplement to breast milk.

Recommendations regarding infant formula

UK NICE guidelines state that healthcare professionals should advise mothers who choose not to breast-feed that there is insufficient evidence to suggest that infant formula based on partially or extensively hydrolysed cow's-milk protein helps to prevent allergies[125]. This, however, is in contrast to the recommendations of the three review papers regarding dietary allergy prevention that are summarised in Table 13.3.

Prebiotics and infant formula

The role of prebiotics on allergy prevention has been investigated in recent studies[126]. Prebiotic supplements were associated with a significantly higher number of faecal bifidobacteria compared with controls but there was no significant difference in *Lactobacillus* counts. Follow-up of these infants at 24 months (n = 134) showed a long-lasting effect of the prebiotic supplement. In the prebiotic group, children were significantly less likely to suffer from eczema, recurrent wheezing and allergic urticaria, and had fewer infections (of any kind), lower antibiotic use and fewer reported fever incidents[127]. Data also showed reduced levels of total IgE and increased levels of secretory IgA in the supplemented groups[128].

It is difficult, however, to relate the findings of these studies to the prebiotics in breast milk, as human-milk oligosaccharides are so heterogeneous. There are more than 200 different human-milk oligosaccharides, and the numbers vary between 30 and 120 from mother to mother.

Despite these data, a recent Cochrane review concluded that there is currently insufficient evidence to determine the role of prebiotic supplementation in infant formula[129].

13.3.5   Weaning and nutrition in early life

There are two issues that should be addressed when dealing with weaning for allergy prevention. First, there is the debate regarding suitable weaning age to ensure optimal nutrition and developmental milestones for the infant, whilst preventing allergic diseases. Second, it is unclear whether there should be different recommendations for weaning onto allergenic (e.g. milk, egg, fish, nuts) and non-allergenic foods.

Weaning age

Weaning age and general health

At present, the World Health Organization recommends that weaning should not be commenced before 6 months of age, based on the health benefits of exclusive breast-feeding for at least 6 months such as less gastrointestinal or respiratory infection in the infant[130]. Furthermore, the Scientific Advisory Committee on Nutrition (SACN) stated in 2001 that there was sufficient evidence that exclusive breast-feeding for 6 months is nutritionally adequate, but that due to current practices in the UK there should be some flexibility in the advice[131]. However, the COMA report (1994) stated that weaning should not be commenced before 4 months of age[132].

Weaning age and allergy prevention

For allergy prevention, the evidence is conflicting, but studies indicate that solids should not be introduced before 4 months of age (ideally 6 months) and that there is no evidence to suggest delaying the introduction of the major allergenic foods beyond 6 months of age[82,133–139]. A recent systematic review looking at complementary feeding before four months of age could find few data linking early solid feeding and allergic conditions, and called for additional trials to look at the relationship between the introduction of solids and allergic risk[140].

Thus, there is no evidence of an allergy-preventing effect of restrictive diets after 6 months of age. Guidelines regarding weaning age and allergy prevention can be seen in Table 13.3.

Which foods when

Tolerance to food allergens appears to be driven by regular early exposure to these proteins during a 'critical early window' of development. Timing of this window for both allergenic and non-allergenic foods is not known at present, but it depends on a very delicate balance of not introducing allergenic foods too early (before gut colonisation and tolerance mechanisms are established), but also not delaying introduction beyond the point of ensuring tolerance to food proteins. Some evidence suggests that this 'window of opportunity' lies between 4 and 6 months of life, but the truth is that we really do not know, and furthermore we do not know if this window differs for allergenic and non-allergenic foods[141]. Some studies also suggest that continued breast-feeding during introduction of complementary foods is important for promoting tolerance.

Until recently, general allergy-preventive weaning advice was based on the studies by Zeiger et al.[54] The weaning advice in this study included a staged delay in introduction of solid foods: non-legume vegetables, rice cereal, meats and non-citrus fruits between 6 and 12 months; cow's milk, wheat, soy, corn and citrus fruits between 12 and 18 months; eggs at 24 months; and peanut and fish at 36 months. However, most guideline documents now realise that there is limited evidence to delay the introduction of allergenic foods to such an extent, and the guidelines have been amended.

In order to shed some light on this issue, there is currently a UK-based randomised controlled trial investigating the regular consumption versus avoidance of peanut protein during infancy. This trial involves infants (4–11 months of age) with egg allergy, severe eczema or both. The intervention group is fed at least 6 g peanut protein weekly, distributed over at least three meals each week. The primary outcome of this study assesses the effects of this intervention on the proportion of children with peanut allergy at 5 years of age[142].

Individual nutrients and allergy prevention

Very little is known regarding the direct effect of specific nutrients in weaning foods on the immune system of the infant.

Observational and intervention studies in early life

Fish intake

Kull et al. recently reported that regular fish intake during the first year of life amongst infants from an unselected population was associated with a reduced risk for allergic disease and sensitisation to food and aeroallergens by 4 years of age[143].

Organic foods

Kummeling et al. were the first group to investigate whether organic food consumption by infants was associated with developing atopic manifestations in the first 2 years, and found that organic dairy products were associated with a lower risk of developing eczema[144].

Vitamin D

Hyppönen et al. found that the prevalence of atopy, allergic rhinitis and asthma was higher in participants who had received vitamin D supplementation regularly during the first year compared to those who did not receive supplements[145]. These results are in contrast to the data presented regarding vitamin D intake in pregnancy and the development of allergic disease in the offspring.

Recommendations regarding weaning

In line with the recommendations summarised in Table 13.3, the ESPGHAN Committee on Nutrition recommends[146]:

- Exclusive or full breast-feeding for about 6 months is a desirable goal.
- Complementary feeding (i.e. solid foods and liquids other than breast milk or infant formula and follow-on formula) should be introduced not earlier than 17 weeks and not later than 26 weeks.

There is no convincing scientific evidence that avoidance or delayed introduction of potentially allergenic foods, such as fish and eggs, reduces allergies, either in infants considered at increased risk for the development of allergy or in those not considered to be at increased risk. This is apart from peanut, where the UK COT report advises avoidance of peanut or peanut-containing foods for the first 3 years of life[48].

It is prudent to avoid both early (< 4 months) and late (≥ 7 months) introduction of gluten, and to introduce gluten gradually while the infant is still breast-fed, inasmuch as this may reduce the risk of coeliac disease, type 1 diabetes mellitus and wheat allergy.

More information is needed regarding the role of individual foods or nutrients during the weaning stage in allergy prevention.

Practical recommendations regarding the weaning diet

- Start with fruit, vegetables and simple starches such as rice and corn (especially if weaning is started before 6 months).
- Increase the variety of diet once the infant is 6 months old, and make sure foods containing vitamins A and D, iron, zinc and selenium are included in the weaning diet.
- Do not start weaning before the age of 4 months, ideally 6 months[147].
- For children at risk of developing allergies the advice (in the UK) is to delay the introduction of peanuts until 3 years of age[48].

13.4   Conclusions

In summary, the immune system starts to develop soon after conception and continues to develop through life. Nutrition and the environment, during pregnancy and early life in particular, can influence the immune system. Follow a healthy balanced diet, with an appropriate amount of calories. Important nutrients include vitamins A, C, E and D, selenium, iron, zinc and LCPUFAs, but pregnant women should not take any supplement without discussing it with a dietitian/midwife/doctor. Other immunologically important nutritional factors include prebiotics (maternal diet, breast milk, infant formula and perhaps the weaning diet) and probiotics (specific strains may be beneficial in prevention of atopic dermatitis).

Concerning allergy prevention per se, a number of studies have examined dietary factors during pregnancy, but no firm conclusions can be made from any of these observational or intervention studies. In the meantime, pregnant women should be advised to follow a healthy, balanced diet which includes recommended intakes of white and fatty fish. For now, pregnant women from high-risk families should be advised regarding the content of the COT report in the UK. There is no evidence to support avoidance of any of the other allergenic foods.

Mothers of newborns should be supported to breast-feed exclusively for at least 4 months, and ideally for 6 months. As with pregnant women, breast-feeding mothers should be advised to follow a healthy, balanced diet including recommended intakes of white and fatty fish. For now, breast-feeding mothers from high-risk families should be advised regarding the content of the COT report in the UK. There is no evidence to support avoidance of any of the other allergenic foods during lactation.

For high-risk mothers who cannot or choose not to breast-feed, an extensively hydrolysed casein formula or a partially hydrolysed whey formula should be suggested. All other mothers could use any cow's-milk-based formula.

Weaning should not be commenced before 6 months, but at least not before 4 months. More information is needed regarding the introduction of allergenic food. Current knowledge suggests that there is no evidence to delay the introduction of highly allergenic foods beyond the age of 6 months. This is apart from peanut, where the UK COT report advises avoidance of peanut or peanut-containing foods for the first 3 years of life.

References

This chapter has been adapted from Venter C, Clayton B and Dean T (2008). Part 2: The role of the midwife in allergy prevention, *British Journal of Midwifery*, vol 16, no 12, 791–803.

1. Austin JB, Kaur B, Anderson HR *et al*. Hay fever, eczema, and wheeze: a nationwide UK study (ISAAC, international study of asthma and allergies in childhood). *Arch Dis Child* 1999; **81**: 225–30.
2. Dennis R, Caraballo L, Garcia E *et al*. Asthma and other allergic conditions in Colombia: a study in 6 cities. *Ann Allergy Asthma Immunol* 2004; **93**: 568–74.
3. Department of Health Allergy Services Review Team. A review of services for allergy: the epidemiology, demand for, and provision of treatment and effectiveness of clinical interventions. London, Department of Health, 2006.
4. Woods RK, Abramson M, Bailey M, Walters EH. International prevalences of reported food allergies and intolerances. Comparisons arising from the European Community Respiratory Health Survey (ECRHS) 1991–1994. *Eur J Clin Nutr* 2001; **55**: 298–304.
5. Zuberbier T, Edenharter G, Worm M *et al*. Prevalence of adverse reactions to food in Germany: a population study. *Allergy* 2004; **59**: 338–45.
6. Jansen JJ, Kardinaal AF, Huijbers G *et al*. Prevalence of food allergy and intolerance in the adult Dutch population. *J Allergy Clin Immunol* 1994; **93**: 446–56.
7. Young E, Stoneham MD, Petruckevitch A, Barton J, Rona R. A population study of food intolerance. *Lancet* 1994; **343**: 1127–30.
8. Osterballe M, Hansen TK, Mortz CG, Høst A, Bindslev-Jensen C. The prevalence of food hypersensitivity in an unselected population of children and adults. *Pediatr Allergy Immunol* 2005; **16**: 567–73.
9. Roehr CC, Edenharter G, Reimann S *et al*. Food allergy and non-allergic food hypersensitivity in children and adolescents. *Clin Exp Allergy* 2004; **34**: 1534–41.
10. Bock SA. Prospective appraisal of complaints of adverse reactions to foods in children during the first 3 years of life. *Pediatrics* 1987; **79**: 683–8.
11. Venter C, Pereira B, Voigt K *et al*. Prevalence and cumulative incidence of food hypersensitivity in the first three years of life. *Allergy* 2008; **63**: 354–9.

12. Pereira B, Venter C, Grundy J *et al.* Prevalence of sensitization to food allergens, reported adverse reaction to foods, food avoidance, and food hypersensitivity among teenagers. *J Allergy Clin Immunol* 2005; **116**: 884–92.

13. Venter C, Pereira B, Grundy J *et al.* Incidence of parentally reported and clinically diagnosed food hypersensitivity in the first year of life. *J Allergy Clin Immunol* 2006; **117**: 1118–24.

14. Venter C, Pereira B, Grundy J *et al.* Prevalence of sensitization reported and objectively assessed food hypersensitivity amongst six-year-old children: a population-based study. *Pediatr Allergy Immunol* 2006; **17**: 356–63.

15. Rhodes HL, Sporik R, Thomas P, Holgate ST, Cogswell JJ. Early life risk factors for adult asthma: a birth cohort study of subjects at risk. J Allergy Clin Immunol 2001; 108(5): 720–725.

16. Sicherer SH, Noone SA, Muñoz-Furlong A. The impact of childhood food allergy on quality of life. *Ann Allergy Asthma Immunol* 2001; **87**: 461–4.

17. Bender B, Leung S, Leung D. Actigraphy assessment of sleep disturbance in patients with atopic dermatitis: an objective life quality measure. *J Allergy Clin Immunol* 2003; **111**: 598–602.

18. Avery NJ, King RM, Knight S, Hourihane J. Assessment of quality of life in children with peanut allergy. *Pediatr Allergy Immunol* 2003; **14**: 378–82.

19. Exl BM, Fritsche R. Cow's milk protein allergy and possible means for its prevention. *Nutrition* 2001; **17**: 642–51.

20. Kjellman NI. Atopic disease in seven-year-old children: incidence in relation to family history. *Acta Paediatr Scand* 1977; **66**: 465–71.

21. Kurukulaaratchy R, Fenn M, Matthews S, Hasan Arshad S. The prevalence, characteristics of and early life risk factors for eczema in 10-year-old children. *Pediatr Allergy Immunol* 2003; **14**: 178–83.

22. Muraro A, Dreborg S, Halken S *et al.* Dietary prevention of allergic diseases in infants and small children. Part I: immunologic background and criteria for hypoallergenicity. *Pediatr Allergy Immunol* 2004; **15**: 103–11.

23. Muraro A, Dreborg S, Halken S *et al.* Dietary prevention of allergic diseases in infants and small children. Part II: evaluation of methods in allergy prevention studies and sensitization markers. Definitions and diagnostic criteria of allergic diseases. *Pediatr Allergy Immunol* 2004; **15**: 196–205.

24. Vance GH, Lewis SA, Grimshaw KE *et al.* Exposure of the fetus and infant to hens' egg ovalbumin via the placenta and breast milk in relation to maternal intake of dietary egg. *Clin Exp Allergy* 2005; **35**: 1318–26.

25. Church MK, Holgate ST, Lichtenstein LM. *Allergy*, 3rd edn. London: Mosby, 2006.

26. Novak R. *Mosby's Crash course in Immunology*. Philadelphia, PA: Mosby/Elsevier, 2006.

27. Warner JO. The early life origins of asthma and related allergic disorders. *Arch Dis Child* 2004; **89**: 97–102.

28. Holt PG, Jones CA. The development of the immune system during pregnancy and early life. *Allergy* 2000; **55**: 688–97.

29. Hayward AR. Ontogeny of the immune system. In: Ulijaszek SJ, Johnston FE, Preece MA, eds. *The Cambridge Encyclopaedia of Human Growth and Development*. Cambridge: Cambridge University Press, 1998; 166–9.

30. Chew BP, Park JS. Carotenoid action on the immune response. *J Nutr* 2004; **134**: 257S–261S.

31. Jason J, Archibald LK, Nwanyanwu OC *et al.* The effects of iron deficiency on lymphocyte cytokine production and activation: preservation of hepatic iron but not at all cost. *Clin Exp Immunol* 2001; **126**: 466–73.

32. Wieringa FT, Dijkhuizen MA, West CE *et al.* Reduced production of immunoregulatory cytokines in vitamin A- and zinc-deficient Indonesian infants. *Eur J Clin Nutr* 2004; **58**: 1498–504.

33. Osendarp SJ, West CE, Black RE. The need for maternal zinc supplementation in developing countries: an unresolved issue. *J Nutr* 2003; **133**: 817S–827S.

34. Jackson MJ, Dillon SA, Broome CS *et al.* Are there functional consequences of a reduction in selenium intake in UK subjects? *Proc Nutr Soc* 2004; **63**: 513–17.

35. Cantorna MT, Zhu Y, Froicu M, Wittke A. Vitamin D status, 1,25-dihydroxyvitamin D3, and the immune system. *Am J Clin Nutr* 2004; **80** (6 Suppl): 1717S–1720S.
36. Calvani M, Alessandri C, Sopo SM *et al*. Consumption of fish, butter and margarine during pregnancy and development of allergic sensitizations in the offspring: role of maternal atopy. *Pediatr Allergy Immunol* 2006; **17**: 94–102.
37. Sausenthaler S, Koletzko S, Schaaf B *et al*. Maternal diet during pregnancy in relation to eczema and allergic sensitization in the offspring at 2 y of age. *Am J Clin Nutr* 2007; **85**: 530–7.
38. Romieu I, Torrent M, Garcia-Esteban R *et al*. Maternal fish intake during pregnancy and atopy and asthma in infancy. *Clin Exp Allergy* 2007; **37**: 518–25.
39. Ushiyama Y, Matsumoto K, Shinohara M *et al*. Nutrition during pregnancy may be associated with allergic diseases in infants. *J Nutr Sci Vitaminol (Tokyo)* 2002; **48**: 345–51.
40. Willers SM, Devereux G, Craig LC *et al*. Maternal food consumption during pregnancy and asthma, respiratory and atopic symptoms in 5-year-old children. *Thorax* 2007; **62**: 773–9.
41. Martindale S, McNeill G, Devereux G *et al*. Antioxidant intake in pregnancy in relation to wheeze and eczema in the first two years of life. *Am J Respir Crit Care Med* 2005; **171**: 121–8.
42. Stazi MA, Sampogna F, Montagano G *et al*. Early life factors related to clinical manifestations of atopic disease but not to skin-prick test positivity in young children. *Pediatr Allergy Immunol* 2002; **13**: 105–12.
43. Devereux G, Turner SW, Craig LC *et al*. Low maternal vitamin E intake during pregnancy is associated with asthma in 5-year-old children. *Am J Respir Crit Care Med* 2006; **174**: 499–507.
44. Litonjua AA, Rifas-Shiman SL, Ly NP *et al*. Maternal antioxidant intake in pregnancy and wheezing illnesses in children at 2 y of age. *Am J Clin Nutr* 2006; **84**: 903–11.
45. Camargo CA Jr, Rifas-Shiman SL, Litonjua AA *et al*. Maternal intake of vitamin D during pregnancy and risk of recurrent wheeze in children at 3 y of age. *Am J Clin Nutr* 2007; **85**: 788–95.
46. Hourihane JO, Dean TP, Warner JO. Peanut allergy in relation to heredity, maternal diet, and other atopic diseases: results of a questionnaire survey, skin prick testing, and food challenges. *BMJ* 1996; **313**: 518–21.
47. Lack G, Fox D, Northstone K, Golding J. Factors associated with the development of peanut allergy in childhood. *N Engl J Med* 2003; **348**: 977–85.
48. Committee on Toxicity of Chemicals in Food, Consumer Products and the Environment. *Peanut Allergy*. London: Department of Health, 1998.
49. Dean T, Venter C, Pereira B *et al*. Government advice on peanut avoidance during pregnancy: is it followed correctly and what is the impact on sensitization? *J Hum Nutr Diet* 2007; **20**: 95–9.
50. Lilja G, Dannaeus A, Fälth-Magnusson K *et al*. Immune response of the atopic woman and foetus: effects of high- and low-dose food allergen intake during late pregnancy. *Clin Allergy* 1988; **18**: 131–42.
51. Fälth-Magnusson K, Kjellman NI. Development of atopic disease in babies whose mothers were receiving exclusion diet during pregnancy: a randomized study. *J Allergy Clin Immunol* 1987; **80**: 868–75.
52. Lovegrove JA, Hampton SM, Morgan JB. The immunological and long-term atopic outcome of infants born to women following a milk-free diet during late pregnancy and lactation: a pilot study. *Br J Nutr* 1994; **71**: 223–38.
53. Vance GH, Grimshaw KE, Briggs R *et al*. Serum ovalbumin-specific immunoglobulin G responses during pregnancy reflect maternal intake of dietary egg and relate to the development of allergy in early infancy. *Clin Exp Allergy* 2004; **34**: 1855–61.
54. Zeiger RS, Heller S, Mellon MH *et al*. Effect of combined maternal and infant food-allergen avoidance on development of atopy in early infancy: a randomized study. *J Allergy Clin Immunol* 1989; **84**: 72–89.
55. Hattevig G, Kjellman B, Sigurs N, Björkstén B, Kjellman NI. Effect of maternal avoidance of eggs, cow's milk and fish during lactation upon allergic manifestations in infants. *Clin Exp Allergy* 1989; **19**: 27–32.

56. Herrmann ME, Dannemann A, Gruters A et al. Prospective study of the atopy preventive effect of maternal avoidance of milk and eggs during pregnancy and lactation. *Eur J Pediatr* 1996; **155**: 770–4.

57. Björkstén B. Effects of intestinal microflora and the environment on the development of asthma and allergy. *Springer Semin Immunopathol* 2004; **25**: 257–70.

58. Penders J, Thijs C, van den Brandt PA et al. Gut microbiota composition and development of atopic manifestations in infancy: the KOALA Birth Cohort Study. *Gut* 2007; **56**: 661–7.

59. Kukkonen K, Savilahti E, Haahtela T et al. Probiotics and prebiotic galacto-oligosaccharides in the prevention of allergic diseases: a randomized, double-blind, placebo-controlled trial. *J Allergy Clin Immunol* 2007; **119**: 192–8.

60. Kalliomaki M, Salminen S, Arvilommi H et al. Probiotics in primary prevention of atopic disease: a randomised placebo-controlled trial. *Lancet* 2001; **357**: 1076–9.

61. Abrahamsson TR, Jakobsson T, Bottcher MF et al. Probiotics in prevention of IgE-associated eczema: a double-blind, randomized, placebo-controlled trial. *J Allergy Clin Immunol* 2007; **119**: 1174–80.

62. Kopp MV, Hennemuth I, Heinzmann A, Urbanek R. Randomized, double-blind, placebo-controlled trial of probiotics for primary prevention: no clinical effects of *Lactobacillus* GG supplementation. *Pediatrics* 2008; **121**: e850–6.

63. Taylor AL, Dunstan JA, Prescott SL. Probiotic supplementation for the first 6 months of life fails to reduce the risk of atopic dermatitis and increases the risk of allergen sensitization in high-risk children: a randomized controlled trial. *J Allergy Clin Immunol* 2007; **119**: 184–91.

64. Kalliomaki M, Salminen S, Poussa T, Arvilommi H, Isolauri E. Probiotics and prevention of atopic disease: 4-year follow-up of a randomised placebo-controlled trial. *Lancet* 2003; **361**: 1869–71.

65. Kalliomaki M, Salminen S, Poussa T, Isolauri E. Probiotics during the first 7 years of life: a cumulative risk reduction of eczema in a randomized, placebo-controlled trial. *J Allergy Clin Immunol* 2007; **119**: 1019–21.

66. Prescott SL, Björkstén B. Probiotics for the prevention or treatment of allergic diseases. *J Allergy Clin Immunol* 2007; **120**: 255–62.

67. Dunstan JA, Mori TA, Barden A et al. Fish oil supplementation in pregnancy modifies neonatal allergen-specific immune responses and clinical outcomes in infants at high risk of atopy: a randomized, controlled trial. *J Allergy Clin Immunol* 2003; **112**: 1178–84.

68. Marks GB, Mihrshahi S, Kemp AS et al. Prevention of asthma during the first 5 years of life: a randomized controlled trial. *J Allergy Clin Immunol* 2006; **118**: 53–61.

69. Kramer MS, Kakuma R. Maternal dietary antigen avoidance during pregnancy or lactation, or both, for preventing or treating atopic disease in the child. *Cochrane Database Syst Rev* 2006; (3): CD000133.

70. Muraro A, Dreborg S, Halken S et al. Dietary prevention of allergic diseases in infants and small children. Part III: critical review of published peer-reviewed observational and interventional studies and final recommendations. *Pediatr Allergy Immunol* 2004; **15**: 291–307.

71. Strachan DP. Family size, infection and atopy: the first decade of the 'hygiene hypothesis'. *Thorax* 2000; **55** (Suppl 1): S2–10.

72. Hällström M, Eerola E, Vuento R, Janas M, Tammela O. Effects of mode of delivery and necrotising enterocolitis on the intestinal microflora in preterm infants. *Eur J Clin Microbiol Infect Dis* 2004; **23**: 463–70.

73. Renz-Polster H, David MR, Buist AS et al. Caesarean section delivery and the risk of allergic disorders in childhood. *Clin Exp Allergy* 2005; **35**: 1466–72.

74. Brandtzaeg P. Mucosal immunity. *Dev Biol (Basel)* 2003; **115**: 111–17.

75. Bailey M, Haverson K, Inman C et al. The development of the mucosal immune system pre- and post-weaning: balancing regulatory and effector function. *Proc Nutr Soc* 2005; **64**: 451–7.

76. Sampson HA. Update on food allergy. *J Allergy Clin Immunol* 2004; **113**: 805–19.

77. Oddy WH. The impact of breastmilk on infant and child health. *Breastfeed Rev* 2002; **10**: 5–18.

78. Fanaro S, Chierici R, Guerrini P, Vigi V. Intestinal microflora in early infancy: composition and development. *Acta Paediatr Suppl* 2003; **91**: 48–55.

79. Oddy WH. A review of the effects of breastfeeding on respiratory infections, atopy, and childhood asthma. *J Asthma* 2004; **41**: 605–21.

80. Das UN. Essential fatty acids as possible enhancers of the beneficial actions of probiotics. *Nutrition* 2002; **18**: 786.

81. Brandtzaeg P. Mucosal immunity: integration between mother and the breast-fed infant. *Vaccine* 2003; **21**: 3382–8.

82. Saarinen KM, Juntunen-Backman K, Jarvenpaa AL *et al*. Supplementary feeding in maternity hospitals and the risk of cow's milk allergy: a prospective study of 6209 infants. *J Allergy Clin Immunol* 1999; **104**: 457–61.

83. Kull I, Wickman M, Lilja G, Nordvall SL, Pershagen G. Breast feeding and allergic diseases in infants: a prospective birth cohort study. *Arch Dis Child* 2002; **87**: 478–81.

84. Oddy WH, Peat JK, de Klerk NH. Maternal asthma, infant feeding, and the risk of asthma in childhood. *J Allergy Clin Immunol* 2002; **110**: 65–7.

85. Arshad SH, Kurukulaaratchy RJ, Fenn M, Matthews S. Early life risk factors for current wheeze, asthma, and bronchial hyperresponsiveness at 10 years of age. *Chest* 2005; **127**: 502–8.

86. Wright AL, Holberg CJ, Taussig LM, Martinez FD. Factors influencing the relation of infant feeding to asthma and recurrent wheeze in childhood. *Thorax* 2001; **56**: 192–7.

87. Sears MR, Greene JM, Willan AR *et al*. Long-term relation between breastfeeding and development of atopy and asthma in children and young adults: a longitudinal study. *Lancet* 2002; **360**: 901–7.

88. Bergmann RL, Diepgen TL, Kuss O *et al*. Breastfeeding duration is a risk factor for atopic eczema. *Clin Exp Allergy* 2002; **32**: 205–9.

89. Pratt HF. Breastfeeding and eczema. *Early Hum Dev* 1984; **9**: 283–90.

90. Saarinen UM, Kajosaari M. Breastfeeding as prophylaxis against atopic disease: prospective follow-up study until 17 years old. *Lancet* 1995; **346**: 1065–9.

91. Yu G, Duchen K, Björkstén B. Fatty acid composition in colostrum and mature milk from non-atopic and atopic mothers during the first 6 months of lactation. *Acta Paediatr* 1998; **87**: 729–36.

92. Jones CA, Holloway JA, Popplewell EJ *et al*. Reduced soluble CD14 levels in amniotic fluid and breast milk are associated with the subsequent development of atopy, eczema, or both. *J Allergy Clin Immunol* 2002; **109**: 858–66.

93. Gdalevich M, Mimouni D, David M, Mimouni M. Breast-feeding and the onset of atopic dermatitis in childhood: a systematic review and meta-analysis of prospective studies. *J Am Acad Dermatol* 2001; **45**: 520–7.

94. Mimouni Bloch A, Mimouni D, Mimouni M, Gdalevich M. Does breastfeeding protect against allergic rhinitis during childhood? A meta-analysis of prospective studies. *Acta Paediatr* 2002; **91**: 275–9.

95. Greer FR, Sicherer SH, Burks AW. Effects of early nutritional interventions on the development of atopic disease in infants and children: the role of maternal dietary restriction, breastfeeding, timing of introduction of complementary foods, and hydrolyzed formulas. *Pediatrics* 2008; **121**: 183–1.

96. Venter C, Pereira B, Voigt K *et al*. Factors associated with maternal dietary intake, feeding and weaning practices and the development of food hypersensitivity in the infant. *Pediatr Allergy Immunol* in press.

97. Dunstan JA, Mitoulas LR, Dixon G *et al*. The effects of fish oil supplementation in pregnancy on breast milk fatty acid composition over the course of lactation: a randomized controlled trial. *Pediatr Res* 2007; **62**: 689–94.

98. Høst A, Husby S, Hansen LG, Osterballe O. Bovine beta-lactoglobulin in human milk from atopic and non-atopic mothers: relationship to maternal intake of homogenized and unhomogenized milk. *Clin Exp Allergy* 1990; **20**: 383–7.

99. Hoppu U, Kalliomaki M, Isolauri E. Maternal diet rich in saturated fat during breastfeeding is associated with atopic sensitization of the infant. *Eur J Clin Nutr* 2000; **54**: 702–5.

100. Duchen K, Casas R, Fageras-Bottcher M, Yu G, Björkstén B. Human milk polyunsaturated long-chain fatty acids and secretory immunoglobulin A antibodies and early childhood allergy. *Pediatr Allergy Immunol* 2000; **11**: 29–39.

101. Kankaanpaa P, Nurmela K, Erkkila A *et al*. Polyunsaturated fatty acids in maternal diet, breast milk, and serum lipid fatty acids of infants in relation to atopy. *Allergy* 2001; **56**: 633–8.

102. Stoney RM, Woods RK, Hosking CS *et al*. Maternal breast milk long-chain n-3 fatty acids are associated with increased risk of atopy in breastfed infants. *Clin Exp Allergy* 2004; **34**: 194–200.

103. Reichardt P, Muller D, Posselt U *et al*. Fatty acids in colostrum from mothers of children at high risk of atopy in relation to clinical and laboratory signs of allergy in the first year of life. *Allergy* 2004; **59**: 394–400.

104. Wijga AH, van Houwelingen AC, Kerkhof M *et al*. Breast milk fatty acids and allergic disease in preschool children: the Prevention and Incidence of Asthma and Mite Allergy birth cohort study. *J Allergy Clin Immunol* 2006; **117**: 440–7.

105. Almqvist C, Garden F, Xuan W *et al*. Omega-3 and omega-6 fatty acid exposure from early life does not affect atopy and asthma at age 5 years. *J Allergy Clin Immunol* 2007; **119**: 1438–44.

106. Laitinen K, Sallinen J, Linderborg K, Isolauri E. Serum, cheek cell and breast milk fatty acid compositions in infants with atopic and non-atopic eczema. *Clin Exp Allergy* 2006; **36**: 166–73.

107. Sjögren YM, Duchén K, Lindh F, Björkstén B, Sverremark-Ekström E. Neutral oligosaccharides in colostrum in relation to maternal allergy and allergy development in children up to 18 months of age. *Pediatr Allergy Immunol* 2007; **18**: 20–6.

108. Høst A, Koletzko B, Dreborg S *et al*. Dietary products used in infants for treatment and prevention of food allergy. Joint Statement of the European Society for Paediatric Allergology and Clinical Immunology (ESPACI) Committee on Hypoallergenic Formulas and the European Society for Paediatric Gastroenterology, Hepatology and Nutrition (ESPGHAN) Committee on Nutrition. *Arch Dis Child* 1999; **81**: 80–4.

109. Høst A, Halken S, Muraro A *et al*. Dietary prevention of allergic diseases in infants and small children. *Pediatr Allergy Immunol* 2008; **19**: 1–4.

110. Hoppu U, Kalliomaki M, Laiho K, Isolauri E. Breast milk – immunomodulatory signals against allergic diseases. *Allergy* 2001; **56** (Suppl 67): 23–6.

111. Ip S, Chung M, Raman G *et al*. *Breastfeeding and Maternal and Infant Health Outcomes in Developed Countries*. Tufts-New England Medical Center Evidence-Based Center. Evidence Report/Technology Assessment 153. AHRQ Publication 07-E007. Rockville, MD: Agency for Healthcare Research and Quality, 2007.

112. Lucas A, Brooke OG, Morley R, Cole TJ, Bamford MF. Early diet of preterm infants and development of allergic or atopic disease: randomised prospective study. *BMJ* 1990; **300**: 837–40.

113. de Jong MH, Scharp-van der Linden VT, Aalberse R, Heymans HS, Brunekreef B. The effect of brief neonatal exposure to cows' milk on atopic symptoms up to age 5. *Arch Dis Child* 2002; **86**: 365–9.

114. Lindfors AT, Danielsson L, Enocksson E, Johansson SG, Westin S. Allergic symptoms up to 4–6 years of age in children given cow milk neonatally: a prospective study. *Allergy* 1992; **47**: 207–11.

115. Chirico G, Gasparoni A, Ciardelli L *et al*. Immunogenicity and antigenicity of a partially hydrolyzed cow's milk infant formula. *Allergy* 1997; **52**: 82–8.

116. Oldaeus G, Anjou K, Björkstén B, Moran JR, Kjellman NI. Extensively and partially hydrolysed infant formulas for allergy prophylaxis. *Arch Dis Child* 1997; **77**: 4–10.

117. Vandenplas Y, Hauser B, Van den Borre C, Sacre L, Dab I. Effect of a whey hydrolysate prophylaxis of atopic disease. *Ann Allergy* 1992; **68**: 419–24.

118. Chan YH, Shek LP, Aw M, Quak SH, Lee BW. Use of hypoallergenic formula in the prevention of atopic disease among Asian children. *J Paediatr Child Health* 2002; **38**: 84–8.

119. Marini A, Agosti M, Motta G, Mosca F. Effects of a dietary and environmental prevention programme on the incidence of allergic symptoms in high atopic risk infants: three years' follow-up. *Acta Paediatr Suppl* 1996; **414**: 1–21.

120. von Berg A, Koletzko S, Filipiak-Pittroff B *et al.* Certain hydrolyzed formulas reduce the incidence of atopic dermatitis but not that of asthma: three-year results of the German Infant Nutritional Intervention Study. *J Allergy Clin Immunol* 2007; **119**: 718–25.

121. Mallet E, Henocq A. Long-term prevention of allergic diseases by using protein hydrolysate formula in at-risk infants. *J Pediatr* 1992; **121**: S95–100.

122. Nentwich I, Michkova E, Nevoral J, Urbanek R, Szepfalusi Z. Cow's milk-specific cellular and humoral immune responses and atopy skin symptoms in infants from atopic families fed a partially (pHF) or extensively (eHF) hydrolyzed infant formula. *Allergy* 2001; **56**: 1144–56.

123. Halken S, Hansen KS, Jacobsen HP *et al.* Comparison of a partially hydrolyzed infant formula with two extensively hydrolyzed formulas for allergy prevention: a prospective, randomized study. *Pediatr Allergy Immunol* 2000; **11**: 149–61.

124. Halken S, Høst A, Hansen LG, Osterballe O. Preventive effect of feeding high-risk infants a casein hydrolysate formula or an ultrafiltrated whey hydrolysate formula: a prospective, randomized, comparative clinical study. *Pediatr Allergy Immunol* 1993; **4**: 173–81.

125. National Institute for Health and Clinical Excellence. *NICE guidelines: Maternal and Child Nutrition*. London: NICE, 2008.

126. Moro G, Arslanoglu S, Stahl B *et al.* A mixture of prebiotic oligosaccharides reduces the incidence of atopic dermatitis during the first six months of age. *Arch Dis Child* 2006; **91**: 814–19.

127. Arslanoglu S, Moro GE, Schmitt J *et al.* Early dietary intervention with a mixture of prebiotic oligosaccharides reduces the incidence of allergic manifestations and infections during the first two years of life. *J Nutr* 2008; **138**: 1091–5.

128. van Hoffen E, Ruiter B, Faber J *et al.* A specific mixture of short-chain galacto-oligosaccharides and long-chain fructo-oligosaccharides induces a beneficial immunoglobulin profile in infants at high risk for allergy. *Allergy* 2008.

129. Osborn DA, Sinn JK. Prebiotics in infants for prevention of allergic disease and food hypersensitivity. *Cochrane Database Syst Rev* 2007; (4): CD006474.

130. Department of Health. *Department of Health Recommendation on Infant Feeding*. London: DOH, 2001. www.dh.gov.uk.

131. Scientific Advisory Committee on Nutrition. *Optimal Duration of Exclusive Breastfeeding and Introduction of Weaning*. SACN 01/07, 2001. www.sacn.gov.uk.

132. Department of Health. *Weaning and the Weaning diet: Report of the Working Group on the Weaning diet of the Committee on Medical Aspects of Food Policy*. Report on Health and Social Subjects 45. London, HMSO, 1994.

133. Kajosaari M. Atopy prophylaxis in high-risk infants: prospective 5-year follow-up study of children with six months exclusive breastfeeding and solid food elimination. *Adv Exp Med Biol* 1991; **310**: 453–8.

134. Kajosaari M, Saarinen UM. Prophylaxis of atopic disease by six months' total solid food elimination: evaluation of 135 exclusively breast-fed infants of atopic families. *Acta Paediatr Scand* 1983; **72**: 411–14.

135. Fergusson DM, Horwood LJ, Shannon FT. Early solid feeding and recurrent childhood eczema: a 10-year longitudinal study. *Pediatrics* 1990; **86**: 541–6.

136. Wilson AC, Forsyth JS, Greene SA *et al.* Relation of infant diet to childhood health: seven year follow up of cohort of children in Dundee infant feeding study. *BMJ* 1998; **316**: 21–5.

137. Morgan J, Williams P, Norris F *et al.* Eczema and early solid feeding in preterm infants. *Arch Dis Child* 2004; **89**: 309–14.

138. Zutavern A, von Mutius E, Harris J *et al.* The introduction of solids in relation to asthma and eczema. *Arch Dis Child* 2004; **89**: 303–8.

139. Zutavern A, Brockow I, Schaaf B *et al.* Timing of solid food introduction in relation to atopic dermatitis and atopic sensitization: results from a prospective birth cohort study. *Pediatrics* 2006; **117**: 401–11.

140. Tarini BA, Carroll AE, Sox CM, Christakis DA. Systematic review of the relationship between early introduction of solid foods to infants and the development of allergic disease. *Arch Pediatr Adolesc Med* 2006; **160**: 502–7.

141. Prescott SL, Smith P, Tang M *et al.* The importance of early complementary feeding in the development of oral tolerance: concerns and controversies. *Pediatr Allergy Immunol* 2008; **19**: 375–80.

142. Ivarsson A, Hernell O, Stenlund H, Persson LA. Breast-feeding protects against celiac disease. *Am J Clin Nutr* 2002; **75**: 914–21.

143. Kull I, Bergström A, Lilja G, Pershagen G, Wickman M. Fish consumption during the first year of life and development of allergic diseases during childhood. *Allergy* 2006; **61**: 1009–15.

144. Kummeling I, Thijs C, Huber M *et al.* Consumption of organic foods and risk of atopic disease during the first 2 years of life in the Netherlands. *Br J Nutr* 2008; **99**: 598–605.

145. Hyppönen E, Sovio U, Wjst M *et al.* Infant vitamin d supplementation and allergic conditions in adulthood: northern Finland birth cohort 1966. *Ann N Y Acad Sci* 2004; **1037**: 84–95.

146. Agostoni C, Decsi T, Fewtrell M *et al.* Complementary feeding: a commentary by the ESPGHAN Committee on Nutrition. *J Pediatr Gastroenterol Nutr* 2008; **46**: 99–110.

147. Food Allergy and Intolerance Interest Group, British Dietetic Association. Position statement: practical dietary prevention strategies for infants at risk of developing allergic diseases. London: BDA, 2004.

14 Management of Allergic Disease

14.1 Allergic rhinitis

Samantha Walker

14.1.1 Introduction

Allergic rhinitis is a common problem which is trivialised by sufferers and health professionals, despite being associated with absence from school and work, and with learning impairment in children. In the UK, seasonal rhinitis is usually caused by high grass-pollen counts, which coincide with national exams and require timely and effective treatments. Perennial rhinitis is less commonly associated with allergy, but can be triggered by persistent exposure to dust mites or furry animals. Nasal steroids and antihistamines are effective treatments when taken regularly, but poor nasal spray technique can result in treatment failure. Short courses of oral steroids are useful in the event of treatment failure or before significant exams or life events, whilst grass-pollen immunotherapy is available sublingually or subcutaneously for those patients with hay fever who are unresponsive to conventional treatment. Rhinitis alone is rarely a manifestation of food allergy, but symptoms commonly coexist. It is therefore important to ask about rhinitis symptoms when investigating food allergy so that appropriate treatment can be given.

14.1.2 Background

Rhinitis is a common problem in Western societies, affecting approximately 24% of the UK adult population[1]. Rhinitis can be defined as a collection of symptoms including a runny and/or blocked nose, sneezing, itching and sometimes postnasal drip (mucus running down the back of the throat) or conjunctivitis, occurring for an hour or more on most days. Symptoms can be seasonal (hay fever), perennial, or perennial with seasonal exacerbations, and have been shown to differ in their allergic (atopic) state, clinical presentation and medical history. In a large study of nearly 3,000 adults, 3% had seasonal symptoms only, 13% had perennial symptoms only, and 8% had perennial symptoms with seasonal exacerbations[1]. The majority (78%) of those with seasonal symptoms had an allergic cause for their symptoms, whereas only 50% of perennial symptoms were allergic in nature. In those with perennial and seasonal symptoms, 68% were allergic. Seasonal rhinitis was characterised by sneezing, itching, and a high prevalence of diurnal variation in symptoms. The most common triggers were dust, pollens and infections. By comparison, perennial rhinitis was characterised by a higher prevalence of nasal blockage and catarrh, and a lower prevalence of diurnal variation and pollen-related triggers. Subjects with seasonal rhinitis were more likely to be atopic (i.e. have positive skin prick tests or serum IgE tests to common aeroallergens) and to have eczema and a family history of hay fever than those without rhinitis. Those with perennial rhinitis were more likely to have past or current eczema or migraine, be wheezy or labelled asthmatic, or have a family history of nose trouble other than hay fever[1].

14.1.3   Impact of allergic rhinitis

Allergic rhinitis (including hay fever) is common and can have a big impact on daily activities. Research has shown that it may adversely affect concentration[2], reduce productivity and impair exam performance[3] in adolescents. The high prevalence of hay fever among adolescents[3], combined with that fact that GSCE and A-level exams take place at the peak of the grass-pollen season, mean it is vital to consider strategies for managing hay-fever symptoms in this age group proactively, and to encourage patients to take advantage of the broad range of treatments available.

14.1.4   What is the role of allergy?

Causes of rhinitis are varied, but for simplicity they can be broadly grouped under headings of allergic and non-allergic. Their symptoms are similar, but allergic rhinitis is characterised by sneezing and itching, whereas the commonest symptoms in non-allergic rhinitis are nasal blockage and postnasal drip. Although rhinitis is easy to treat using a structured approach, it is helpful to differentiate between allergic and non-allergic rhinitis, as the treatments may be different. In practice, simple questions can help you to discover the most likely cause and select the most appropriate treatment.

Accurate history taking is of primary importance in establishing the role of allergy. However, a positive response to the question 'do you get hay fever?' correlates to a positive allergy test (skin prick test or measurement of serum specific IgE) approximately 75% of the time[3].

In general, rhinitis is more likely to be allergic in nature if a trigger can be identified, if symptoms include sneezing and itching, and if there are associated eye symptoms.

Treatment is, in the majority of sufferers, extremely effective. However, care needs to be taken to get the combination of treatments right and to ensure patients take them correctly and regularly. Pollen avoidance may also help.

14.1.5   Mechanisms

Allergic rhinitis is caused by inhalation of allergen (e.g. grass pollen) which results in a classic sequence of events caused by an inappropriate immune response to otherwise harmless substances[4]. The classic signs of allergy (itching, redness and swelling) and its time course (immediate symptoms, usually occurring within 15 minutes of exposure) are caused mainly by the release of histamine, a potent chemical that causes itching due to irritation of nerve endings, redness due to vasodilation of blood vessels, and swelling due to increased vascular permeability via immunoglobulin E (IgE). The signs of itching, redness and swelling mark the cornerstone of allergy diagnosis and, at a simplistic level, allow the differentiation between allergic and non-allergic symptoms.

Other causes of rhinitis symptoms include infection (viral, bacterial), structural problems of the nose (e.g. deviation of the nasal septum and polyps) and, less commonly, endocrine problems (hypothyroidism) and iatrogenic disease (e.g. the combined oral contraceptive pill).

14.1.6   Diagnosis

The medical history, related to the nature and timing of the symptoms, trigger factors, and evidence of personal and family history of allergic disease, should guide the need for, and the choice of, diagnostic test[7]. Where avoidance is both effective and possible (in the case of food or drug allergy) or an allergen-specific treatment such as immunotherapy is being considered, then identification of the specific allergen trigger is essential, although accurate history taking is of primary importance in establishing the role of allergy and interpreting test results. The probability of rhinitis symptoms being allergic in nature is significantly increased, if symptoms are triggered by animals or pollen, or if the patient has a personal history or a family history of allergy[3].

However for many individuals, identifying the underlying allergenic trigger may have little or no bearing on the management of the condition, especially as it is not always possible to avoid exposure to allergen triggers. The need for a diagnostic test should therefore depend on whether or not the identification of an allergen trigger will influence the treatment decision[6]. A pragmatic approach may be to opt for empirical treatment as an initial step for rhinitis patients with a convincing history of allergy, that is, patients with a personal or family history of asthma, eczema or hay fever who have symptoms which occur within minutes of exposure and fit the pattern of histamine release in one or more target organs (i.e. redness, itching or swelling). For many patients treatment is based on managing specific symptoms that include nasal blockage, discharge and sneezing. The most effective treatments are oral antihistamine and topical nasal corticosteroids[5].

14.1.7   Management

Allergen avoidance

Airborne allergens such as grass pollen, house-dust mite and cat allergen are difficult to avoid. The effectiveness of allergen avoidance measures in adults[5,8], has not yet been definitively shown, whereas complex interventions based on individual allergen sensitivities have shown some benefit in high-risk children[9].

Pharmacological management of rhinitis

Guidelines recommend a combination of non-sedating antihistamines, long-acting topical nasal corticosteroids and anti-inflammatory eye drops[10]. Part of the management strategy should also be to arrange adequate follow-up and to encourage patient self-management for optimal symptom control.

- Patients with persistent nasal symptoms (particularly nasal blockage, itching and sneezing) should be treated with a nasal corticosteroid; once-daily preparations may aid compliance.
- Possible side effects include nose bleeds and nasal crusting, and these are generally related to method of administration. Prescription of topical nasal sprays should always be accompanied by an explanation of device technique (Table 14.1); sniffing hard during administration should be avoided.
- Patients should be advised of the need for regular steroid treatment and advised that benefit may not be immediate.
- Regular (daily) use is superior to use as the need arises (PRN use), although PRN use is superior to placebo.
- Watery rhinorrhea tends to respond to topical anticholinergic drugs better than to nasal corticosteroids.
- In patients whose symptoms remain uncontrolled, consider adding a non-sedating antihistamine.
- Antihistamines are less effective in the treatment of nasal blockage, although newer antihistamines such as desloratidine or fexofenadine may be helpful.
- Antihistamines are effective at reducing associated eye symptoms.
- In patients with seasonal symptoms, treatment should begin at least 2 weeks before symptoms are expected to start for maximal effect.
- Topical sodium cromoglycate should be added for uncontrolled eye symptoms (its use is contraindicated in contact-lens wearers); topical H_1-antagonists should be considered in patients with isolated eye/nose symptoms; corticosteroid eye drops should not be used unless supervised by an ophthalmologist because of the risks of side effects.

Table 14.1 Using nasal sprays.

Advice when prescribing aqueous sprays should include
• Stand up, fixing the eyes on a point on the floor about 3 feet away
• Using the right hand for the left nostril and vice versa, insert the tip of the nasal spray as far as is comfortable
• Use the required number of sprays according to instructions
• Do not sniff – this may result in the drug going to the stomach instead of the nose; sniffing may be the primary cause of treatment failure

- Patients with rhinitis should be investigated for asthma and treated with bronchodilators and inhaled corticosteroids as appropriate.
- A follow-up visit allows identification of side effects which may affect compliance with treatment.

The main reasons for treatment failure are likely to be poor compliance, poor nasal spray technique, or inadequate dosing. If symptoms persist despite optimal pharmacotherapy, or if the patient has exams or an important event coming up, a number of options are available.

Managing severe or uncontrolled symptoms

A short course of oral corticosteroids (e.g. 20 mg prednisolone daily for 5 days) may be effective for severe hay-fever symptoms, although evidence is limited and unacceptable systemic side effects occur with prolonged use.

Although depot steroid injections are effective in controlling symptoms of severe hay fever[6], there remains concern over their safety. Reported side effects include local effects such as post-injection flare, facial flushing and skin and fat atrophy; systemic complications are rare but include tissue atrophy[5,8,9,11,12]. Moreover, a persistent effect on bones or eyes cannot be excluded. Depot corticosteroid treatment for hay fever was found to cause avascular necrosis of both hips[10], and fatalities related to intramuscular and intra-articular injections have been reported[11].

Medico-legal issues related to the use of intramuscular corticosteroid treatment have arisen, and using these drugs to treat a condition for which alternative safe and effective treatments exist should be considered with caution.

Immunotherapy, or desensitisation, retains a role in the treatment of those with hay fever who are unresponsive to or cannot tolerate conventional pharmacotherapy. Subcutaneous immunotherapy has been shown to reduce symptoms by half and medication use by 80%[12]. Long-term efficacy of immunotherapy following 3 years of treatment has also been demonstrated[13].

Success depends on appropriate patient selection, that is, clinically monosensitive patients with identifiable IgE-mediated disease who do not respond to a combination of nasal steroids and antihistamines. Subcutaneous immunotherapy is only available from trained staff based in specialist centres. Sublingual immunotherapy is a safe and effective alternative[13] that can be prescribed in general practice, although careful patient selection is again required.

Who and when to refer

Referral for a specialist allergy opinion should occur for patients in whom there is diagnostic uncertainty, or those for whom allergen-specific therapy is being considered, as well as those patients who have potentially life-threatening symptoms, or – particularly in children – concomitant food allergy and asthma. Other patients who may benefit from referral to an allergist or appropriate specialist include:

- patients who are not responding to treatment;
- patients who require doses or drugs that are unlicensed for a particular condition;
- patients who require skin prick testing with non-aeroallergens which are not available as a specific IgE test (e.g. fruits, vegetables, drugs);
- adults who have had anaphylaxis with cardiac or respiratory involvement;
- patients who are candidates for specific allergen immunotherapy;
- patients who require food challenges.

14.1.8 Summary

Allergic rhinitis is one of the most common allergic conditions, affecting a quarter of the UK population and often coexisting with food allergy. It is often trivialised by health professionals, although symptoms have been associated with impaired concentration and learning ability. It is treatable in the majority of cases, but success depends on recognition, appropriate treatment selection, patient education and regular follow-up. Adolescents particularly should be assessed and treated carefully to prevent poor school and exam performance.

References

1. Sibbald B, Rink E. Epidemiology of seasonal and perennial rhinitis: clinical presentation and clinical history. *Thorax* 1991; **46**: 895–901.
2. Juniper EF, Guyatt GH. Development and testing of a new measure of health status for clinical trials in rhinoconjunctivitis. *Clin Exp Allergy* 1990; **21**: 77–83.
3. Walker S, Khan-Wasti S, Fletcher M *et al*. Seasonal allergic rhinitis is associated with a detrimental impact on exam performance in United Kingdom teenagers: case–control study. *J Allergy Clin Immunol* 2007; **120**: 381–7.
4. Coombs RRA, Gell PGH. The classification of allergic reactions underlying disease. In: Gell PGH, Coombs RRA, eds. *Clinical Aspects of Immunology*. Oxford: Blackwell, 1963: 317–37.
5. Gøtzsche PC, Johansen HK. House dust mite control measures for asthma. *Cochrane Database Syst Rev* 2008; (2): CD001187.
6. Walker S, Morton C, Sheikh A. Diagnosing allergy in primary care: are the history and clinical examination sufficient? *Prim Care Respir J* 2006; **15**: 219–21.
7. Gendo K, Larson EB. Evidence-based diagnostic strategies for evaluating suspected allergic rhinitis. *Ann Intern Med* 2004; **140**: 278–89.
8. Sheikh A, Hurwitz B. House dust mite avoidance measures for perennial allergic rhinitis: a systematic review of efficacy. *Brit J Gen Pract* 2003; **53**: 318–22.
9. Morgan WJ, Crain EF, Gruchalla RS *et al*. Inner-City Asthma Study Group. Results of a home-based environmental intervention among urban children with asthma. *N Eng J Med* 2004; **351**: 1068–80.
10. Price D, Bond C, Bouchard J *et al*. International Primary Care Respiratory Group (IPCRG) guidelines: management of allergic rhinitis. *Prim Care Respir J* 2006; **15**: 58–70.
11. Dyment PG. Local atrophy following triamcinalone injection. *Pediatrics* 1970; **46**: 136–7.
12. Jacobs MB. Local subcutaneous atrophy after corticosteroid injection. *Postgrad Med J* 1986; **80**: 159–60.
13. Dahl R, Kapp A, Colombo G *et al*. Efficacy and safety of sublingual immunotherapy with grass allergen tablets for seasonal allergic rhinoconjunctivitis. *J Allergy Clin Immunol* 2006; **118**: 434–40.

14.2   Asthma

Jane Leyshon

14.2.1   Introduction

Asthma is a common chronic respiratory disease which can begin at any age, although onset in childhood is most common. Asthma symptoms can vary in frequency and severity over time and between people. At present there is no permanent cure for asthma, but, for the majority of people with asthma, modern treatments can effectively abolish symptoms. Unfortunately some people with symptoms are not identified as having asthma, or when diagnosed do not receive correct treatment. This can result in persistent symptoms causing significant limitations to daily activities, absences from school or work, increased risk of acute episodes and associated hospital admissions, and potentially a greater risk of death or long-term damage to the airways.

Asthma is considered part of the family of allergic diseases that include eczema, rhinitis (hay fever) and food allergy. Symptoms are commonly triggered by inhaled allergens such as pollens, animal dander or house-dust mite. Not all asthma symptoms, however, are allergic in origin, and symptoms can result from inhaling irritant fumes, exercise, viral infection – or may have no clear trigger at all. Asthma symptoms are not commonly triggered by food allergy, but the two conditions often coexist. Children with asthma and food allergy are at increased risk of fatal reactions to food[1], and should be referred to an allergy specialist. It is therefore important to ask about asthma symptoms when investigating food allergy so that appropriate referral and treatment can be given.

14.2.2   Background

Asthma currently affects approximately 5.2 million people in the UK, with about 1.1 million being children[2]. This equates to 1 in 12 adults and 1 in 10 children (2–15 years) with current disease[2], although the number who will have received a diagnosis from a doctor at some time in their lives is much higher, at 15% of adults and 21% of children[3]. In recent years awareness of asthma by both the public and health professionals has been growing, and there have been pharmaceutical advances and continued refinement of clinical guidelines[4]. Despite this, asthma continues to cause considerable morbidity, with poorly controlled asthma limiting every aspect of some individuals' lives. Of the over 5 million people in the UK with asthma it is estimated that less than a tenth have severe or difficult-to-control asthma, and that the rest have asthma that should be able to be well controlled using current treatments[5]. Two-thirds of people with asthma, however, report difficulty in running for a bus or enjoying exercise, and half report disturbed sleep due to nocturnal symptoms[5]. Poor control results in people being unable to perform their usual daily activities, including paid work, and results in more intensive use of health-service resources with increased consultations and hospital admissions. It is therefore important to improve asthma control in order to improve the individual's quality of life and to reduce the burden on society overall.

14.2.3 Disease process

When a person with asthma inhales an allergen to which they are sensitised it sets off a chain of events leading to airway inflammation, triggered through the actions of the antibody immunoglobulin E (IgE). The main mechanisms that result in narrowing of the airways (bronchoconstriction) are:

- smooth-muscle constriction (bronchospasm);
- increased mucus production;
- oedema causing swelling of the airway wall.

Frequent exposure to allergens results in chronic inflammation and increased sensitivity of the airways, making them more reactive to triggers. If asthma is not well controlled longer-term airway damage can occur as a result of damage to the lining of the airways and thickening of the smooth muscle in response to chronic inflammation. For this reason accurate diagnosis and appropriate treatment are essential.

14.2.4 Diagnosis

Asthma is typified by variable airway obstruction which results in symptoms such as wheeze, shortness of breath, chest tightness and cough with or without sputum production[4]. The variable nature of asthma means that patients can present with seemingly episodic symptoms of varying degrees of frequency and severity, which might at first appear to be a series of acute illnesses. A high index of suspicion must be raised if an individual presents with regular or frequent consultations for respiratory symptoms, particularly in the presence of other allergic conditions. If asthma is suspected then referral for full assessment is indicated.

A detailed and comprehensive history should be taken to eliminate other potential causes of symptoms such as other respiratory or cardiac conditions. A personal or family history of eczema, rhinitis (hay fever) or other allergic reactions can indicate an increased likelihood of asthma. Clues that the common respiratory symptoms of cough, wheeze and chest tightness may be caused by asthma include[4]:

- symptoms are variable;
- symptoms are intermittent;
- symptoms are worse at night and/or in the early morning;
- symptoms are made worse by specific trigger factors, including exercise.

Where possible, this clinical history should be supported with objective evidence of variable airflow obstruction using lung function tests. Investigations such as chest x-ray or blood and sputum tests are normally only required when diagnostic doubt exists. The majority of people with asthma can be assessed and treated in primary care, but if diagnostic uncertainty remains, particularly if there is little or no response to asthma therapy, then specialist referral may be indicated[4].

Triggers

Most people with asthma will have more than one trigger factor for their asthma symptoms. Trigger factors are not the same for all people with asthma, and what provokes symptoms in one person may not present a problem to another. The most common trigger factors for asthma include:

- viral or bacterial infections including the common cold;
- house-dust mite;
- pollens and spores;
- animals (e.g. cats, dogs, horses, birds);
- exercise;
- cold air;
- drugs (beta-blockers; aspirin; non-steroidal anti-inflammatory drugs such as ibuprofen).
- occupational agents (exposure at work is an important and often overlooked cause of adult-onset asthma).

Asthma triggered by food is relatively uncommon, and tends to occur in people with more than one allergic disorder. Foods that can trigger asthma by way of an allergic reaction include:

- peanuts;
- nuts;
- sesame;
- fish and shellfish;
- dairy products and eggs.

Certain preservatives and food additives may also trigger asthma symptoms, but not via an allergic reaction. These include the dye tartrazine (E102), which is found in many foods and some medicines, the preservative benzoic acid (E210), found in fruit products and soft drinks, and the sulphites (E220–228), which can be found in wine, home-made beer, fizzy drinks and some prepared meals and salads.

14.2.5 Management

In the treatment and management of asthma the aim is to enable people with asthma to fully participate in all aspects of their daily lives. Individual patients may have different goals and different attitudes to the potential risk/benefit profile of taking the actions required to achieve 'perfect' control, so it is not appropriate to define a fixed level of symptom control or lung function that must be achieved. British asthma guidelines[4] suggest that in general the following should be considered markers of good control:

- minimal symptoms day and night;
- minimal need for reliever treatment;
- no exacerbations;
- no limitation of physical activity;
- normal lung function.

Allergen avoidance

It would seem to make sense that if the trigger for asthma could be identified then avoidance of that trigger could form an effective method of eliminating symptoms. For the majority of people with asthma, however, they will have multiple triggers that cannot easily be avoided. There is little evidence to support allergen avoidance measures in adults[6], although complex interventions based on individual allergen sensitivities have shown some benefit in high-risk children[7].

Pharmacological management of asthma

The British guidelines for asthma management are regularly updated and provide the basis for clinicians in providing evidence-based asthma management[4]. There are two main groups of drugs that are used in asthma management: *bronchodilators*, which help to open up the airways and are often referred to as relievers, and *anti-inflammatory treatments*, which reduce or prevent inflammation of the airways and are often referred to as preventers.

The guidelines adopt a stepwise approach to the pharmacological management of chronic asthma[4]. For those with very mild and infrequent symptoms (less than three times a week) it is possible to treat symptomatically with the use of intermittent bronchodilators alone. The majority of people with asthma, however, will require the use of regular anti-inflammatory treatment, usually in the form of inhaled corticosteroids to control airway inflammation, and the intermittent use of bronchodilators to control breakthrough symptoms. It is important to remember that people with asthma may also have rhinitis, and if this is treated appropriately with nasal steroids and antihistamines it can contribute to an overall improvement in symptom control and quality of life.

In cases of poor control on low doses of inhaled corticosteroids, then diagnosis, inhaler technique and compliance should all be checked before increasing therapy. Only if they are found to be satisfactory should treatment be stepped up by the addition of other agents. Current guidelines provide a hierarchy for the addition of therapeutic agents such as long-acting beta-2 agonists (LABA), leukotriene receptor antagonists (LTRA), increased inhaled corticosteroid and methylxanthines[4]. Where inhaled corticosteroids and long-acting bronchodilators are used together they may be combined in one device, which may be helpful in simplifying treatment regimes and promoting compliance.

To control symptoms in severe disease, higher-dose inhaled steroids may be required along with the addition of multiple other agents and possibly regular oral steroids. At any step of the current guidelines a short course of oral steroids may be required to treat an acute exacerbation and regain control[4].

Asthma exacerbations

Asthma exacerbations or acute attacks can occur, even in normally well-controlled asthma, as the result of a viral infection or increased exposure to a trigger factor. Sometimes, however, they can be indicators of a failure of long-term management, and frequent exacerbations would indicate suboptimal therapy. This may be due to inadequate doses of medication, poor inhaler technique or lack of compliance with regular therapy.

Acute episodes of asthma are treated with increased doses of bronchodilators and a short course of oral corticosteroids, and depending on severity may require hospital admission[4]. Follow-up is essential to monitor the response to treatment, to identify where possible the reason for the acute episode, and to optimise therapy in order to try to reduce the likelihood of future attacks[4].

Using inhaler devices

The majority of asthma treatments are delivered straight to the lung by inhalation. For inhaled therapy to be effective the required dose of the correct medication must reach the lungs consistently and reliably[8]. In order for it to do this the individual must be not only technically able to operate the device but also willing to do so. So treatment decisions are much more complex than simply selecting the correct drug, because the selection of a suitable inhaler device is also crucial for a successful outcome.

The wide range of currently available inhaler devices vary in shape and size, have different features such as dose counters, and require different inhalation techniques and different levels of manual dexterity to operate. Although the British guidelines provide a clear framework for healthcare professionals for their treatment decisions[4], it is important to remember that each person with asthma is an individual and will have different needs. Before an inhaler device is prescribed, the patient must be shown how to use the device, and his or her ability to use it must be assessed. If technique is poor with one device then an alternative device must be considered. Regular teaching and checking of technique at every visit is essential, to maintain ongoing effectiveness of therapy[4].

Follow-up

An important part of the management of asthma is regular follow-up, to monitor response to treatment and to encourage patient self-management. It is important that people with asthma clearly understand the need for regular steroid treatment and are advised when starting therapy that benefit may not be immediate. It should be explained that inhaled steroids must be continued even in the absence of symptoms in order to prevent acute episodes and long-term airway damage. It is also important that the patient is made aware of signs of deteriorating control which may indicate a need for increased medication or medical advice. Signs of worsening asthma include[4]:

- increased symptoms, cough, wheeze or shortness of breath;
- waking at night with cough, wheeze or shortness of breath;
- reduced exercise tolerance;
- increased use of reliever inhaler;
- reliever inhaler not as effective as usual.

14.2.5   Summary

Asthma is a common respiratory condition which can often coexist with other allergic conditions such as eczema, rhinitis and food allergy. It is treatable, and in the majority of cases successful treatment can abolish symptoms almost entirely. Successful management relies on effective recognition of symptoms, appropriate treatment including inhaler device selection, patient education and regular follow-up. Although asthma symptoms are rarely triggered by food allergy, the presence of both conditions in children indicates a high risk of fatal reactions to food. Where asthma is suspected in children with food allergy, early referral for confirmation of diagnosis is crucial, and when asthma diagnosis is confirmed specialist allergy advice is essential.

References

1. Colver AF, Nevantaus H, Macdougall CF, Cant AJ. Severe food-allergic reactions in children across the UK and Ireland, 1998–2000. *Child Care Health Dev* 2005; **31**: 741–2.
2. Asthma UK. *Where Do We Stand? Asthma in the UK Today*. London: Asthma UK, 2004. www.asthma.org.uk.
3. British Thoracic Society. *The Burden of Lung Disease*, 2nd edn. London: British Thoracic Society, 2006. www.brit-thoracic.org.uk.
4. British Thoracic Society, Scottish Intercollegiate Guidelines Network. *British Guideline on the Management of Asthma*, revised edition. Guideline 101. Edinburgh: SIGN, 2007. www.sign. ac.uk/guidelines/fulltext/101/index.html.
5. Asthma UK. *Living on a Knife Edge*. London: Asthma UK, 2004. www.asthma.org.uk.
6. Gøtzsche PC, Johansen HK. House dust mite control measures for asthma. *Cochrane Database Syst Rev* 2008; (2): CD001187.
7. Morgan WJ, Crain EF, Gruchalla RS *et al.* Inner-City Asthma Study Group. Results of a home-based environmental intervention among urban children with asthma. *N Eng J Med* 2004; **351**: 1068–80.
8. Crompton G, Barnes P, Broeders M *et al.* The need to improve inhalation technique in Europe: a report from the Aerosol Drug Management Improvement Team. *Respir Med* 2006: **100**: 1479–94.

14.3   Atopic eczema

Helen Cox

14.3.1   Introduction

Atopic eczema is one of the most common skin disorders seen in infants and children. It is a chronic, itchy, inflammatory disorder of the skin which presents in the first 2 years of life in the majority of infants. It typically follows an episodic course with periods of exacerbations or flares, lasting from a few days to weeks, with spontaneous resolution of eczema in 50% by their teenage years and in 65% by the age of 16 years[1]. There has been a fourfold increase in the prevalence of atopic eczema over the past 40 years, and this has mirrored the increase in other allergic disorders such as asthma and allergic rhinitis[2]. Having a child with eczema can have a profound effect on many aspects of family life (Table 14.2). In particular, the detrimental effects of sleep disturbance on the child's psychological functioning and quality of life should not be underestimated. Fortunately the majority of children with eczema have only mild skin disease (80%) which follows an intermittent course and is more likely to resolve spontaneously. The remaining 20% of children have moderate (18%) or severe (2%) eczema, with fewer periods of remission and a tendency to persist into adult life[3].

There is a strong association with other allergic diseases, with up to a half of infants with eczema developing asthma and two-thirds developing allergic rhinitis in subsequent years. This association of diseases is frequently referred to as the allergic march[1,3,4]. Furthermore, in a subset of infants and young children with moderate or severe atopic eczema, food allergy is present in one-third[5-8].

Table 14.2   Severity of eczema.

Skin/physical severity		Impact on quality of life	
Clear	Normal skin, no evidence of atopic eczema	None	None
Mild	Areas of dry skin, infrequent itching	Mild	Little impact on everyday activities, sleep and psychosocial wellbeing
Moderate	Areas of dry skin, frequent itching, redness (with or without excoriation or skin thickening)	Moderate	Moderate impact on everyday activities and psychosocial wellbeing, frequently disturbed sleep
Severe	Widespread areas of dry skin, incessant itching, redness (with or without excoriation) extensive skin thickening, bleeding, oozing, cracking and alteration of pigment)	Severe	Severe limitation of everyday activities and psychosocial functioning, nightly loss of sleep

14.3.2 Management

The management of atopic eczema requires a holistic approach which takes into account the severity of the eczema and its impact on the individual's quality of life, everyday activities, sleep and psychosocial functioning[9]. This allows for more effective treatment decisions based on an overall clinical impression of the severity of the eczema (mild, moderate or severe). A detailed history needs to include the timing of eczema onset, the duration, pattern and severity of eczema, and response to previous and current treatments.

The treatment of eczema requires a two-pronged approach: firstly the identification and avoidance of potential trigger factors, and secondly the control of skin inflammation through topical and/or systemic therapies. Education on both avoidance and the application of topical creams plays a significant role in determining the effectiveness and success of any treatment strategy. Ideally verbal education should be accompanied by a written care plan and a practical demonstration of how to apply topical treatments.

14.3.3 Identification and avoidance of trigger factors

A number of potential trigger factors for eczema have been postulated. These include irritant factors (e.g. detergents, soap, wool), contact allergens (e.g. perfumed creams), inhalant allergens, food allergens, dietary factors, infection, climate and environmental factors (e.g. hard water, tobacco smoke, pollution)[9]. All of these factors have the potential to contribute to epidermal barrier dysfunction. Whilst some of these factors lead to damage specifically to the skin barrier, other factors (allergic triggers and infection) are capable of inducing both skin and systemic responses.

Soaps and detergents

Optimal barrier function is maintained by the skin having an acidic pH of 5.4–5.9. The acid mantle protects the skin from microbial invasion and is important for integrity of the stratum corneum. Surfactants found in soaps, detergents and certain creams can damage the skin, provoking dryness and thinning of the stratum corneum, thereby exacerbating atopic eczema. Avoidance of soaps and detergents and the frequent application of non-surfactant-containing creams form the cornerstone of eczema management[9].

Microbes

Bacterial colonisation of the skin with *Staphylococcus aureus* and group A *Streptococcus* is a frequent feature of atopic eczema, with isolates of *S. aureus* being present in 90% of eczematous skin compared with 30% of skin samples from unaffected individuals[10]. The density of *S. aureus* tends to increase with the severity of atopic eczema lesions, and it can contribute to acute flares of eczema[11]. Recognition and treatment of bacterial infection with appropriate antibiotics forms an important and integral part of eczema management. However, the signs of infected eczema are not always clinically obvious. Infection is usually suspected in the presence of weeping, pustules, crusts, fever or malaise. These features are not invariable, and infection should be considered when there is a rapid deterioration in eczema or when eczema is poorly responsive to treatment, even in the absence of overt clinical signs of infection[9]. Treatment is usually with systemic antibiotics for 1–2 weeks. Topical antibiotics should only be used to treat local areas of infection for no longer than 2 weeks. Understanding the mechanism for increased *S. aureus* colonisation and infection is an area of active investigation.

Infection with the herpes simplex virus (eczema herpeticum) can be potentially dangerous and is an indication for urgent same-day referral if clinically suspected. It can arise in normal-looking skin without evidence of atopic eczema, leading to the formation of blisters which rapidly erode to form 'punched out' lesions on the skin. The severity can range from localised disease to widespread dissemination, and very rarely herpetic encephalitis and death[12]. Systemic treatment with acyclovir should be initiated immediately if herpes simplex infection is clinically suspected[9].

Food allergens

The role of food allergens in the pathogenesis of atopic eczema is controversial (see also Chapter 2). However, there is now considerable evidence at a clinical, cellular and molecular level to support the role of food allergy as an important trigger in eczema pathogenesis. Double-blind placebo-controlled food challenges have demonstrated that food allergens induce immediate hypersensitivity reactions in 35–56% of children with moderate to severe eczema[5–8]. Up to 90% of patients reacting positively on challenge developed skin rashes with intense pruritis, erythema, and a macular, morbilliform or urticarial rash within 0–2 hours of challenge, followed by a delayed eczematous response in 50%.

The foods most commonly implicated in atopic eczema are cow's milk, hen's egg, peanuts and tree nuts, which account for 75% of all positive challenge tests. Reactions to wheat, soya, fish, shellfish, sesame and kiwi occur less commonly. Although all foods are potentially capable of provoking an allergic response the above foods account for 90% of all food allergic reactions[5–8]. Removal of proven food allergens from a patient's diet can lead to significant clinical improvement in the eczema[13].

The association between breast-feeding and atopic eczema has been controversial. In most studies a protective effect of breast-feeding has been demonstrated[14]. Rarely infantile eczema can be aggravated by the transmission of food proteins within breast milk with the potential to cause protein-losing enteropathy with diarrhoea, marked weight loss, hypoalbuminaemia and severe eczema[15]. In the recent NICE guideline for atopic eczema in children, the importance of early recognition and treatment of food allergy in young infants with moderate to severe eczema is emphasised[9]. Clinicians are asked to consider food allergy in children with eczema who have reacted previously with immediate symptoms or in infants and young children with moderate or severe eczema, particularly if associated with gut dysmotility (colic, vomiting, altered bowel habit) or failure to thrive. The guideline states further that a 6–8 week trial of an extensively hydrolysed or amino-acid formula should be offered in place of cow's-milk formula to infants less than 6 months of age with moderate to severe eczema.

Regular follow-up and reassessment is important, as the natural history is for the majority of patients to acquire tolerance over time to most allergens, particularly when the binding epitopes are held together in a conformational structure, rendering them less stable and more susceptible to heat degradation (e.g. milk, egg, wheat, soya). Other allergens, however, are more likely to persist due to the presence of linear binding epitopes (e.g. nuts, fish)[16].

Aeroallergens

Several studies have demonstrated the ability of aeroallergens to provoke eczematous flares. Intranasal and bronchial inhalation challenge with house-dust mite or animal dander can lead to worsening of eczema skin lesions[17]. Epicutaneous application of aeroallergens such as cat dander or house-dust mite can elicit eczematous reactions, with isolation of house-dust-mite-specific T cells from patch tests sites.

Studies utilising covers impenetrable to house-dust mite have produced controversial results, with some studies demonstrating benefit whilst others do not[18]. The issue of pets is another area of controversy, with limited data to guide us on the issue of avoidance. A paradoxical relationship has been shown between exposure to animal dander and subsequent development of atopic sensitisation, with early exposure favouring the development of immune tolerance through stimulation of Th1 responses. In contrast, exposure to animal dander at later time points does not seem to be associated with any protective effects on the immune system, and indeed might promote the development of allergic sensitisation[19].

14.3.4   Treatment to control skin inflammation

Emollients

The application of topical creams forms the most important part of eczema management. In particular, the application of emollients should form the basis of any treatment strategy and should continue even when the eczema has cleared. Emollients form a protective film over the skin to keep moisture in, by occluding water loss, and to keep irritants out, by directly adding water to the dry outer layer of skin. In this way they are a highly effective treatment for atopic eczema provided they are used liberally and frequently. The use of large quantities of emollients can be markedly steroid-sparing, with up to a 75% reduction in the need for topical steroids. All patients therefore require an essential package of emollient therapy. This would normally include:

- a bath oil;
- a soap substitute for cleansing (with or without antimicrobial activity);
- large quantities of a non-perfumed leave-on emollient (250–500 g per week).

A variety of different emollient wash products and leave-on preparations is available (creams, ointments, lotions, gels). Ointments are greasy in nature, whereas creams and lotions contain water and are often more acceptable cosmetically. It is important to offer patients a choice of emollients, as 'one size does not fit all'[9].

Topical corticosteroids

Topical corticosteroids are derived from the naturally occurring corticosteroid, cortisol, which is secreted by the adrenal cortex. Corticosteroids have anti-inflammatory and immunosuppressant effects and exert local effects on the skin, inhibiting the proliferation of fibroblasts and synthesis of collagen, as well as causing local vasoconstriction. They are available as both cream and ointment preparations and are categorised as mild, moderate, potent and very potent.

A stepped approach to management is recommended in the recent NICE guideline for atopic eczema, with treatment being tailored to eczema severity[9]. The guideline stresses the importance of emollient therapy for everyday use, with the addition or cessation of topical steroids or other anti-inflammatory treatments depending on eczema severity. During eczema flares the potency of topical treatments is 'stepped up', whilst once control is achieved the treatment is 'stepped down' accordingly. In general, topical steroids of mild potency are used to treat mild eczema, moderate-potency steroids for moderate eczema and potent steroids for severe eczema. In children with eczema of differing severity affecting different parts of the body, the potency of topical steroid used is tailored to the individual site being treated (e.g. mild topical steroids for mild eczema on body, potent topical steroids for severe eczema on hands and feet.) In general, topical corticosteroids are only applied to affected eczematous skin. However, in children with frequent recurrent flares (two or three per month), topical corticosteroids can be used for two consecutive days per week applied to normal skin at the usual sites of eczema, as a strategy for flare prevention. This is often referred to as 'weekend therapy', and it has been shown to be effective in maintaining eczema control[20].

Although topical corticosteroids are highly effective at treating skin inflammation in eczema, concerns regarding their possible adverse effects are expressed by the majority of parents. This frequently leads to under-treatment of the eczema. Despite the fact that topical corticosteroids have been around since 1962, limited data are available on their long-term side effects. Clinical consensus suggests that long-term usage within clinically recommended doses appears to be safe. Inappropriate use, however, does have the potential to cause several adverse effects including damage to the epidermal barrier (skin thinning, skin atrophy, telangiectasia, acne) and cutaneous absorption of corticosteroid with adverse systemic effects (adrenal suppression, growth suppression). In light of this, certain precautions are necessary when applying topical corticosteroids[9]:

- Topical corticosteroids should only be applied to affected eczematous skin (with the exception of weekend therapy).

- The face and neck should only be treated with mild-potency topical corticosteroids, apart from severe flares, where topical corticosteroids of moderate potency can be used for up to 5 days.
- Moderately potent or potent topical corticosteroids can be used on areas of thin skin such as the axillae and groin for 7–14 days only.
- Potent topical corticosteroids should not be used in infants < 12 months without specialist dermatological advice.
- Very potent topical corticosteroids should not be used without specialist dermatological advice.

The finger-tip unit is a validated method to help guide the application of cream in safe quantities. One finger-tip unit is a squeeze of cream along the index finger from the tip to the first finger joint. This equates to half a gram and will cover the surface area of two adult hands including the fingers[21].

Calcineurin inhibitors

Both pimecrolimus and tacrolimus are topical immunosuppressants which act by binding to and inhibiting the action of a protein called calcineurin, involved in the activation of T cells. The main effect of calcineurin inhibitors is to inhibit the production of cytokines, produced by T cells, which contribute to the skin inflammation that leads to an eczematous flare. Topical tacrolimus is available in two strengths, 0.03% and 0.1%, with only the weaker strength being licensed for use in children aged 2–16 years. Pimecrolimus is a 1% cream that is licensed for use in children aged 2 years or over[22].

One of the main advantages of topical calcineurin inhibitors over topical corticosteroids is that topical calcineurin inhibitors do not cause thinning of the skin or skin atrophy. They are therefore particularly useful for treating delicate skin sites such as the face, periorbital areas and neck.

Wet-wrap therapy

Various types of dressings can be used in the management of eczema. 'Wet-wrap therapy' refers to the process of applying a wet bandage layer (soaked in tepid water) to the skin immediately after the skin application of emollients and/or topical corticosteroid. A dry bandage layer is then applied over this. Wet-wrap therapy can be a useful adjunct to therapy in children with severe eczema that is either very dry or failing to respond to conventional topical therapies. However, as the absorption of topical corticosteroids increases under occlusion, the use of wet wraps together with topical corticosteroids should be restricted to 7–14 days[9,23,24].

Antihistamines

Antihistamines block the activity of histamine at receptor sites in the skin, alleviating itching and reducing the wheal and flare response in urticaria. Older antihistamines tend to be more sedating and short-acting (6–12 hours) whilst the new-generation antihistamines bind more selectively to H_1 histamine receptors and are mostly non-sedating and longer-acting (about 24 hours). Although the evidence base surrounding their use is rather weak, the review on which the current NICE guideline is based concluded that they were helpful in some circumstances, e.g. in the eczematous child with frequent urticaria. A reasonable approach is to offer patients with severe itching or urticaria a 1-month trial of a non-sedating antihistamine, which can safely be extended for longer periods if found to be of benefit. The use of sedating antihistamines should be restricted to short-term use (7–14 days) for eczematous flares causing debilitating sleep disturbance[9].

Other systemic treatments

Phototherapy and other immunomodulating systemic treatments (cyclosporine, azathioprine) have been used to treat severe eczema which is poorly responsive to topical therapies. These treatments should only be offered under close supervision in specialist centres experienced and trained in their use, as they require close monitoring for safety aspects.

References

1. Williams HC, Strachan DP. The natural history of childhood eczema: Observations from the British 1958 birth cohort study. *Br J Dermatol* 1998; **139**: 834–9.
2. Burr ML, Wat D, Evans C, Dunstan FDJ, Doull IJM, on behalf of the British Thoracic Society Research Committee. Asthma prevalence in 1973, 1988 and 2003. *Thorax* 2006; **61**: 296–9.
3. Ben-Gashir MA, Seed PT, Hay RJ. Predictors of atopic dermatitis severity over time. *J Am Acad Dermatol* 2004; **50**: 349–56.
4. Ninan TK, Russell G. Respiratory symptoms and atopy in Aberdeen schoolchildren: evidence from two surveys 25 years apart. *BMJ* 1992; **304**: 873–5.
5. Sampson H. Role of immediate food hypersensitivity in the pathogenesis of atopic dermatitis. *J Allergy Clin Immunol* 1983; **71**: 473–80.
6. Sampson H, McCaskill C. Food hypersensitivity and atopic dermatitis: evaluation of 113 patients. *J Pediatr* 1985; **107**: 669–75.
7. Burks A, James J, Hiegel A *et al*. Atopic dermatitis and food hypersensitivity reactions. *J Pediatr* 1998; **132**: 132–6.
8. Niggemann B, Reibel S, Roehr C *et al*. Predictors of positive food challenge outcome in non-IgE mediated reactions to food in children with atopic dermatitis. *J Allergy Clin Immunol* 2001; **108**: 1053–8.
9. National Institute for Health and Clinical Excellence. *Atopic Eczema in Children: Management of Atopic Eczema in Children from Birth up to the Age of 12 Years*. Guideline 57. London: NICE, 2007. www.nice.org.uk/CG057.
10. Hoare C, Li Wan Po A, Williams H. Systematic review of treatments for atopic eczema. *Health Technol Assess* 2000; **4**: 1–191.
11. Ricci G, Patrizi A, Neri I, Bendandi B, Masi M. Frequency and clinical role of *Staphylococcus aureus* overinfection in atopic dermatitis in children. *Pediatr Dermatol* 2003; **20**: 389–92.
12. Lai YC, Shyur SD, Fu JL. Eczema herpeticum in children with atopic dermatitis. *Acta Paediatr Taiwan* 1999; **40**: 325–9.
13. Fiocchi A, Bouygue GR, Martelli A, Terracciano L, Sarratud T. Dietary treatment of childhood atopic eczema/dermatitis syndrome (AEDS) *Allergy* 2004: **59** (Suppl 78): 78–85.

14. Saarinen UM, Kajosaari M. Breast feeding as prophylaxis against atopic disease: prospective follow up study until 17 years old. *Lancet* 1995; **346**: 1065–9.
15. Hill DJ, Cameron DJS, Francis DM, Gonzales-Andaya AM, Hosking CS. Challenge confirmation of late-onset reactions to extensively hydrolysed formulas in infants with multiple food protein intolerance. *J Allergy Clin Immunol* 1995; **96**: 386–94.
16. Sampson HA. Update on food allergy. *J Allergy Clin Immunol* 2004; **113**: 805–19.
17. Tupker RA, De Monchy JG, Coenraads PJ *et al.* Induction of atopic dermatitis by inhalation of house dust mite. *J Allergy Clin Immunol* 1996; **97**: 1064–70.
18. Tan BB, Weald D, Strickland I *et al.* Double blind controlled trial effect of housedust-mite allergen avoidance on atopic dermatitis. *Lancet* 1996; **347**: 15–18.
19. Holt PG, Macaubas C. Development of long term tolerance versus sensitisation to environmental allergens during the perinatal period. *Curr Opin Immunol* 1997; **9**: 782–7.
20. Berth-Jones J, Damstra RJ, Golsch S *et al.* Twice weekly fluticasone propionate added to emollient maintenance treatment to reduce risk of relapse in atopic dermatitis: randomised, double blind, parallel group study. *BMJ* 2003; **326**: 1367.
21. Long CC, Finlay AY. The finger-tip unit: a new practical measure. *Clin Exp Dermatol* 1991; **16**: 444–7.
22. National Institute for Clinical Excellence. *Tacrolimus and Pimecrolimus for Atopic Eczema.* Technology Appraisal 82. London: NICE, 2004. www.nice.org.uk/TA082.
23. Hindley D, Galloway G, Murray J *et al.* A randomised study of 'wet wraps' versus conventional treatment for atopic eczema. *Arch Dis Child* 2006; **91**: 164–8.
24. Schnopp C, Holtmann C, Stock S *et al.* Topical steroids under wet-wrap dressings in atopic dermatitis: a vehicle-controlled trial. *Dermatology* 2002; **204**: 56–9.

14.4   Anaphylaxis

Samantha Walker

14.4.1   Introduction

Anaphylaxis is an acute potentially life-threatening medical condition that is commonly due to a systemic allergic reaction to an allergen, e.g. a food, drug or insect sting. Its onset is immediate and rapid. In patients who have experienced an episode of anaphylaxis there is an increased risk of recurrence, but in far too many of these episodes patients fail to receive potentially life-saving treatment with adrenaline[1]. Recent estimates suggest that anaphylaxis is responsible for between 20 and 30 deaths each year in the UK[2], many of which are potentially preventable. Although patients with acute symptoms rarely present in outpatient or community settings, it is essential that all health professionals are familiar with managing acute symptoms. Equally important, and perhaps more relevant for long-term care, is the need to consider anaphylaxis not only as an acute episode but as a chronic condition requiring long-term follow-up and detailed health education[3].

14.4.2   Mechanisms

Although anaphylaxis is the term commonly used to describe all acute, severe allergic-type emergencies, in fact there are two main mechanisms involved, namely *anaphylactic* (allergic or IgE-mediated) and *anaphylactoid* (pseudoallergic or non-IgE-mediated) reactions. In both anaphylactic and anaphylactoid reactions, a very similar clinical picture develops requiring identical immediate management; the precise mechanism involved may be important, however, in guiding investigations in order to identify possible trigger(s), as IgE-mediated disease (but not non-IgE-mediated disease) can be investigated using skin prick testing and measurements of serum specific IgE.

14.4.3   Clinical features

Crucial to effective management is quick and accurate diagnosis and being able to identify those at greatest risk of adverse outcomes. Any of a number of organ systems may be affected, the most important of which are the respiratory and cardiovascular systems. Early signs of anaphylaxis (which are often ignored or misinterpreted) include flushing and systemic urticaria. Death is usually due either to cardiovascular collapse or to suffocation (especially in younger children). Treatment may be delayed due to non-recognition of early signs, and delayed administration of adrenaline is associated with increased mortality.

Symptoms typically begin within minutes of exposure, and as a rule of thumb the quicker that symptoms begin, the more severe the clinical reaction is likely to be. Latex-induced anaphylaxis is known to develop more slowly, however – normally over a period of about 30 minutes or so. The main clinical features that characterise anaphylaxis are summarised in Table 14.3, and differential diagnoses are shown in Table 14.4.

Symptoms typically differ according to the type of exposure, i.e. whether the offending substance has been inhaled, ingested or injected. Food exposure is more likely to result in respiratory symptoms[2], whereas patients who experience injected- or venom-induced anaphylaxis are more likely to experience cardiovascular symptoms. It should be recognised, however, that anaphylaxis is a dynamic event during which multiple symptoms may come and go but which, once recognised, should be treated promptly with adrenaline to prevent the development of potentially life-threatening symptoms.

Table 14.3   Clinical features of anaphylaxis.

Organ	Symptoms and signs
Skin	Pruritis, flushing, urticaria and angio-oedema
Respiratory	Rhinitis, sneezing, stridor and hoarseness as features of upper-airway inflammation and oedema Cough, wheezing and dyspnoea due to lower-airway obstruction; if untreated, cyanosis and asphyxia may develop
Cardiovascular	Vasodilatation, tachycardia, hypotension, circulatory collapse, leading to shock and infarction of tissues
Gastrointestinal	Tingling and swelling of the lips and tongue, palatal itch, nausea, vomiting, abdominal cramps and diarrhoea
Neurological	Anxiety, headache, convulsions and loss of consciousness

Table 14.4 Differential diagnosis of anaphylaxis.

Condition	Comment
Vasovagal attack	Bradycardia not tachycardia No urticaria, pruritis, angio-oedema, upper respiratory obstruction Pallor instead of flushing Nausea without abdominal pain
Serum sickness	Slower onset (over days instead of minutes) No upper respiratory obstruction, brochospasm or hypotension
Mastocytosis	No upper respiratory obstruction Slower onset Chronic low-level symptoms between attacks
Angiodema and C1-esterase inhibitor deficiency	No flushing, pruritis, urticaria, bronchospasm or hypotension History of C1-esterase inhibitor deficiency
Globus hystericus	No clinical evidence of upper respiratory obstruction No flushing, pruritis, urticaria, angio-oedema, bronchospasm, hypotension
Acute or chronic urticaria	Generalised rash without respiratory symptoms or hypotension

14.4.4   Diagnosis

Diagnosis of specific triggers may be possible using skin prick tests (not recommended in primary care for reasons of safety) or measurement of specific IgE antibodies in the blood. Measurement of specific IgE in the blood can be arranged via a local laboratory. Measurement of total IgE is not related to specific IgE and so is not helpful for diagnosis. In non-IgE-mediated reactions, however, there are no tests which are able to identify specific triggers, and the diagnosis must be made from taking a detailed history of the reaction.

Raised serum tryptase levels can be observed in approximately 50% of patients presenting with acute allergic reactions, and may be helpful in providing evidence of histamine release if measured at the time of the reaction[4]. Results should be interpreted with caution, as raised tryptase levels have been identified in patients without respiratory, cardiovascular or abdominal signs.

14.4.5   Risk factors

Age

Risk of food-induced reactions is greatest in children. There is some evidence to suggest that peanut-induced anaphylaxis is an increasing problem in young children[5]. Although current recommendations advise families with an allergic history to avoid peanuts during pregnancy and lactation, and that children should avoid peanuts and peanut-containing products until the age of 3 years[6], in fact there is little evidence to support this advice, and each case should be considered individually. Children with asthma and food allergy are at increased risk of fatal reactions to food, and should be referred to an allergy specialist.

Overall, the risk of death from anaphylaxis is highest in females and the elderly[7]. Young atopic males react more severely to foods, whereas there is a tendency for older non-atopic females to react more severely to idiopathic, drug, or venom reactions[8]. Risk of drug-induced anaphylaxis increases with age, peaking in the elderly, presumably because of the increased proportion of people regularly using one or more drugs.

Concurrent disease and medication

Those with pre-existing ischaemic heart disease or asthma, and those on beta-blockers, are at increased risk of serious adverse outcomes[9].

It is important to be aware that parenteral use of drugs, especially if given by the intravenous route, increases the risk of anaphylaxis. Reactions that occur following parenteral use are also likely to be more severe. It is therefore advisable that, whenever possible, the oral route for drug administration is preferred.

14.4.6   Triggers

The life-threatening nature of anaphylaxis makes it important that all sufferers are reviewed by an allergy specialist or, if unavailable, an organ-based specialist with a particular interest in allergy. An important consideration is identification of the trigger factor(s) and providing patients with detailed advice on avoiding these agent(s). Familiarity with some of the most commonly encountered triggers (foods, drugs and venom) is therefore important.

Foods

Whilst almost any foods may cause anaphylaxis, those most commonly implicated are dairy products (egg, milk and cheese), nuts (peanuts and tree nuts), pulses, fruits (e.g. strawberry and kiwi fruit) and seafood. Oral allergy syndrome (OAS) (see Chapter 7), a condition common in those sensitive to tree pollen and characterised by itchy lips, mild lip and mouth swelling on exposure to stoned fruits, is very rarely a precursor of anaphylaxis. However, patients with a history of OAS should be carefully questioned to ensure that anaphylaxis is not being overlooked. OAS alone does not justify a prescription for injected adrenaline, although this may be considered in patients who get severe throat or tongue swelling.

Drugs

Penicillin-induced anaphylaxis is relatively common, and reactions may also be triggered by penicillin derivatives. Approximately 10% of those with penicillin allergy will also be allergic to cephalosporins (the problem being most common with first-generation cephalosporins), an important example of the phenomenon of cross-sensitivity. It is important to formally identify true IgE-mediated allergy to antibiotics, as lifelong avoidance is often necessary. The majority of rashes which occur during antibiotic therapy are not mediated by IgE and do not recur on subsequent exposure.

In a hospital setting, anaesthetic agents (particularly muscle relaxants) are relatively common culprits. Peptide hormones such as insulin and antidiuretic hormone, and enzymes such as streptokinase, can also induce anaphylaxis. More important in general practice, however, is the risk of anaphylaxis in those using aspirin and other non-steroidal anti-inflammatory drugs[10]. Opioid analgesics are well recognised for being able to precipitate anaphylaxis.

In children, immunisations represent the most important therapeutic risk. Those members of the primary-care team involved in immunising children should therefore be made aware of the early presenting features of anaphylaxis and its immediate management.

Insect venoms

Venoms from the sting of bees and wasps are an important cause of anaphylaxis during the spring, summer and autumn months. Bees tend to provoke symptoms earlier on in the year whereas wasps are more abundant in the late summer and autumn. Differentiating the two is important, because allergen immunotherapy (an effective form of treatment involving regular injections of the venom involved) is an option in this group[11].

Latex

IgE-mediated allergy to latex rubber is an increasingly important trigger of anaphylaxis, particularly amongst medical personnel who have become sensitised through the use of latex gloves[12]. Anaphylaxis may also occur in sensitised patients when examined with the gloved hand.

Other triggers

Blood, plasma, immunoglobulins, and in very rare cases seminal fluid exposure (during coitus), have been identified as triggers of anaphylaxis reactions. Less common causes include physical stimuli such as exercise and exposure to cold weather. Idiopathic anaphylaxis also occurs, although mastocytosis and the carcinoid syndrome should be excluded as occult causes.

14.4.7 Acute and longer-term care

Treatment of anaphylaxis can be considered as a two-stage process: immediate treatment and longer-term care. In primary care, immediate treatment consists of:

- basic and advanced life support (if required);
- restoring blood pressure (by lying the patient flat and raising the feet);
- adrenaline given by intramuscular injection: the dose of adrenaline that should be given is 0.3–0.5 ml of 1 : 1,000 in adults, but varies with age and body weight in children[13];
- administering high-flow oxygen (if available);
- arranging emergency admission to hospital.

It is important to give adrenaline promptly, as delayed administration is associated with an increased risk of mortality. Doses of adrenaline may be repeated every 10 minutes, according to blood pressure and pulse, until improvement occurs. In those who are moribund, and if there is doubt about the adequacy of the circulation, a dilute solution of adrenaline (1 : 10,000) may need to be given by the intravenous route. Intravenous administration should only be given while the patient is undergoing cardiac monitoring, because of the risk of cardiac arrhythmias.

Additional treatment measures that should be considered in those failing to respond include chlorphenamine 10–20 mg by slow intravenous or intramuscular injection and hydrocortisone 100–300 mg by intravenous or intramuscular injection. Other treatments that may be of value in resistant cases include intravenous fluids, nebulised adrenaline and/or salbutamol and vasopressors.

A protocol can help primary-care professionals respond quickly and efficiently to anaphylaxis in a crisis situation. An algorithm based on the Resuscitation Guidelines[13] is useful. The protocol should be explicit, explaining how to recognise symptoms, advising precisely when to administer adrenaline in response to which symptoms, and stating what dose of adrenaline to give. It should also include a reminder to dial 999 and to transfer the patient to hospital.

Longer-term care should involve identification of the trigger, advice on avoidance and instructions on the immediate management of further episodes. Identification of the triggers most likely to be responsible for provoking anaphylaxis in different age groups may prevent future reactions by making allergen avoidance possible. An anaphylaxis management plan has been shown to reduce the number and severity of reactions in children with peanut or nut allergy[14], and such plans should be developed and tailored to individual patient use.

14.4.8   Other considerations

Many health professionals prescribe adrenaline auto-injectors while the patient waits for an appointment with an allergist. This may be unnecessary[15], as it may be later discovered that the patient did not have anaphylaxis, or had a reaction for which adrenaline is no protection. Where possible, prescription of an auto-injector should wait until a firm diagnosis has been made. Patients in whom an allergic trigger has been identified may benefit from a Medic-Alert bracelet which gives details of their allergy to others in an emergency.

14.4.9 Conclusions

Many of the deaths from anaphylaxis are considered preventable. Patients treated in casualty departments often receive no follow-up or advice on management of future reactions. It is vital, therefore, that the health professionals responsible for assessing and/or managing patients with anaphylaxis are equipped to provide long-term management strategies for their patients.

Living with anaphylaxis is for many people an extremely stressful experience. A detailed management plan, developed in collaboration with the patient, provides practical, structured advice about symptom management and may reassure the patient concerning his or her ability to manage reactions competently. Anxieties and concerns, especially in the case of children, are likely to be high, and one of the key roles of the primary-care practitioner is to explore and tackle such issues, thereby helping those prone to anaphylaxis to live with their condition with confidence and a sense of self-control.

References

1. Mullins RJ. Anaphylaxis: risk factors for recurrence. *Clin Exp Allergy* 2003; **33**: 1033–40.
2. Pumphrey RS. Lessons for management of anaphylaxis from a study of fatal reactions. *Clin Exp Allergy* 2000; **30**: 1144–50.
3. Walker S, Sheikh A. Managing anaphylaxis: effective emergency and long term treatment are necessary. *Clin Exp Allergy* 2003; **33**: 1015–18.
4. Lin RY, Schwartz LB, Curry A *et al.* Histamine and tryptase levels in patients with acute allergic reactions: an emergency department-based study. *J Allergy Clin Immunol* 2000; **106**: 65–71.
5. Ewan PW. Clinical study of peanut and nut allergy in 62 consecutive patients: new features and associations. *BMJ* 1996; **312**: 1074–8.
6. Committee on Toxicity of Chemicals in Food, Consumer Products and the Environment. *Peanut Allergy*. London: Department of Health, 1998.
7. Alves B, Sheikh A. Age specific aetiology of anaphylaxis. *Arch Dis Child* 2006; **85**: 348.
8. Pumphrey RS, Stanworth SJ. The clinical spectrum of anaphylaxis in north-west England. *Clin Exp Allergy* 1996; **26**: 1364–70.
9. Toogood JH. Complications of topical steroid therapy for asthma. *Am Rev Respir Dis* 1990; **141**: S89–96.
10. Vervloet D, Durham SR. ABC of allergies: adverse reactions to drugs. *BMJ* 1998; **316**: 1511–14.
11. Bousquet J, Lockey R, Malling HJ. Allergen immunotherapy: therapeutic vaccines for allergic diseases. A WHO position paper. *J Allergy Clin Immunol* 1998; **102**: 558–62.
12. Cullinan P, Brown R, Field A *et al.* Latex allergy: a position paper of the British Society of Allergy and Clinical Immunology. *Clin Exp Allergy* 2003; **33**: 1484–99.
13. Chamberlain D. Resuscitation Council (UK) Project Team. Anaphylaxis management in primary care. *Prof Nurse* 2001; **16**: 1214–15.
14. Ewan PW, Clark AT. Long term prospective observational study of patients with peanut and nut allergy after participation in a management plan. *Lancet* 2001; **357**: 111–15.
15. Unsworth DJ. Adrenaline syringes are vastly overprescribed. *Arch Dis Child* 2001; **84**: 410–11.

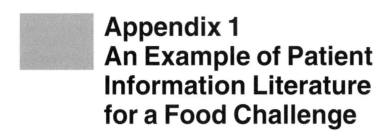

Appendix 1
An Example of Patient
Information Literature
for a Food Challenge

1. Certain medications must be stopped (this may differ from centre to centre)

	Avoid for _____ before challenge
Pirition (Chlorpheniramine), *Vallergan, Phenergan*	48 hours
Ketotifen, Zirtek (Ceterizine), *Clarityn* (Loratadine)	72 hours
Hismanal (Astemizol)	1 month

(If not possible to avoid completely, tailor the antihistamines down to the lowest effective dose)

On the day of challenge, do not take or use:

- Anti-cholinergics (ipratropium bromide – *Atrovent*)
- B-agonist bronchodilators (*Ventolin* and *Bricanyl*)
- Cromolyn (*Intal* or *Nalcrom*)
- Nasal sprays and oral decongestants
- Steroids – discuss the use of all steroids with the doctor/nurse/dietician responsible for the challenge.

2. The challenge should be done on an almost empty stomach, so you (your child) should eat only a **light breakfast** *before you come in.*

3. What will happen during the day?

You will sign a consent form for the challenge.
A doctor and nurse will see you (your child) before the challenge. They will also monitor any changes in your (your child's) condition during the challenge.
Your (your child's) blood pressure, pulse rate, respiration and peak flow will be monitored if and when appropriate.

(Then, for open challenge) We start the challenge by wiping the inside of the lip with the suspected allergen (e.g. milk/egg/soya) whilst observing you (your child) closely (some centres may wish to omit this step). If no reaction occurs you (your child) will

be asked to undergo an oral food challenge test, which involves eating or drinking a very small quantity of the suspected food or drink in increasing amounts. This could be milk hidden in another fluid, cake or biscuits for an egg challenge, or flapjacks for a nut challenge. If you (your child) is a fussy eater, discuss this with the dietician.

(Or, for blind challenge) You (your child) will receive two sets (some centres may prefer to give 3 or more sets of food) of food or drink on the day of challenge. One will contain the suspected allergen (e.g. cow's milk) and the other placebo (dummy substance). The challenge begins by wiping the inside of the lip with either the suspected allergen or a placebo whilst observing you (your child) closely. If no reaction occurs, you (your child) will be asked to undergo an oral food challenge test which involves eating or drinking increasing amounts of the food or drink containing the suspected food or placebo. This could be milk hidden in another fluid, cake or biscuits for an egg challenge, or flapjacks for a nut challenge. Please discuss any food preferences with the dietician.

The first challenge, which could contain either the suspected allergen or the placebo, will be performed in the morning, and the next challenge (allergen or placebo) follows at a later time as discussed with the study doctor.

Neither the doctor nor the nurse involved in the study knows which food or drink contains the active substance or the placebo.

The challenge may take several hours, so be prepared to spend most of the day at the hospital/allergy centre.

If you (your child) has a reaction at any stage, the challenge will be stopped and treatment given.

Before you go home the doctor will ensure that you (your child) is well.

There is tea and coffee available, and we can provide a sandwich lunch or you can obtain lunch from the canteen. You are welcome to bring along any foods/drinks you (your child) likes and would normally have for when you (your child) gets hungry/thirsty. No other food will be allowed for the first 2 hours of the challenge.

(For children) Although there are toys available to entertain young children, it is a good idea to bring some activities or toys along.

4. On discharge, you (your child) should remain quiet for the remainder of the day as strenuous exertion could induce a delayed reaction.

5. Should you experience a delayed reaction, please inform the ward. The dietician and/or doctor will be in contact with you regularly during the week following the challenge.

6. For any further information, please do not hesitate to contact . . .

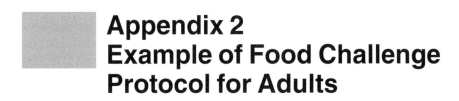

Appendix 2
Example of Food Challenge
Protocol for Adults

Objectives

1. To prove that a certain food allergen plays a role in individual clinical symptoms, or to exclude a food allergy in order to prevent unnecessary food restrictions[1].
2. To assess whether an adult has 'outgrown' a childhood food allergy such as milk, egg or peanuts[2].
3. To assess whether sensitisation to a food as evidenced by positive skin prick or specific IgE tests is clinically relevant[2,3].

Inclusion/exclusion criteria[3]

Inclusion

For those with a history of adverse food reactions who are actively avoiding those foods:

- Establish/exclude diagnosis where there is a negative specific IgE and/or skin prick test or results which are well below the diagnostic cut-off point (although we only have these for children and also only for certain foods).
- Determine threshold value or degree of food sensitivity where there are concerns about exposure and reactions to trace amounts of food allergens.

For those without a history of adverse food reactions but who are actively avoiding food(s):

- Establish/exclude diagnosis where chronic symptoms are suspected by the patient to be food-related.
- Establish/exclude diagnosis where patient is on self-imposed improper exclusion diet and is at nutritional risk.
- Determine the clinical relevance of sensitisation due to cross-reactivity where tolerance is unknown or where there are positive skin prick or specific IgE tests to foods but no symptoms.

Exclusion

- People with a strong reported history to a food they are actively avoiding who also have positive specific IgE or skin prick tests (usually above the cut-off point).

- Patients with ongoing disease, e.g. infection, unstable angina, and those who are pregnant.
- Patients taking medication which may enhance, mask or delay/prevent evaluation of any reaction.
- Patients with reported oral allergy syndrome who have severe reactions should not be challenged in allergen season if relevant.
- NB: European Academy of Allergology and Clinical Immunology (EAACI) guidelines also suggest that patients with a history of anaphylaxis should not be challenged. However, we do currently challenge such people but will always weigh the risk of challenge against the risk of misinterpreting a skin prick or specific IgE test and the misery of an unnecessary dietary exclusion.

Material

1 Fresh foods brought in by patients will be used, as this is known to produce better results for both skin prick testing and oral food challenge[4,5].
2 If the food causing the symptoms is unknown then the composite food should be brought in, being the exact type and brand of food the patient reported symptoms to.
3 Foods will either be raw or cooked as appropriate. If required raw for skin prick testing, foods will be cooked prior to consumption as appropriate (e.g. fish and shellfish).

Procedures (include timing, preparation of dilutions, processing samples, equipment, etc.)

1 Referral made to specialist allergy registrar
2 Specialist allergy registrar discusses cases with specialist allergy dietician
3 Appointment sent – patients are requested to bring the foods they consider to be involved in their reactions
4 Patient admitted and observations taken by nursing staff
5 Seen and assessed by specialist allergy registrar and specialist allergy dietician
6 Written consent obtained
7 PEFR and BP measured
8 Prick-by-prick testing performed with appropriate fresh foods
9 Medical assessment and cannulation as appropriate
10 Oral challenge commences with a maximum of one or two foods being challenged on any one admission

Open challenges

1 Labial challenge (outer lip) – food rubbed on outer lip and then removed with a wet tissue
2 Wait 10 minutes

3   Labial challenge (inner lip) – food rubbed on inner lip
4   Wait 10 minutes
5   Chew and spit – food chewed and disgorged (fruit and vegetables), or hold on tongue – food held on tongue and disgorged (all other foods)
6   Wait 15 minutes
7   Swallow – a pinhead-sized piece of the food is swallowed
8   Wait 10–15 minutes (depending on clinical history)
9   If there are no reported symptoms, give the next dose, which is double the size of the previous dose
10   Follow the above until the patient has taken what is considered to be a normal portion, e.g. one apple or one bag of nuts
11   If there are any reported or observed symptoms at any stage, the challenge will be stopped and BP and PEFR measured
12   An assessment will be made whether this symptom is related to the food challenge or not and a positive challenge will be declared where there is:

- Observable lip or tongue oedema
- Obvious laryngeal oedema, or vocal cord dysfunction
- 20% fall in PEFR or severe wheezing
- Severe facial flushing, rash or hives
- Vomiting/diarrhoea (this may require confirmation through blind challenge)
- Faintness or dizziness accompanied by a fall in BP

13   If the symptoms do not meet the criteria for a positive challenge then the challenge will be paused until symptoms have subsided, following which the same challenge dose as that which caused the symptoms will be administered with caution
14   If the symptoms do not return the challenge will continue as per the protocol, but if symptoms return then a blind challenge will need to be performed
15   All patients will have the result of their challenge recorded both in the clinical notes and in the food-challenge lever arch file

Blind challenges

These will follow the same protocol but there will be two challenges, preferably held on two different days. The test food will either be in a flapjack (nuts, legumes and seeds), a vegetable puree (wheat), or a blackcurrant puree (fruits and vegetables). The dosages will be prepared by the dietician and administered by the registrar or nurse specialist, using the protocol above.

Safety precautions (for patients and doctors)

- All patients will give written consent.
- All patients will be cannulated if they have previously experienced anaphylaxis, severe angio-oedema, dizziness, fall in blood pressure, vomiting or a systemic reaction.

- The anaphylaxis box will be placed on the patient's bedside table.
- All personnel involved in food challenge testing have been trained to recognise the signs of anaphylaxis and can administer epinephrine.
- There is an agreed protocol on the management of anaphylaxis.

Advice to patients after procedures

All patients will have a letter sent to their general practitioner (GP) informing the GP of the outcome of the challenge.

Patients who have a positive challenge will be:

- given written information on the avoidance of the food, advice about food labels, eating out and holidays;
- prescribed medication as appropriate, including epinephrine, and given advice on how to administer the medication and what to do if they think they are having a reaction;
- given information on MedicAlert bracelets if they have not received this previously;
- sent an appointment to come back to the clinic in 6–12 months' time but advised to return sooner if they should experience any further reactions.

Patients who have had a negative challenge will be:

- given advice on how to normalise their diet;
- advised to try to include the tested food back in their diet where possible;
- given advice about the medications they may have been taking or carrying, such as an epinephrine auto-injector pen, and whether this is still necessary;
- told to make an appointment should they develop any further symptoms, but otherwise they will be discharged from the clinic.

References

1. Niggemann B, Rolinck-Werninghaus C, Mehl A *et al*. Controlled oral food challenges in children: when indicated, when superfluous? *Allergy* 2005; **60**: 865–70.
2. Ewan PW, Clark AT. IgE mediated food allergy: when is food challenge needed? *Arch Dis Child* 2005; **90**: 555–6.
3. Bindslev-Jensen C, Ballmer-Webber BK, Bengtsson U *et al*. Standardization of food challenges in patients with immediate reactions to foods: position paper from the European Academy of Allergology and Clinical Immunology. *Allergy* 2004; **59**: 690–7.
4. Anhaj C, Backer V, Nolte H. Diagnostic evaluation of grass- and birch-allergic patients with oral allergy syndrome. *Allergy* 2001; **56**: 548–52.
5. Rancé F, Juchet A, Brémont F, Dutau G. Correlations between skin prick tests using commercial extracts and fresh foods, specific IgE, and food challenges. *Allergy* 1997; **52**: 1031–5.

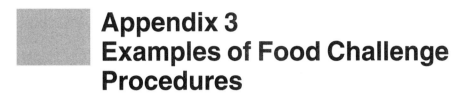

Appendix 3
Examples of Food Challenge Procedures

Food	Challenge material	Labial challenge	Dosage
Milk or soya	For infants < 6 months, any cow's milk/soya formula All other children and adults, skimmed cow's milk or unflavoured soya milk	Place 1 drop of milk on lower oral mucosa	0.5 ml, 1 ml, 2 ml, 5 ml, 10 ml, 15 ml, 25 ml, 40 ml Final dose: 100–200 ml milk/formula or 100–200 ml yoghurt
Egg	40 g cooked egg (10 g dried product)	Rub the mucosa of the lower lip with cooked egg	1 g, 2 g, 5 g, 10 g, 22 g Final dose: children < 1 year, 1 medium egg children > 1 year, 1 large egg adults, 1–2 large eggs
Peanut	Peanut May wish to use chocolate-coated peanuts or peanuts baked into a flapjack	Rub the mucosa of the lower lip with a peanut (not salted or with chocolate)	1/4 peanut, 1/2 peanut, 1, 2, 3.5 peanuts Children: eat 10 peanuts altogether during the whole challenge Adults: eat another 10 peanuts in addition to those consumed in the challenge
Fish or prawns	60 g poached fish (13 g dried product) or 35 g cooked prawn (10.5 g dried product)	Rub the mucosa of the lower lip with the fish or prawn	1 g, 2 g, 5 g, 10 g, 15 g, 27 g poached fish or 1 g, 2 g, 3 g, 5 g, 10 g, 14 g prawn Final dose for children: 100 g poached fish to be consumed openly or < 3 years, 1–2 fish fingers 3–5 years, 2–3 fish fingers > 5 years, 3–4 fish fingers Final dose for adults: 100–200 g fish to be consumed openly
Wheat	1/2 Weetabix/Shredded Wheat (9.4 g dried product) or 30 g cooked pasta (10 g raw) for challenge (9 g dried product)	1 drop of Weetabix/Shredded Wheat mixed with water on lower lip or 1 drop of wheat flour mixed with water on lower lip	1/4 teaspoon, 1/2 tsp, 1 tsp, 2 tsp, 5 tsp Weetabix/Shredded Wheat Final dose: children 1 Weetabix/Shredded Wheat, adults 2 Weetabix/Shredded Wheat or 1 g, 2 g, 5 g, 8 g, 10 g pasta Final dose: children 80 g, adults 200–290 g cooked pasta
Kiwi	100 g of kiwi (8 g dried product)	Rub the mucosa of the lower lip with kiwi	1 g, 2 g, 5 g, 10 g, 15 g, 25 g, 40 g kiwi Final dose for adults and children: 60–100 g of kiwi

NB. The observation period between dosages and after the challenges will vary according to the patient history. The usual period for immediate reactions is 10 minutes between the labial and oral challenge, 10–30 minutes between challenge doses, and 1–2 hours between the last dose of challenge (e.g. 40 ml of milk) and the final dose (e.g. 100–200 ml of milk/formula or yoghurt).

Appendix 4
Examples of Prolonged Open Food Challenge Procedures

Milk challenge

For children < 1 year

For the prolonged challenge, we would like you to provide your child with **the equivalent of 20 oz of cow's milk formula per day.** You can use the formula to make custard or use it on cereal.

For children > 1 year

For the prolonged challenge, we would like you to provide your child with **2–3 portions of cow's milk or cow's milk products per day.** The following foods are all equal to 1 portion of milk:

- 8 fl oz of cow's milk infant formula
- 8 fl oz of cow's milk
- 8 oz of custard
- 1 yoghurt or fromage frais
- 1 oz cheese

For adults

For the prolonged challenge, we would like you to consume **3–4 portions of cow's milk or cow's milk products per day.** The following foods are all equal to 1 portion of milk:

- 8 fl oz of cow's milk infant formula
- 8 fl oz of cow's milk
- 8 oz of custard
- 1 yoghurt or fromage frais
- 1 oz cheese

Soya challenge

For children < 1 year

For the 7-day/prolonged challenge, we would like you to provide your child with **20 oz of soya milk formula per day.** You can use the formula to make custard or use it on cereal.

For children over 1 year (1–2½ years)

For the 7-day/prolonged challenge, we would like you to provide your child with **the equivalent of 20 oz of soya milk per day**. The following foods are all equal to 1 oz of soya milk:

- 1 oz of soya milk infant formula
- 1 oz of soya milk (up to a maximum of 5 oz mixed in with food) not suitable as a main source of milk intake in children younger than 2 years
- 1 oz of custard made with soya milk using custard powder
- ¼ soya yoghurt
- 1 oz soya cheese

For children over 2½ years and adults

For the prolonged challenge, we would like you (your child) to consume **2–4 portions of soya milk or soya milk products per day**. The following foods are all equal to 1 portion of soya milk:

- 8 fl oz of soya milk
- 8 oz of custard made with soya milk
- 1 soya yoghurt or soya dessert
- 1 oz of soya cheese

Wheat challenge

For the 7-day/prolonged challenge, we would like you (your child) to consume the following amounts of **wheat-containing foods** on a daily basis:

Children aged 6 months to 2 years	2–3 portions
Children aged 2–3 years	4 portions
Children aged 4–6 years	4–5 portions
Children over 6 years and adults	4–6 portions

You could give half-portions of a larger variety of wheat-containing foods as well, e.g. to provide three portions to a 1-year-old child, you could give six half-portions. The following foods are all equal to 1 wheat portion:

- 1 slice of bread
- 3 tablespoons of cereal (not rice cereals or corn cereals)
- 1 Weetabix or Shredded Wheat type cereal
- 1 biscuit
- 1 slice of cake
- 1 tablespoon of pasta

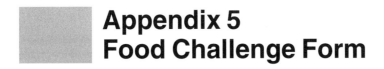

Appendix 5
Food Challenge Form

CHALLENGE PROCEDURE

Food to be challenged:		**Date:**	

Type of challenge	Open		Double-blind placebo-controlled	
	To be completed <u>only</u> when code is broken		Active	Placebo

Patient's name & address	DOB	
	Age at challenge	yr mth
	IW No	
	Weight at challenge	

Other relevant allergies/illness (asthma etc)　　Yes　　No
If yes

Relevant medication taken in last 3 days　　Yes　　No
If yes

Supervising Doctor

Supervising Nurse

Supervising dietician

Overall result of challenge

Negative	Positive	Not completed	Reason

Reactions	Yes	No	N/A	If yes

Medication given	Yes	No	N/A	If yes

Medication　　　　　　　　　　　　　Dose

Doctor's signature _____　　　Date _____

FOOD CHALLENGE CLINICAL MANIFESTATION
For 1-day challenge

Method of challenge: | Labial | | Oral | | Topical | |

Name | | No. |
DOB | | Weight |

Time								
T								
P								
R								
BP								
Peak flow								
Erythematous rash								
Eczema								
Pruritis								
Urticaria								
Angio-oedema								
Rash								
Sneezing/Itching								
Nasal congestion								
Rhinorrhoea								
Laryngeal								
Wheezing								
Abdo pain								
Nausea								
Vomiting								
Diarrhoea								
Pallor								
Headache								
Other								

Change in behaviour, mood, activity – describe:

Other – describe:

Time given	Vehicle/ food	Dose	Time evaluated	Reaction (additional notes on reverse)

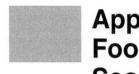

Appendix 6
Food Challenge Symptom
Score Chart

Skin

Erythematous rash – % area involved

Pruritis

0 = Absent
1 = Mild – occasional scratching
2 = Moderate – scratching continuously for > 2 min at a time
3 = Severe – hard continuous scratching – excoriations

Urticaria

0 = Absent
1 = Mild – < 3 hives
2 = Moderate – < 10 hives but > 3
3 = Severe – generalised involvement

Angio-oedema

0 = absent
1 = 1 area affected (e.g. lips)
2 = 2 areas affected (e.g. lips and tongue)
3 = 3 or more areas affected (e.g. lips, tongue, throat, eyes)

Rash

0 = Absent
1 = Few areas of faint erythema
2 = Moderate – areas of erythema, macular and raised rash
3 = Severe – generalised marked erythema (> 50%), extensive raised lesions (25%),
vasculation and/or piloerection)

Upper respiratory

Sneezing

0 = Absent
1 = Mild – rare bursts
2 = Moderate – bursts < 10, intermittent rubbing of nose, and/or eyes
3 = Severe – continuous rubbing of nose and/or eyes, periocular swelling and long bursts of sneezing

Nasal congestion

0 = Absent
1 = Mild – some hindrance to breathing
2 = Moderate – nostrils feel blocked, breathes through mouth most of time
3 = Severe – nostrils occluded

Rhinorrhoea

0 = Absent
1 = Mild – occasional sniffing
2 = Moderate – frequent sniffing, requires tissues
3 = Severe nose runs freely despite sniffing and tissues

Laryngeal

0 = Absent
2 = Mild – occasional sniffing
4 = Moderate – hoarseness, frequent dry cough
6 = Severe – Inspiratory stridor

Lower respiratory

Wheezing

0 = Absent
2 = Mild – expiratory wheezing to auscultation
4 = Moderate – dyspnoea, inspiratory and expiratory wheezing
6 = Severe – dyspnoea, use of accessory muscles, audible wheezing

Gastrointestinal

Subjective

Nausea

0 = Absent
1 = Mild – frequently complains of nausea + decreased activity

2 = Moderate – frequently complains of nausea > 30 min + decreased activity + pallor

3 = Severe – patient in bed, notably distressed

Abdominal pain

0 = Absent

1 = Mild – frequently complains of abdominal pain + decreased activity

2 = Moderate – frequently complains of abdominal pain > 30 min + decreased activity + pallor

3 = Severe – patient in bed, notably distressed

Objective

Vomiting

0 = Absent

1 = Mild – 1 episode of emesis

2 = Moderate – 2–3 episodes of emesis

3 = Severe – > 3 episodes of emesis

Diarrhoea

0 = Absent

1 = Mild – 1 episode of diarrhoea

2 = Moderate – 2–3 episodes of diarrhoea

3 = Severe – > 3 episodes of diarrhoea

Pallor

0 = Absent

1 = Mild

2 = Moderate

3 = Severe

Headache

0 = Absent

1 = Mild – complains of headache

2 = Moderate – frequently complains of headache > 30 min

3 = Severe – patient in obvious distress, crying

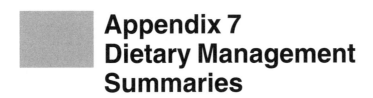

Appendix 7
Dietary Management
Summaries

This appendix contains a summary of the main points from each chapter in Part 2 (Chapters 5–10). Each summary gives the key points for each food group, including prevalence, population group affected, foods involved, diagnosis and management.

Milk allergy

Who is affected

Hypersensitivity reactions to cow's milk are seen both in children and in adults. Cow's-milk protein allergy (CMPA) has a prevalence of 2–3% in the first three years of life. In adulthood the most common CMPA is non-immune-mediated, with 4.8% reporting a variety of symptoms.

Lactose intolerance is often confused with CMPA. It is distinctly different, in that it is not immune-mediated and is due to an intolerance to the carbohydrate lactose in cow's milk, caused by the absence or deficiency, to a varying degree, of the enzyme lactase in the gastrointestinal tract.

Which foods are involved

Cow's milk and any other mammalian milks (e.g. goat, sheep, donkey and buffalo) and milk products should be avoided.

Presenting symptoms

CMP can induce both acute (IgE-mediated) and delayed (non-IgE-mediated and mixed) reactions. The clinical spectrum ranges from acute anaphylactic manifestations to atopic dermatitis, urticaria, food-associated wheeze, rhinitis, infantile colic, gastro-oesophageal reflux, enterocolitis, food-associated proctocolitis and constipation.

How to diagnose

Positive specific IgE antibody skin prick or serum tests and a positive history are usually sufficient to make a diagnosis of CMPA. Food challenge is used to diagnose resolution of the allergy.

Management

The mainstay of treatment is the avoidance of cow's-milk protein in addition to other mammalian milks and milk products. Dietary exclusion must be complete, including traces of milk, and measures to reduce accidental exposure from cross-contamination should also be implemented. The management of lactose intolerance depends on the level of lactase deficiency and therefore may vary from total avoidance of milk and milk products to avoidance of dairy products high in lactose only (e.g. fresh milk).

Egg allergy

Who is affected

Hypersensitivity reactions to hens' eggs are seen both in children and in adults. Egg allergy has a prevalence of 1.6% in the first three years of life. Egg allergy follows a similar trend to cow's-milk protein allergy in adults.

Which foods are involved

Clinically relevant allergens are found in both egg yolk and egg white, but egg-white allergy is more commonly seen. Research has found a difference in allergenicity between cooked and raw egg. It is therefore not uncommon for egg-allergic individuals to tolerate well-cooked egg, but not loosely cooked or raw egg.

Presenting symptoms

Atopic dermatitis represents the main clinical manifestation of egg allergy in infancy, although several authors have reported urticaria, angio-oedema, acute vomiting, violent diarrhoea or even anaphylaxis on first known exposure to egg in infants' weaning diets.

How to diagnose

Positive specific IgE antibody skin prick or serum tests and a positive history are usually sufficient to make a diagnosis of egg allergy. History will often reveal if the allergy is to all egg or just certain forms of egg (e.g. cooked egg). Food challenge is used to diagnose resolution of the allergy.

Management

The treatment for egg allergy consists of avoiding egg and all egg-related products. Those who can tolerate well-cooked egg can eat this but should continue to avoid loosely cooked and raw egg.

Seafood allergy

Who is affected

Both children and adults can have fish allergy, whereas allergy to crustaceans tends to occur mainly in older children and adults. Seafood allergy is also more likely to occur in people who are atopic and sensitised to other aeroallergens, or have rhinitis or asthma.

Which foods are involved

Fish allergy can involve both fresh- and salt-water fish as they are cross-reactive. Fish do not normally cross-react with crustaceans but there is the risk of contamination. Crustacean allergy is more common than mollusc allergy, and the commonest allergen is the shrimp or prawn allergen. There is cross-reactivity between crustaceans (prawns, lobster, crab, crayfish) and molluscs (mussels, squid, clams, octopus), but also between crustaceans and house-dust mite, and cockroaches.

Presenting symptoms

Usually only associated with immediate symptoms related to an IgE-mediated food hypersensitivity response. Reactions to both fish and shellfish are potentially severe and cross-reactivity is common.

How to diagnose

Positive specific IgE antibody skin prick or serum tests and a positive history are usually sufficient to make a diagnosis. However, due to the often very severe reported symptoms, and the possibility of a differential diagnosis, a negative specific IgE screen needs confirmation by an oral food challenge.

Differential diagnoses include scombroid poisoning, allergy to fish roe and allergy to the nematode worms which can be found in several fish species including cod and herring.

Management

Avoidance of all fish/seafood is often required due to cross-reactivity or contamination. Although they are all now required by European Union (EU) legislation to be labelled, fish, crustaceans and molluscs can appear in some unusual foods (Worcestershire sauce and Gentleman's Relish) and due to the longevity of shrimp allergens, contamination can be a major problem, especially when eating out.

Fruit and vegetable allergy

Who is affected

Primary fruit/vegetable allergy – is a condition where the sufferer has a primary sensitisation to a fruit or vegetable allergen. It usually affects older children and adults, but is becoming an increasing problem in younger children, especially to particular foods such as kiwi. The prevalence is unknown, although in adults this type of fruit and vegetable allergy is thought to be more common in southern Europeans than in the UK or northern Europe.

Oral allergy syndrome (OAS) – does not involve a primary sensitisation to a plant food allergen, but is caused by a cross-reaction between pollen antibodies and plant food allergens. OAS is most common in people who are sensitised to birch-tree pollen, and therefore often have seasonal rhinitis in the spring from March to May. The condition usually affects teenagers and adults, and is thought to affect 5% of northern Europeans.

Which foods are involved

Primary fruit/vegetable allergy – can be provoked by any raw or cooked fruit or vegetable, although apple, peach, kiwi and celery cause the most severe reactions.

OAS – triggered by many different plant foods, most commonly apple, stone fruit, tree nuts, strawberry, kiwi, tomato, melon and citrus fruits. Reactions are usually to the raw fruit or vegetable, with cooked, canned or microwaved foods tolerated.

Presenting symptoms

Primary fruit/vegetable allergy – symptoms usually are moderate to severe and involve immediate reactions to the food, in any form, often resulting in urticaria, angio-oedema and systemic symptoms including anaphylaxis.

OAS – usually sensitised to tree pollens and may have rhinitis in the spring and/or summer time. Their food symptoms are characterised by immediate-onset mild symptoms, typically involving pruritis, tingling, and oedema of the oropharynx, which usually resolve within half an hour, often without any medication.

How to diagnose

Primary fruit/vegetable allergy – best made using skin prick and specific IgE estimation, although negative tests need to be confirmed by a prick-to-prick test with the suspected food followed by an oral challenge, especially if symptoms are severe.

OAS – take a careful clinical history, which can be confirmed by skin prick testing with the suspected raw food using the prick-to-prick method.

Management

Primary fruit/vegetable allergy – it is essential to avoid all forms of the food, raw or cooked, in even small amounts.

OAS – avoid the trigger food in it raw state, but there is no need to avoid botanical relatives of that food unless they also precipitate symptoms.

Peanut, legume, seed and tree-nut allergy

Who is affected

Affects both children and adults, although peanut, soya bean, nut and sesame seed allergy are more common in young children. The prevalence of peanut allergy is rising, and it is thought to affect 1.4% of all children. Also on the increase, especially among the very young, are cashew-nut and sesame-seed allergies.

Which foods are involved

Peanut and soya-bean allergy are the most common legume allergies. Peanut allergy is infrequently outgrown (only in 20%) whereas soya-bean allergy is a transient childhood allergy rarely seen in adulthood. Lentil and chickpea are by contrast more common in adulthood. In the UK, the commonest tree-nut allergies are to almond, Brazil nut and hazelnut, with cashew-nut allergy becoming more of a problem in childhood. The commonest seed allergy in the UK involves sesame seeds, which are capable of causing severe reactions. Mustard, the other common seed allergen, occurs predominantly in adulthood.

Presenting symptoms

Nuts and seeds can provoke a full range of moderate to severe allergic symptoms including urticaria, atopic eczema, angio-oedema and projectile vomiting. Peanut allergy is the commonest cause of reported food-induced fatal anaphylaxis.

How to diagnose

Positive skin prick tests (SPT) and high specific IgE levels in blood alongside a clear clinical history are necessary for an accurate diagnosis of these food allergies. Food challenges should be used when these tests prove equivocal or contradict clinical history. In childhood, diagnostic predictive values for both SPTs and specific IgE levels have been developed for peanut allergy, thus allowing the clinician to be more certain of the diagnosis.

Management

Because of the severity of allergic reactions provoked by legumes, nuts and seeds, complete avoidance, even to trace amounts in the diet, is necessary. Particular care must be taken to reduce the risk of cross-contamination, and thorough cleaning of hands and cooking and eating surfaces is essential, given the hardy nature of these allergens.

Coeliac disease

Who is affected

CD affects 1% of the population in the UK, although only 1 in 8 cases are diagnosed. CD can present and be diagnosed at any age.

Which foods are involved

Gluten-containing cereals, e.g. wheat, rye and barley (and in some cases oats), need to be avoided. The most obvious sources of gluten in the diet are breads, flour, pasta, pizza bases, biscuits, cakes and pastries.

Presenting symptoms

Possible symptoms include bloating, abdominal pain, nausea, diarrhoea, excessive wind, heartburn, indigestion, constipation, any combination of iron, vitamin B_{12} or folic-acid deficiency anaemias, tiredness, headaches, weight loss (but not in all cases), recurrent mouth ulcers, hair loss, dermatitis herpetiformis, defective tooth enamel, osteoporosis, depression, infertility, recurrent miscarriages, joint or bone pain, neurological problems such as ataxia and neuropathy.

Infants may present after weaning onto gluten with symptoms such as failure to thrive, diarrhoea, vomiting, abdominal distension, constipation, muscle wasting and irritability.

How to diagnose

Antibody blood test, IgA tTG and/or EMA, followed by small-bowel biopsy. Biopsy is mandatory in all cases (both adults and children). Anyone being tested for CD must be on a normal gluten-containing diet prior to testing. A GF diet should not be started until diagnosis of CD is established. Therapeutic trials of a GF diet are not warranted if CD is suspected; clinical response to either withdrawal or reintroduction of gluten has no role in the diagnosis of CD.

Management

A lifelong GF diet involving complete exclusion of the cereals wheat, rye and barley. Some people also need to avoid oats. Because of the increased risk of osteoporosis, adults with CD may need additional calcium.

Wheat and cereal allergy

Who is affected

More common in children, and may affect 0.4% of the population. Rare in adults, in whom it is usually linked to exercise-induced anaphylaxis (WDEIA).

Which foods are involved

Wheat staples such as bread, pasta and breakfast cereals, but can also involve a diverse range of foods such as wheat beer, tortilla chips (corn), bitter beer (barley), malted foods (barley) or Breton *galettes* (buckwheat).

Presenting symptoms

Children may present with mild symptoms of atopic dermatitis, and adults with pruritis and erythema. However severe symptoms can be quite common and so anyone presenting with anaphylaxis or severe angio-oedema linked to foods other than peanuts and seafood, especially if it is their first episode, should be screened for an allergy to wheat or other cereals.

How to diagnose

History, skin prick and specific IgE tests are not very useful. The best method is to perform an open or blinded food challenge. It is important to ensure that those with grass-pollen allergy who have a positive SPT or specific IgE to wheat are further tested, because of the high cross-reactivity between grass and wheat.

Management

Avoidance of wheat requires expert advice on wheat substitutes, and depending on the quality of the diet may necessitate supplementation of vitamins and minerals. Exclusion of other cereals will also require expert intervention to assess the individual's diet, to ensure that all forms of the offending cereal are removed. Food labels have to declare the presence of all gluten-containing cereals (wheat, barley, rye and oats), but corn and rice are not required to be labelled as an allergen on food product labels.

Food additives

Who is affected

Reported prevalence much greater than confirmed prevalence, which is in the region of 0.1–1% in adults. Prevalence in specific subjects is likely to be higher: 1–3% of those with chronic idiopathic urticaria and 2–5% of asthmatics could be affected by food additives.

Which additives and foods are involved

Food additives are present in a wide range of foods and include food colourings such as cochineal or carmine, annatto, turmeric and saffron and azo dyes, preservatives such as benzoates and sulphites, flavour enhancers such as monosodium glutamate (MSG) and others.

Presenting symptoms

Chronic urticaria has been linked to the consumption of both benzoates and tartrazine, rhinitis with benzoates and sulphites, and asthma with sulphites. Hyperactive disorders and behavioural changes in children have also been linked to both azo dyes and benzoates. MSG has been linked with headache but has also been reported to provoke symptoms in asthmatics.

How to diagnose

Skin prick and specific IgE tests are not useful due to the lack of IgE-mediation thought to characterise hyerpsensitivity to most food additives, although a skin prick test using natural colourings may provoke an antibody response. A careful history will help, but reactions may be dose-related and therefore not happen every time the additive is consumed. The best method of diagnosis will be careful elimination of the suspected additive, followed by reintroduction and oral food challenge if available.

Management

Avoidance of all foods containing the additive may be required, although if the reaction is dose-dependent then a limited amount of the additive may be safely consumed. All additives have an E number, and some such as sodium metabisulphite have to be declared on the food label if present above a certain level.

Pharmacologic food reactions: salicylates, vasoactive amines, coffee and alcohol

Who is affected

There are little or no prevalence data for this type of food hypersensitivity. Aspirin-sensitive asthmatics are more likely to suffer from salicylate hypersensitivity, and histamine-containing foods may exert a greater effect on those suffering from migraine. Surveys suggest that alcoholic drinks may affect up to 14% of the population, with those who have asthma or allergic rhinitis more likely to experience hypersensitivity reactions to different forms of alcohol.

Which foods are involved

Salicylates are present in a great many fruits and vegetables, being particularly high in wine, dried herbs, tea, coffee, black pepper, tomatoes, strawberries and foods containing oil of wintergreen or spearmint flavouring. Histamine is found naturally in strong cheese, red wine, tuna and mackerel. The commonest alcoholic drinks to cause reported reactions are red and white wine. Wine, beer and lager can provoke an IgE-mediated reactions; they also contain sulphites.

Presenting symptoms

Symptoms of salicylate hypersensitivity can be very varied, non-specific and dose-dependent. The main symptoms of hypersensitivity to vasoactive amines are flushing and headache, although a range of other symptoms can also be reported.

How to diagnose

Skin prick and specific IgE tests are not helpful unless an IgE-mediated reaction to wine or beer is suspected. If salicylate sensitivity is suspected, then confirmation of aspirin hypersensitivity is an important diagnostic step. Careful evaluation of the history of the reactions and symptoms elicited will give the best clue as to what is causing the problem. Elimination of the offending foods and objective symptom scoring is the only way to diagnose hypersensitivity to food additives. It can be difficult to undertake oral provocation tests due to difficulties in quantifying the dose present in the food.

Management

Avoidance of salicylates is very difficult, and it is important to establish thresholds, as many people only need to avoid high-salicylate foods. If someone is very sensitive to salicylates, then expert dietary advice will be needed in order to ensure that nutritional deficiency does not arise. There are no specific nutritional issues involved in the avoidance of vasoactive amines, coffee or alcohol.

Food-dependent exercise-induced anaphylaxis (FDEIA)

Who is affected

Prevalence is unknown, but studies suggest that 13% of cases of anaphylaxis could be caused by FDEIA, and that 80% of cases of anaphylaxis linked to exercise are precipitated by food.

Which foods are involved

Wheat, crustaceans and tomatoes are all commonly reported to cause this condition. However, FDEIA can be precipitated by a wide range of foods including maize, soya, peanuts, celery, cheese, strawberries and alcohol. Aspirin can also precipitate FDEIA in the absence of exercise.

Presenting symptoms

There may be severe systemic symptoms including urticaria, angio-oedema and anaphylaxis, on or soon after taking exercise in close proximity to eating a particular food or foods.

How to diagnose

A good history is very important, recording fully those foods taken before exercising, when these foods may be consumed without getting reactions, type of exercise and proximity to eating. If wheat is suspected, then an estimation of IgE antibody levels of omega-5 gliadin, the key allergen involved in wheat-dependent exercise-induced anaphylaxis, can be diagnostic when correlated with a good history. If other foods are suspected it is important to look for specific IgE antibodies, although a negative result does not rule out FDEIA. Neither does the type of exercise involved. Jogging is the most common type to elicit a reaction, but much more mild exercise such as sweeping up can also be a trigger. The final diagnostic test is exercise with/without prior consumption of the food within 2 hours of the exercise taking place.

Management

Avoidance of the trigger food 4–6 hours before exercising, or taking aspirin if that is a known augmentation factor, is the main advice. Rarely do patients need to avoid the food altogether, unless the condition is being precipitated frequently due to a low threshold for exercise. In some people just walking upstairs can be sufficient to cause an attack. Patients should also wear medical identification jewellery and carry adrenaline. An exercise 'buddy' is also advisable, especially if patients are exercising in a remote place.

Index

AAP, 278, 289, 290
abdominal symptoms, 7, 37, 46, 49, 70, 78, 344
acacia, 172
acetylsalicylic acid, 25, 221, 222
ACR20, 83
Actinidiaceae, 150
active immunity, 280, 284
Addison's disease, 187
additives, 14–16, 25, 33–4, 48, 58–9, 61, 65, 107, 112, 148, 210–12, 215, 216, 218–21, 228
ADHD, 59, 63
Adoxaceae, 150
adrenaline, 132, 170, 231, 265, 323, 325, 327, 354
adrenaline auto-injectors, 170, 327
Advisory Committee on Borderline Substances, 195, 267
aeroallergens, 279, 293, 304, 308, 318, 347
albumin seed storage proteins, 108, 167
alcohol, 8, 34, 39, 41, 65, 70, 77, 107, 142, 183, 189, 197, 225, 227–31, 352–3, 354
alcohol-soluble prolamins, 183
aldehyde dehydrogenase, 227
algae oil, 143
allergens, 22, 27, 33–5, 38, 107–12
    allergen labelling, 195
    allergen nomenclature, 108
allergic march, 24
allergic rhinitis, 32, 149, 216, 227, 278, 293, 303–4, 308, 315, 352
allergy prevention, 241, 278–9, 283–4, 287–94
Alliaceae, 150
allura red (E129), 215
almond, 123, 151, 154, 167, 176–9, 268, 349

α-lactalbumin, 118
α-livetin, 129
Alternaria, 157
amaranth (E123), 214
amaretto, 179
American Academy of Pediatrics, 278, 289
American College of Rheumatology's scoring system for signs and symptoms of RA, 83
amino acids, 6, 48, 109, 167
amino-acid-based formula, 93, 124, 260, 318
Anacardiaceae, 150, 178
anaemia, 185, 187, 196, 244, 262
anaphylactoid, 322
anaphylaxis, 6, 9, 22, 31, 96–7, 111–12, 119, 128, 132, 138, 140, 148, 152–3, 157, 166, 170–1, 174–5, 177–8, 203–6, 211–12, 214, 217–18, 226, 228–31, 265, 266, 269, 273–5, 308, 322–8, 332–46, 348–9, 351, 353–4
    idiopathic anaphylaxis, 326
anchovies, 138, 140, 142, 225
angio-oedema, 6–8, 22–5, 95, 128, 139, 157, 206, 216–17, 342
    hereditary, 24
angular cheilitis, 54
animals, 303, 305, 311
    dander, 309, 318
    food allergens, 109
Anisakis, 139–40
anise, 219
annatto (E160b), 174, 211, 214, 352
antibody, 6, 7, 83, 109, 111, 129, 137, 141, 147, 185, 197, 230
anticholinergic drugs, 306
anti-fungal drugs, 72
Antigen Leukocyte Cellular Antibody Test, 91

antigens, 6, 7, 27, 38, 47–8, 55, 69, 83, 107, 109, 184, 212, 286
antihistamines, 76, 303, 305–7, 312, 320–1, 329
antimicrobial agents, 216
anti-tissue transglutaminase, 185
anxiety, 63, 226
Apiaceae, 150, 156
apples, 15, 27, 41, 78, 148–9, 152, 154–9, 161, 205, 223, 257, 268, 333, 348
  apple allergens (Mal d 2, Mal d 3), 152–3, 156
apricots, 152, 217
Aqua libra, 176
arachidonic acid, 221
Arecaceae, 150
arrhythmia, 224
arthralgia, 70
Arthropods, 109, 138
artificial food colours, 7, 58–61, 65, 67, 210, 214–15
Asian food, 170
Asparagaceae, 150
aspartame, 65, 77, 79
Aspergillus, 157
aspirin, 212, 215, 217–18, 221–2, 229–31, 311, 326, 352–4
Asteraceae, 150
asthma, 31–5, 95, 120, 136, 139, 204–5, 211–18, 224, 227–9, 276, 278, 285, 288, 293, 305, 307, 309–15, 325, 347, 352
atopic dermatitis, 22, 25–7, 111, 119, 124, 157, 167, 168, 204, 206–7, 212, 215, 248, 289, 294, 345, 351
atopy, 26, 31, 60, 69, 285, 288, 293
Attention-deficit/hyperactivity disorder, 59
aubergines, 151, 153, 223–5
aura, 74, 78
autism and autistic spectrum disorders, 63–6
autoantibodies, 24–5, 29
autoimmune thyroid disease, 187
avenins, 193
avocado, 157
avoidance diets, 243, 260, 262
azathioprine, 46
azo dyes, 214–15, 217, 352

B cells, 281
B vitamins, 251, 257
bacteria, 8, 48, 65, 110, 127, 140, 149, 216, 279, 280–2, 284–7
baked beans, 123
baker's asthma, 31, 205
Balsam of Peru, 219, 220
bananas, 16, 39, 64, 78, 124, 148, 152, 155, 157, 222
barley, 27, 29, 64, 183, 190–5, 197, 204–7, 228, 255, 268, 350–1
barnacles, 139
basophils, 6
bean sprouts, 156
beans, 16, 148, 154, 167, 172–3, 190, 204, 223, 225, 230, 251, 253, 256
beef, 82
beer, 142, 191, 204–7, 216, 225, 228–9, 311, 351, 353
beeswax, 47
behaviour, 243, 255
behavioural disorders, 58
behavioural therapy, 59
benzoates, 8, 33, 55–7, 211–13, 211, 215–17, 229, 311
berries, 24, 56, 216
beta-2 agonists, 312
β-lactoglobulin, 83, 118, 122
beta-phenylethylamine, 77
Betula verrucosa, 148
bhetki, 137
bifidobacteria, 285, 287, 291
bilberries, 56, 222
biochemical markers, 244, 248
biogenic amines, 7, 74, 76, 223, 227–8
biotin, 251
birch, 27, 32, 110, 147–9, 152, 154–6, 158, 160–1, 178
birch pollen allergens
  Bet v 1, 108, 110–11, 149, 153, 155–6, 159–60, 178
  Bet v 2, 155–6, 159
biscuits, 41, 64, 100, 129, 175, 186, 190, 207
Bixa orellana, 214
black pepper, 222
blackcurrants, 222
bloating, 40, 41, 46, 70–1, 117, 127, 184, 188, 197, 350

blood tests, 85, 91
blood–brain barrier, 77
blueberry, 150, 152, 223
Body Ecology Diet, 65
bonito, 137, 140
botanical classification of plant foods, 149–50
bottled sauces, 207
bowel biopsy, 185–7, 197, 350
bradikynin, 6
bran, 39, 191
brandy, 228
Brassicaceae, 150
Brazil nuts, 123, 150–1, 155, 167, 176–7, 349
breads, 64–5, 173, 175–6, 188, 190, 193, 253, 256, 350
breakfast cereals, 64, 123, 207, 255
breast milk, 247, 249, 279, 284, 287–91, 294, 317
breast-feeding, 108, 117, 119, 122, 124, 198, 247, 249, 283, 287–92, 294–5, 317
British Dietetic Association, 126, 247
British National Formulary, 259
Bromeliaceae, 150
bronchodilators, 212, 217, 307, 312–13, 329
brownies, 170, 179
buckwheat, 151, 191, 195, 204, 207, 256, 351
butter, 64, 121, 169, 196, 214
butylated hydroxyanisole, 212, 219
butylated hydroxytoluene, 212, 219

cabbage, 153
cacao nut, 226, 227
caffeine, 42, 67, 71, 77, 82, 225–6
caffeine in different beverages and foods, 226
cakes, 57, 100, 126, 170, 175, 179, 190, 207
calcineurin inhibitors, 320
calcium, 67, 121–5, 189, 196, 207, 244, 246–50, 253, 254, 258–60, 350
  calcium-rich foods, 123, 250
  homeostasis, 124
  non-dairy calcium sources, 250
  recommendation, 189

  requirement, 123, 246, 249, 250
  supplements, 67, 249, 250, 253, 259
Candida, 41, 42, 72
Capparaceae, 150
carageenan (E407), 219
caraway, 150, 156
carbohydrate, 40, 42, 255, 261, 345
carmine, 211, 213–14, 352
carmoisine (E122), 55, 214
carnauba wax, 47
carotenoids, 214, 257
carrageenan, 47
carrots, 27, 148, 152, 154–5, 156, 158, 160, 223
casein, 64–5, 107–10, 118, 121
cashew nuts, 150, 166, 176–8
cashew nut allergens
  Ana o 1, 151, 175, 177, 178
  Ana o 2, 151, 177
  Ana o 3, 177
cassava, 157, 207
celery, 17, 112, 148, 150, 152–60, 230, 348, 354
centipedes, 138
cephalosporins, 325–6
cereals, 16, 41, 56, 64, 82, 112, 148, 183, 190–6, 198, 203, 204, 206–7, 213, 253, 254–6, 338, 350–1
  prolamins, 149, 204–5
  α-amylase inhibitors, 205
challenge – see food challenge
cheese, 39, 64, 65, 74, 76, 121–2, 126–7, 128, 130, 190–1, 213–14, 218, 224–5, 230, 250, 268, 325, 337–8, 353–4
cheesecake, 207
Chenopodiaceae, 150
cherry, 151–2, 154, 155, 158, 223
chestnut, 150, 154, 157, 177, 179, 223
chewing gum, 41, 57, 222, 223
chickpeas, 150, 154, 171–2, 207, 349
Chinese food, 179, 213, 218
Chinese restaurant syndrome, 218
chitinases, 156
chocolate, 14–15, 55, 57, 64, 74, 77, 124, 210, 224–7
  cacao nut, 226, 227
  cocoa, 14, 39, 42, 55, 225–6
chronic fatigue syndrome/ME, 68–72

chronic idiopathic urticaria, 210, 215–16, 218, 224
cider, 191, 217, 223, 225, 228–9
ciguatera poisoning, 140
cinnamaldehyde, 55, 56
cinnamon, 55–7, 150, 213, 216, 219
citrus, 8, 14, 24, 39, 74, 76, 82, 155, 224
Cladosporium, 157
clams, 138, 143, 347
class 1 allergens, 108–9
classification, 3, 109, 119, 128, 149, 167, 177
  cow's milk protein-induced immune reactions, 119
  egg-containing foods, 130
  gut damage in celiac disease, 186
clinical history, 85, 120
cloves, 213, 216, 219
cochineal (E120), 214, 352
cockroaches, 138–9, 347
cocoa, 14, 39, 42, 55, 225–6
coconut, 65, 122, 128, 150, 177, 223
cod, 14, 110, 136–8, 142
Codex standard, 193
Codex wheat starch, 194
coeliac disease, 16, 28, 66–7, 78, 107, 127, 183, 188, 203, 205, 207, 247, 256, 294, 350
Coeliac UK, 183, 190, 194, 198, 270
coffee, 39, 42, 65, 191, 222, 226, 271, 330, 352–3
cola drinks, 226
colitis, 119, 128, 188
colonic microbiota, 38–40, 42
complementary and alternative medicine, 90
complementary feeding, 294
compliance, 257–60, 306–7, 312–13
component-based diagnosis, 159
conjunctivitis, 303
constipation, 37, 66, 70–1, 119–20, 185, 255, 345, 350
contact dermatitis, 29
contact hypersensitivity, 55, 118, 216
contact urticaria, 24
Convolvulaceae, 150
cookies, 170, 179
coriander, 150, 153, 156

corn, 16, 39, 65, 82, 148, 190–1, 194, 205, 207, 228, 268, 293–4, 338, 351
corticosteroids, 46, 48, 50, 55
  inhaled, 307, 312–14
  intramuscular, 307
Corylaceae, 150
co-sensitisation, 178, 206
cosmetics, 57, 132, 213, 216
COT, 283–4, 294, 295
cottonseed, 174
courgette, 150, 153–4, 157, 223
couscous, 191, 207
cow's milk, 9, 13, 25, 33, 49, 64, 67, 82–3, 100, 110, 117–18, 121, 127, 243, 245, 247–8, 250, 253, 261, 268, 289, 291, 293, 317, 330, 337, 345
  allergy, 248–50, 260–2, 290–1, 345
  alternatives, 250
  enterocolitis, 119
  formulas, 290
  substitutes, 248–50
  CM-free diet, 246, 248, 249, 253
  CM-free enteral feeds, 261
  CM-free supplements, 260
Cox's Orange, 161
COX-1, COX-2, 221
crab, 38, 137–8, 143, 225, 347
cranberry, 150, 216, 223
cream, 121, 122
Crocus sativus, 214
Crohn's disease, 46–50, 55
croissants, 126, 179
cross-contamination, 196, 266
cross-reactivity, 32, 108–11, 126, 136–9, 143, 149, 152, 155–8, 160, 167, 172, 177–9, 207, 217
crustaceans, 17, 109, 112, 136, 138–9, 141–3, 230–1
Cucurbitaceae, 150
cupin superfamily, 110, 149
curcumin, 214
curd, 121
custard powder, 214, 338
cutaneous, 17, 22–5, 28–9, 55, 108, 119, 203–4, 206
cyclic prostenoids, 221
cycling, 230
cyclooxygenase, 212, 221

Cyperaceae, 150
cypress, 154

Dactylopius coccus, 214
dairy products, 33, 39–40, 55, 59, 82, 124,
    246, 293, 311, 325, 346
dapsone, 187
delayed hypersensitivity, 6, 55
Department of Health, 269–70, 275
dermatitis, 22, 28–9, 119, 128, 139, 212,
    214, 216, 219–20, 248, 346, 350
dermatitis herpetiformis, 28–9, 184, 186
desensitisation, 307
DEXA (dual x-ray absorptiometry) scan,
    189
diagnosis, 7, 16, 24–6, 39, 47, 63, 85–6,
    90, 92, 94, 96, 110–11, 117, 119,
    120–1, 127, 129, 140–2, 157–60, 168,
    172, 175, 177–9, 184–9, 196–8, 203,
    206, 216, 218, 229–31, 305, 310, 324,
    354
diagnostic decision points, 87, 90, 121, 168
diagnostic exclusion diets, 92
diamine oxidase, 75, 224
diarrhoea, 37, 40–1, 46, 49, 66–7, 70–1,
    117, 126–7, 128, 185, 188
Dietary
    adequacy, 243–5, 247, 250, 257–60
    dietary advice, 243, 246, 257, 353
    assessment, 94
    fibre, 39
    histamine, 224
    management, 71, 345
    manipulations, 247
    methylxanthines, 225
    migraine triggers, 74
    supplements, 65, 258
dietitian, 39, 42, 66, 71, 72, 171, 180, 248,
    267, 271, 285, 294
differential diagnoses, 140, 347
dill, 150, 156
disaccharidase, 8
diverticular disease, 255
d-limonene, 219
donkey, 118, 121, 345
dopamine, 223, 225
double-blind, placebo-controlled food
    challenge (DBPCFC), 9, 14–16, 33,

60–1, 77–8, 85, 94–102, 159, 203–4,
    206, 210–11, 215–16, 218–19, 226,
    228
Down's syndrome, 187
dried fruit, 217
duo-test/paired comparison test and
    triangle test, 100
dyspepsia, 7

earth nuts, 169
eating out, 271, 273
eczema, 9, 22, 25–7, 96–7, 101, 119–20,
    122, 212, 271, 276, 278, 283, 285,
    288, 291, 293, 304–5, 309–10,
    314–21, 349
    non-atopic eczema, 26
EF-hand proteins, 109
egg, 9, 13–17, 24–5, 27, 31, 39, 55, 59, 83,
    89, 92, 100–12, 117, 124, 128–32,
    137, 141, 148, 171, 174, 190, 203,
    224, 228, 245, 251, 267–8, 270, 275,
    292–3, 311, 317–18, 325, 329–31,
    346
    allergy, 27, 111, 117, 128–9, 131–2, 346
    dried, 130
    egg-free products, 131
    exclusion, 129
    loosely cooked, 130
    powder, 130
    proteins, 128
    replacers, 131
    white, 128, 131, 225, 346
    whole-egg replacers, 131
    yolk, 128, 130
elemental
    amino-acid-based formula, 125
    protein hydrolysate formula diets, 93
    diet, 48, 58–9, 82, 85, 87, 121, 216,
        244–6
    formula, 56
    sip feeds, 93
elimination diets, 24, 60, 78, 82, 121, 244
emollients, 318, 319
encephalopathy, 69, 82
endomysial antibody, 185
energy, 244, 247, 249–51, 253, 255, 257,
    260
enteral nutrition, 46, 48–50

enterocolitis, 6, 119, 122, 124
enteropathy-associated T-cell lymphoma,
      186, 188–9
environmental triggers, 184
enzyme, 6–8, 4, 39, 48, 64, 65, 76, 89, 126,
      188, 205, 221
eosinophilic oesophagitis, 119
eosinophils, 7
epidermal-barrier dysfunction, 27
epilepsy, 63
epitopes, 6–7, 108–9, 111–12, 118, 147,
      149, 154, 158, 167, 169, 172, 175,
      177–8, 206
   conformational, 109, 111, 167, 207
   sequential (linear) epitopes, 109, 111,
      167, 206
Ericaceae, 150
erythema, 23, 54, 206, 317, 342, 351
erythematous rash, 342
erythrosine, 211, 215
essential oils, 212
ethanol, 14, 224, 227–8
EU food labelling laws, 272–3
European Academy of Allergy and Clinical
      Immunology (EAACI), 278, 332
European ingredient rule (Directive
      2003/89/EC), 112
European Society for Paediatric Allergology
      and Clinical Immunology, 289
European Society of Paediatric Allergy and
      Clinical Immunology, 124
European Society of Paediatric
      Gastroenterology, Hepatology and
      Nutrition, 124, 289, 290, 293
exclusion diets, 49, 55, 244, 245, 250, 260,
      269, 331, 332, 346, 350
exercise, 309–11, 314, 326, 351, 353–4
   food-dependant, exercise-induced
      anaphylaxis (FDEIA), 229–31, 353–4
extensively hydrolysed formulae, 124, 125,
      290–1, 295
eye drops, 306

faba beans, 172
Fabaceae, 150, 156, 167, 172
faddy eating, 66
Fagaceae, 150
faltering growth, 243–4, 260–1
fat, 251, 254, 261, 285, 287–8, 307

fatty fish, 254
fatty-acid, 283, 289, 290
FcεRIα receptor, 24
Feingold diet, 58, 65
fennel, 150, 156, 219
fenugreek, 150, 171–173
fermentation, 47, 76, 172
few-foods diet, 93
fibre, 39, 42, 49–50, 191, 196–7, 251,
      254–7, 285
fibromyalgia, 82
figs, 123, 225
filaggrin, 26, 27
fish, 3, 9, 13–15, 17, 24, 27, 31, 33, 35, 74,
      83, 109–10, 112, 124, 136–43, 148,
      190, 203, 206, 214, 217, 224, 228,
      246, 251, 254–5, 268, 283, 285,
      292–5, 311, 317–18, 332, 347
   allergy, 136
   bait, 140
   fish-oil capsules, 143
fizzy drinks, 35, 191, 221, 223, 311
flavour enhancer, 7, 65, 218
flour, 14, 169, 171–2, 190, 193–4, 204,
      207
flushing, 7, 119, 139, 140, 218, 224, 227,
      307, 323–4, 333, 353
flying, 272
FODMAPS, 47
folate, 130, 196–8, 257
food additives, 29, 33–4, 47–8, 55, 58–61,
      65, 78, 107, 210–13, 215–16, 219,
      221, 258, 311, 351–3
Food Allergen Cellular Test, 91
food allergens, 9, 14, 22, 27, 82–3, 86, 107,
      109–12, 147, 149, 152, 154, 160–1,
      167, 172, 175, 178, 211, 218, 243,
      247, 266, 278, 292, 316–17, 331,
      348
food and symptom diary, 85
food challenge, 3, 8, 9, 13–16, 24–5, 32–3,
      38, 82, 85, 87–9, 93–8, 100–1, 103,
      121, 126, 129, 132, 141–2, 159, 173,
      175, 178, 203, 206, 210, 220, 227,
      231, 265, 329–30, 333, 334–5, 337,
      339–40, 347, 351–2
   challenge dose, 99
   challenge duration, 99
   interpretation of results, 101

management strategies after the
    challenge, 103
observation period, 97
open food challenges, 9, 15, 96
performing the challenge, 98
protocol, 331
single-blind placebo-controlled food
    challenges, 95
symptom score chart, 342
vehicle used for masking the food, 100
food colourings, 60, 64, 214
food exclusion, 3, 55, 64, 66–7, 92
food labelling, 112
food manufacturers, 245, 266
food preferences, 246, 257, 330
food preservatives, 216
food proteins, 6, 287
food reintroduction, 93
Food Standards Agency (FSA), 61, 71, 171,
    195, 212, 247, 266, 276
food substitutes, 247, 257
food triggers, 234
food associated proctocolitis, 119, 345
food-dependent exercise-induced
    anaphylaxis, 229, 353
food-protein-induced enterocolitis, 119
foods containing
    fish and seafood, 143
    legumes, 173
    tree nuts, 179
    seeds, 176
foods high in
    fructose, 41
    salicylates, 223
    vasoactive amines, 225
    rich in histamine/tyramine, 75
foods that
    trigger migraine, 74
    commonly cause OAS, 155
    cross-react to pollen and latex, 154
fried food, 65
frog's legs, 138
frozen chips, 191, 217
fructans, 40–1
fructose, 40–1, 188
Fruit, 8, 13–15, 24, 31, 39–41, 56, 64–5,
    74, 76, 78, 82, 86, 93, 147–9, 152,
    154–61, 177, 190, 197, 214, 216–17,
    219, 222–3, 229–31, 257

fruit & vegetable allergy, 348
fruit and vegetables, 257
fruitcake, 179
fruit juices, 216, 223
fungi, 110, 149, 157

galettes, 204
garlic, 150, 153, 156, 191
gastroenteritis, 69, 127, 140, 184, 287
gastrointestinal, 6, 7, 9–10, 17, 22, 24, 31,
    37, 38, 39, 41, 42, 46, 47, 48, 66–7,
    71, 110, 119, 126–8, 140, 147, 157,
    197, 203, 230, 323, 343
gastrointestinal allergies, 10
gastro-oesophageal reflux, 119, 345
gelatine, 132, 140, 142, 211
Gell–Coombs, 6, 33
genetic susceptibility, 184
ghee, 121
giardiasis, 127
gin, 228
ginger, 214, 223
gliadins, 29, 83, 111, 183, 205–6, 230, 231
glottal oedema, 157
gluten, 16, 17, 28–9, 64–5, 67, 78, 83, 107,
    112, 183–6, 188, 190–1, 193–8, 205,
    207, 268, 350
    challenge, 186
    gluten-free and casein-free diet for
        autism, 64
    gluten-free and gluten-containing foods,
        191
glutenin, 183, 205
glycaemic index, 188
glycerinated food extracts, 86
goat, 40, 64, 67, 110, 118, 121
going on holiday, 272
Golden Delicious, 161
gomashio, 176
gout, 81
Granny Smith, 161
grape, 152, 217, 219, 222–3, 228
grass, 27, 110, 147, 154–5, 158, 160,
    205–6, 230
Greek, 175–6
grossulariaceae, 150
ground nuts, 169
ground rice, 207
groundnut oil, 169

growth failure, 260
guar, 150, 172, 219
gut, 280–1, 284–7, 292, 317
gut bacterial overgrowth, 65

H₁-antagonists, 306
haemolytic anaemia, 187
hair analysis, 91
halvah, 176
hamburgers, 35
hapten, 107, 212, 220
hard sweets, 219
haricot beans, 172
hay fever, 32, 278, 303–4, 305, 307,
    309–10
hazelnut, 15, 27, 154–6, 158, 176–9, 349
HbAlc, 188
headache, 7, 74–8, 95, 218, 224–5, 323,
    344, 352–3
health-and-safety regulations, 270
healthcare professionals, 69, 119, 195, 198,
    267, 291, 313
healthy eating, 197
Heiner's syndrome, 33, 119–20
herbal remedies, 38, 169
herbs, 156, 191, 222–3, 229, 353
hereditary angio-oedema, 24
herpes simplex virus, 317
herring, 137, 138, 140, 225, 254, 347
Hevea brasiliensis, 156–7
high-fibre foods, 50
high-risk infant, 278, 291
hilsa, 137
hip fracture, 189
histamine, 6–8, 14–15, 24, 33, 42, 61,
    74–6, 86, 87, 140–1, 154, 211–12,
    223–4, 227, 230, 305, 320–1, 324,
    352–3
    N-methyltransferase gene, 61
    -induced headache, 76
histidine, 75, 140, 224
history, 96, 243, 278, 288, 303–5, 310,
    316, 318, 324–5, 331–3, 336, 345–9,
    352–4
hives, 22, 139, 333, 342
HLA DQ2/DQ8, 184
hordeins, 183, 205
horse, 118

house-dust mite, 27, 138, 139, 141, 230,
    305, 309, 311, 318, 347
human leucocyte antigen, 184
human-milk oligosaccharides, 291
hummus, 173, 176
hydrogen breath test, 90, 127
hydrogen gas, 127
hydrolysed formulae
    hydrolysed casein, 121, 291, 295
    hydrolysed vegetable protein, 218
    non-milk-based extensively hydrolysed
        formulas, 125
    partially hydrolysed formulas, 124
    partially hydrolysed whey formula, 291,
        295
hymenoptera venom[126], 227
hyperactivity, 58–61, 63, 65, 215
hyperkinesis, 58, 59
hypoallergenic formulas, 124–6, 279
hypoglycaemia, 77
hypotension, 139, 224, 227, 323, 324

ibuprofen, 311
ice cream, 57, 64, 122, 219
immunoglobulins, 281, 287, 326
immunoglobulin A (IgA)
    antibodies, 29, 77, 83, 185, 187
    deficiency, 185
immunoglobulin E (IgE)
    antibodies, 3–4, 6–10, 12–15, 22–7, 29,
        31–3, 38, 59–61, 69, 77–8, 82–3,
        85, 86–94, 97, 102, 107–8, 110–12,
        117–26, 128–9, 132, 136–43, 147,
        149, 154–5, 158–9, 166–9, 172–5,
        178–9, 203–6, 211–12, 214, 219–20,
        224, 227–8, 230–1, 266, 269, 272,
        281–3, 291, 304–5, 307, 308, 310,
        322–4, 326, 331–2, 345–9, 351–4
    -mediated food allergy, 4, 6, 7, 9–14,
        22–3, 25, 29, 31–3, 38, 59, 61, 69,
        77, 82, 85–7, 90, 107, 110, 117–20,
        125–6, 129, 149, 174, 214, 220
immunoglobulin G (IgG)
    antibodies, 6, 7, 38, 77, 78, 83, 91, 92,
        118, 185, 282
    testing, 7, 91
    IgG₃, 24
immunoglobulin M (IgM), 77, 83

immune system, 279–87, 293–4, 318
immune tolerance, 108
immunisations, 326
immunomodulatory components, 287
immunosuppression, 55
immunotherapy, 161, 169, 303, 305, 307, 308, 326
infant formulae, 117, 119, 124, 247–50, 254, 262, 290–1, 294, 337–8
infantile colic, 119, 345
infantile gut, 286
inflammatory bowel disease, 46, 221
inflammatory polyarthritis, 83
influenza, 69, 131
inhalation, 33–4, 107, 118, 139, 203, 205, 212, 220, 304, 313, 318
inhaler devices, 313
insect venoms, 326
insects, 109, 111, 138
interleukin
  IL-1β, 82, 83
  IL-4, 27
  IL-5, 27
  IL-13, 27
  IL-31, 27
Intestinal biopsy, 185
intestinal immune system, 286
invertebrate tropomyosin, 139
iodine, 254
Iridaceae, 150
iron, 120, 125, 184, 196, 207, 244, 257–8, 262, 285, 294, 350
irritable bowel syndrome (IBS), 7, 37–40, 42–3, 49, 70–1, 82, 92, 117, 127, 184, 203, 275–6
isinglass, 142, 228
isoflavines, 253, 254
ispaghula, 39

jogging, 230, 354
Junglandaceae, 150
junk food, 65

kamut, 191, 195
kinesiology, 91
kiss-induced reactions, 118
kiwi, 14–16, 148, 152, 155–6, 159, 317, 325, 348

krill, 137
kwashiorkor, 244

labial rub, 99
lactase, 8, 117, 126–7
Lactobacillus, 285, 287, 291
lactoglobulin, 118, 121
lactose, 40, 90, 121, 126–7, 188, 345
  congenital lactose intolerance, 126
  lactose intolerance, 8, 40, 50, 90, 107, 117, 126–8, 188, 345
  low-lactose foods, 128
lager, 191, 213, 217, 228–9, 353
Lamiaceae, 150
lamina propria, 185
Langerhans cells, 27
laryngeal, 343
laryngeal oedema, 31
latex, 97, 110, 147, 153, 155, 156, 158, 160, 178, 276, 323, 326
  latex–food cross-reaction, 147
  latex–food syndrome, 156
Lauraceae, 150
LCPUFAs, 284, 287, 294
leaky gut, 64
Lecythidaceae, 150
Leguminosae, 150, 159, 166–7, 171–3, 246, 251, 285, 293, 333, 349
lemon/lime juice, 217
lentils, 150, 167, 171–2, 190, 207, 251
lettuce, 152, 154
leukotrienes, 6, 24, 212, 216
leukotriene receptor antagonists, 312
L-glutamate, 218
lifestyle Issues, 265
lima bean, 150, 172
limpets, 139
linseed, 143, 174–6, 255
lip swelling, 54, 55
liquorice, 150, 172, 223
live yoghurts, 127
lobster, 138, 143, 225, 347
LOFFLEX, 49
logan fruit, 152
long-chain polyunsaturated fatty acids, 254, 279, 284
low sugar low yeast anti-Candida diet, 72
lung function, 310, 312

lupin, 17, 112, 171, 172, 173
lychee, 151, 152
lymphocytes, 7, 107, 188, 281
lysozyme, 118, 129, 130

macadamia nuts, 177
macaroons, 207
mackerel, 110, 137–8, 140, 254, 353
magnesium, 247, 257, 285
maize, 39, 154, 190, 204–5, 207, 230,
    255–6, 353
malabsorption, 8, 46, 183, 185, 187, 189
malt extract, 194, 197
malt vinegar, 194
Malvaceae, 150
mammalian milks, 110, 118, 121, 345–6
management of food hypersensitivity, 241,
    303, 305, 311, 316, 345–7, 349,
    350–4
  management of egg allergy, 130
  management of peanut allergy, 168
mandarin, 152
mango, 152, 154, 177
MAOI drugs, 224
mare's milk, 110
margarines, 64
marlin, 140, 254
marmalade, 191, 196, 219, 223
marzipan, 179, 191
mast cells, 6, 24, 32–3, 38, 77, 82, 86, 154,
    212, 224
maternal diet, 283–5, 288, 294
mayonnaise, 129, 130, 131, 191, 275
ME, 68–9, 72
meadowsweet, 221
meat, 246, 285
medical identification jewellery, 231, 354
Mediterranean, 152
Melkersson–Rosenthal syndrome, 54
melon, 154–5, 158, 348
menthol, 14, 219, 223
mercury, 254
methotrexate, 46
microflora, 280, 286–7
micronutrients, 244, 246, 250, 258, 260
  micronutrient requirements, 258
  micronutrient supplementation, 250,
    257–9, 260
migraine, 7, 74–9, 224–6, 304, 352

abdominal migraine, 78
milk, 13–17, 24–5, 27, 33–4, 38–40, 50,
    64, 67, 82, 89, 92, 94, 96, 100–1,
    107–8, 110–12, 117–28, 141, 148,
    171, 174, 190–1, 198, 203, 206, 226,
    231, 244, 246–50, 253, 260–2, 266,
    268, 270–1, 278, 287–92, 295, 318,
    325, 329, 330–1, 337–8, 345–6
  milk solids, 121
  milk–mucus belief, 33
  milkshake, 124, 250
mineral, 48, 65, 122, 248–9, 251, 254,
    256–7, 258–9, 283, 285, 351
mint, 223
miso soup, 225
mites, 138, 153, 204, 303
MMR, 131, 132
molluscs, 17, 109, 112, 136–9, 142–3, 230
monkey nuts, 169
monoamine oxidase, 76, 224
monosodium glutamate (MSG), 7, 34, 55,
    65, 77–8, 211, 215, 218, 219, 352
Moraceae, 150
morbilliform rashes, 23, 119, 317
moulds, 157
mouth ulcers, 184–5, 350
mucosal damage, 185–9, 196
mucosal immune system, 286
mucus, 22, 33, 310
muesli, 123, 170, 179, 191
mugwort, 147, 154–6, 160
mung bean, 150, 172
Musaceae, 150
musculoskeletal disorders, 81
mushrooms, 157, 223
mussels, 137–8, 143, 225, 347
mustard, 17, 112, 174–5, 214
mustard seed, 150, 174
myalgia, 70
myalgic encephalomyelitis, 69
myocardial infarction, 7
Myrtaceae, 151

n-3 polyunsaturated fatty acids, 255, 285
nasal
  nasal congestion, 224, 343
  nasal corticosteroids, 306
  nasal polyps, 216
  nasal sprays, 306

nasal steroids, 303
nasal symptoms, 306
natural food colourings, 214
natural latex rubber, 156
nausea, 7, 70–1, 74, 78, 95, 218, 227, 324, 343
neomycin, 132
neurological disorders, 68, 74
neuropeptides, 27
neutrophils, 7
niacin, 121, 196
NICE guidelines, 39, 317, 319, 321
nickel, 8
nitrates and nitrites, 217
NOAEL, 211
nomenclature, 3–4, 9–10, 12, 13, 108, 128
non-allergic food hypersensitivity, 4, 7, 9, 90, 107
non-Hodgkin's lymphoma, 189
non-IgE-mediated reactions, 9, 119, 129
non-specific lipid transfer proteins (nsLTP), 108, 110, 147, 149, 152–3, 156, 158–61, 204–7, 228
non-starch polysaccharide, 256
non-steroidal anti-inflammatory drugs, 24, 215, 221
no-observed-adverse-effect level, 211
noodles, 130, 204, 207
norepinephrine, 223
nougat, 179
nucleotides, 287
nutrition, 49, 262, 278, 289–90, 293–4
nutritional
    nutritional adequacy, 196, 244–8, 250–1, 257, 292
    nutritional consequences, 243, 246–8, 251, 253, 257
    nutritional deficiencies, 120, 171, 197, 244–7, 253, 257, 353
    nutritional impact, 245–7, 251, 253
    nutritional intake, 244, 257
    nutritional management, 243
    nutritional requirements, 244, 246, 248, 249–50, 260
    nutritional status, 48, 63, 72, 131, 180, 243, 244, 245, 246, 249, 262
    nutritional supplements, 94, 247, 260, 267, 268

nuts, 13–14, 24–25, 27, 39, 59, 94, 108, 112, 131, 154–5, 160, 166, 169, 170–1, 176–80, 231, 245–6, 251, 274, 285, 292, 311, 317–18, 325, 333, 348–9
    almonds, 123, 151, 154, 167, 176–9, 268, 349
    alternative names for some nuts, 179
    Brazil nuts, 123, 150–1, 155, 167, 176–7, 349
    cashew nuts, 150, 166, 176–8
    ground nuts, 169
    groundnut oil, 169
    hazelnut, 15, 27, 154–6, 158, 176–9, 349
    macadamia nuts, 177
    nut milks, 122
    nut-free products, 274
    peanuts – see peanuts
    pecan, 150, 177, 178
    pine nut, 177, 179
    pistachio nut, 150, 177–9
    walnut, 176, 177, 178, 255
nystatin, 41

oats, 39, 64, 83, 190–1, 193, 195, 197, 207, 255, 350–1
    oat allergy, 204
    oat milk, 122
    oatmeal, 24, 255
occupational agents, 311
occupational allergies, 139
occupational asthma, 204, 205
occupational lung disease, 31
octopamine, 76
octopus, 138, 143, 347
oesophageal cancer, 189
oil of wintergreen, 222–3, 353
oily fish, 254, 255
Oleaceae, 151
oligosaccharides, 40
omega-3 fatty acids, 48, 65, 255, 288
omega-5 gliadin, 205, 206, 231, 354
omega-6, 48
onions, 39, 156, 217
oral allergy syndrome, 9, 32, 99, 140, 111, 147–9, 152–61, 177–8, 325, 348–9
oral corticosteroids, 307, 313
oral immunotherapy, 103

oral mucosa, 99, 108, 154–5
oral steroids, 303, 313
oranges, 64, 76, 123, 152, 154, 158,
    213–14, 223, 229
Orchidaceae, 151
organic foods, 293
orofacial granulomatosis, 54–5, 57
oropharyngeal cancer, 189
osteoarthritis, 81
osteopenia, 189
osteoporosis, 184, 189, 276, 350
otitis media, 31–2
ovalbumin, 128–30
ovomucin, 129–30
ovomucoid, 108, 111, 129
ovotransferrin, 129
oysters, 138, 143

palpitations, 102, 140
pancreatic insufficiency, 188
pantothenic acid, 251
parabens, 216, 220
para-hydroxybenzoate, 211
para-hydroxybenzoic acid, 212, 216
paralytic shellfish poisoning, 140
parmesan cheese, 218
parvalbumins, 110, 137
passive immunity, 284
pasta, 41, 64, 188, 190, 194, 197, 207
pastries, 56, 64, 173, 176, 190, 207, 350
patch testing, 55, 90, 121, 129, 220
pathogenesis-related (PR) proteins, 110,
    149
Patum Peperium, 142
pea, 122–3, 128, 150, 172, 261
pea milk, 122, 123
peaches, 41, 148, 151–2, 154, 155–6,
    158–9, 205, 222–3, 348
peach nsLTP, 152
peanut, 3, 9, 13–17, 24–5, 27, 55, 89, 94,
    108, 110–12, 125, 141, 148–9, 154,
    155–6, 160, 166–80, 203, 206, 223,
    228, 251, 265–6, 283, 285, 293–5,
    311, 317, 324–5, 327, 349, 351, 354
  Arachis hypogaea, 169
  arachis oil, 169
  Ara h 1, 108, 111, 156, 166, 167, 171,
    172, 174, 177, 178
  Ara h 2, 108, 111, 112, 156, 167

Ara h 5, 111, 156
Ara h 6, 112
Ara h 8, 111
Ara h 9, 153, 167
common foods which may contain
    peanuts, 170
frying and boiling peanuts, 167
monkey nuts, 169
peanut allergens, 111
peanut allergy diagnosis, 168
peanut oil, 167, 169, 170
peanut, legume, seed and tree-nut allergy,
    349
raw peanuts, 167
roasted peanuts, 111, 167
pears, 41, 152, 156
peas, 39, 167, 190, 223, 251
pecan, 150, 177, 178
Pedaliaceae, 151, 174
penicillin, 325
peppers, 151–2, 154, 156–7, 191, 222–3,
    353
peppermint oil, 219
peptides, 6, 27, 64, 124
perennial rhinitis, 216, 303–4
peripheral neuropathy, 72
peripheral vasodilation, 227
pervasive development disorder, 63
Peyer's patches, 47
pH of the stools, 90
pharmacologic food reactions, 7, 221, 352
phenol sulphotransferase enzymes, 76
phenolic flavinoids, 75
phenolic-compound diet, 64
phenylethylamine, 7, 223–5
phosphate, 247, 248
phosphorous, 121, 254
phototherapy, 321
phyto-oestrogen, 253, 254
pickles, 191, 194, 196, 213, 216, 223
pigeon pea, 150, 172
pimecrolimus, 320
Pinaceae, 151
pine nut, 177, 179
pineapple, 24, 157
Piperaceae, 151
pistachio nut, 150, 177–9
pizza, 64, 143, 173, 176, 190, 207, 268,
    350

placenta, 128
plaice, 137–8
plant defence system, 110, 149
plant food allergens, 110
   plant food superfamilies: cupins and
      2S-albumins, 151
   plant food superfamilies: prolamins, plant
      defence system and profilins, 153
plant foods, 108, 110, 147, 149, 152, 154,
   156, 158, 219
platelet activation factors, 6
play therapists, 97
plums, 41
pollack, 137–8
pollen, 14, 27, 32, 107–8, 110–11, 147–9,
   152–6, 158–9, 160, 161, 178, 205,
   206, 227, 230, 303, 304, 305, 325,
   348, 351
pollen–food syndrome (PFS), 149, 154–61
pollen-related foods, 14
Polygonaceae, 151
pomfret, 137
ponceau, 215
poppy seed, 174
pork, 14, 83
porridge, 123
potassium, 257
potatoes, 16, 39, 78, 148, 153, 156–7,
   190–1, 207, 217, 229, 256
poultry, 190–1, 213, 285
PR proteins, 110, 149, 153, 155–7
praline, 179
prawns, 123, 141, 143, 347
prebiotics, 38, 279, 284–5, 287, 289, 291,
   294
pregnancy, 198, 255, 279, 282, 283, 284,
   285, 289, 293, 294, 324
preservatives, 7, 34, 39, 55, 57–8, 65, 67,
   212, 216–17, 311, 352
prevalence, 3, 9, 13–17, 24, 27, 31–2, 54,
   59, 69, 72, 90, 117, 128, 136–7,
   147–9, 154–5, 157, 166, 171, 174,
   176, 184–5, 187, 189, 203–4,
   210–11, 215, 219, 221
   prevalence of CFS/ME, 69
   prevalence of coeliac disease (CD) in
      those with other autoimmune
      disorders, 187
   prevalence of FHS in adults, 13

prevalence of FHS in children, 14
prevalence of peanut allergy, 166
prevalence of reported allergy to seafood,
   136
prevalence of seronegative CD, 185
prevalence studies, 15, 25
primary biliary cirrhosis, 187
primary lactose intolerance, 127
primary prevention, 279
primary sensitisation, 147
probiotics, 38, 65, 279, 284–5, 287, 294
proctocolitis, 119
prodromes, 74
profilin, 108, 110–11, 149, 153–7
prolamin superfamily, 110, 149, 174
prostaglandins, 6, 24, 212
Proteaceae, 151
protein, 6–8, 26–7, 48–9, 64, 76, 93, 95,
   107–11, 117–18, 121–2, 125, 128–32,
   136, 138, 143, 147, 149, 153, 155,
   156–7, 161, 167, 169, 171–5, 178,
   180, 183, 185, 195, 204–7, 212, 214,
   217–18, 220, 226, 228, 244, 246–51,
   253–5, 285, 287, 290–1, 293, 317,
   320, 345–6
proteolysis, 110, 149, 152, 155, 178
Pru p 3, 152–3, 159
prunes, 213, 216, 223, 229
pruritis, 22–3, 26, 157, 206, 216, 217, 224,
   226, 317, 323–4, 342, 348, 351
pseudoallergic food reaction, 76
psychostimulants, 59
psyllium, 39
pulmonary haemosiderosis, 33
pulse testing, 91
Punicaceae, 151
purified allergen reagents, 158
pyrexia, 46

quality of life, 266, 310, 312, 315–16
quinoa milk, 122
quinoline yellow (E104), 214

radio-allergo-sorbent tests (RAST), 89
ragweed, 147, 154–5
raised plasma histamine levels, 76
rash, 342
raspberry, 151, 216, 223
razor-shell, 137

recipes, 267, 269, 270, 273, 275
recombinant allergens, 110, 158, 231
recombinant DNA, 109, 110
red kidney beans, 123
red wine, 74
reducing substances, 127
refractory coeliac disease, 188
reintroduction of foods, 265
rescue medications, 266
resistant starch classification, 40
resources for health professionals, 276
respiratory, 9, 12, 17, 22, 26, 31–3, 35,
    108, 119–20, 157, 220
restricted diet, 250, 265, 270, 272, 274–5
resuscitation training, 97
rheumatoid arthritis, 81–2
rhinitis, 25, 31–5, 136, 149, 204, 212,
    216–17, 219, 278, 303–10, 303, 312,
    314, 323, 345, 347–8, 352
rhinoconjunctivitis, 31–2, 119, 224
rhinorrhea, 306, 343
riboflavin, 121, 130, 196, 207, 251
rice, 78, 82, 122, 190, 194, 198, 122,
    204–5, 207, 214, 248–50, 255, 256,
    268, 293–4, 338, 351
  rice cakes, 207
  rice milk, 122–3, 248–50
  rice noodles, 207
  rice paper, 207
  rice pudding, 207
rickets, 120, 244, 248
roast potatoes, 217
Rosaceae, 151, 156, 158
Royal Gala, 161
royal icing, 129–30
Rutaceae, 151
rye, 27, 29, 39, 64, 183, 190, 193, 195, 205,
    207, 255, 268, 350–1

saffron, 150, 214, 352
sago, 207
salicylates, 8, 16, 64, 65, 107, 221–2, 352,
    353
salmon, 110, 137–9, 142
Samter's triad, 221–2
Sapindaceae, 151
sarcoidosis, 54
sardines, 123, 138, 140, 225, 254

Scientific Advisory Committee on Nutrition,
    255, 292
scombroid fish, 224
scombroid poisoning, 140, 218, 224, 347
scorpions, 138
scurvy, 161
sea urchin, 137
seafood, 16, 136–43, 254–5, 285, 325,
    347, 351
Seafood allergy, 347
seal meat, 113
seasonal rhinitis, 303–4, 348
secalins, 183, 205
secondary lactose intolerance, 127
secretory IgA, 286, 287, 291
seed storage proteins, 149
seeds, 166, 174, 251, 254, 333, 349
selenium, 251, 285, 294
semolina, 191, 207
sensitisation, 6, 25, 27, 33, 35, 74, 108–10,
    118, 139–40, 147–9, 152, 154,
    156–60, 172, 178, 204, 206–7, 227,
    230, 278–9, 288, 291, 293, 318, 331,
    348
serine protease inhibitors, 109
serological antibody tests, 184, 185, 186
sesame seeds, 16–17, 27, 112, 123, 174–6,
    251, 311, 317, 349
sesame oil, 174, 175, 176
sheep, 40, 64, 118, 121
shellfish, 9, 13–14, 16, 17, 27, 110, 112,
    136–43, 148, 230, 254, 268, 311, 317,
    332, 347
shitake mushrooms, 157
shrimp, 13–16, 38, 136–42, 225, 347
Sjögren's syndrome, 187
skin, 9, 13–16, 22–9, 31, 35, 41, 78, 82,
    85–90, 102, 117–18, 122, 140–1, 148,
    157–60, 168, 178, 186–7, 203–4,
    206, 216, 219, 220, 227, 229, 231
  skin disorders, 12, 22
skin prick testing (SPT), 16, 24, 25, 78, 82,
    86, 87, 89, 90, 93, 97, 112, 117, 120,
    126, 128, 129, 132, 141, 158, 160,
    161, 168, 172, 175, 178, 203, 228, 231
skipjack, 140
skipper, 137
small bowel disorders, 183

small intestinal bacterial overgrowth, 188
small intestine, 127, 183, 187
smoking, 74, 189
snack foods, 213, 221
snails, 138–9, 143
sneezing, 343
soaps and detergents, 316
sobakawa hulls, 204
sodium benzoate, 34, 61, 212, 215–16, 228
sodium caseinate, 121
sodium cromoglycate, 306
sodium metabisulphite, 33–4, 211–12, 217,
    219–21, 227–9, 311, 352–3
  sulphur dioxide, 33, 107, 112, 212, 217
  maximum permitted level (MPL) of
    sulphur dioxide, 217
soft drinks, 41, 42, 57, 213, 216, 226, 311
Solanaceae, 151, 156
soluble fibre, 39, 193, 255, 256
sorbates, 212
sorbet, 129, 130
sorbitol, 41
soups, 190–1, 207, 213–14, 222, 272
soy sauce, 173, 191, 218
soya, 9, 13–15, 17, 25, 27, 38, 65, 83, 112,
    125–6, 131, 156, 167, 172–4, 203–4,
    225, 230, 245, 248–51, 253, 261, 268,
    317–18, 329, 337–9, 354
  soya bean, 123, 172
  soya cheese, 122–3, 128
  soya fermentation, 172
  soya formulas, 125
  soya fruit drink, 123
  soya milk, 122–3, 250, 338
  soya oil, 172
  soya sauce, 172
  soya yoghurt, 122
spearmint oil, 219
specialised formula milks, 267
Specific Carbohydrate Diet, 65
specific IgE, 25, 32, 86, 89–90, 97, 126,
    132, 136, 141, 154, 158, 168, 205–6,
    220
specific IgE tests, 89
spelt, 191, 195
spices, 8, 24, 29, 57, 86, 156, 160, 212,
    219, 220, 222, 229
spiders, 138

spinach, 123, 224–5
squid, 138, 143, 347
Staphylococcus aureus, 316
Starking apples, 161
Sterculiaceae family, 226
steroid-dependent asthmatics, 211
Stevens–Johnson syndrome, 22
stone fruits, 155
strawberries, 124, 148, 151–2, 156, 222–5,
    230, 325, 348, 353–4
sublingual immunotherapy, 307
sugar, 40–2, 47, 58, 65, 72
sulphite, *see* sodium metabisulphite
Sunderland protocol, 65
sunflower, 123, 150, 154, 174–6
sunset yellow (E110), 55, 214–15
sushi, 140
sweets, 179, 211, 213–14, 221, 223, 253,
    274
synephrine, 76
systemic antibiotics, 317

T cells, 6, 7, 27, 188, 281, 318, 320
tachycardia, 139, 227, 323, 324
tacrolimus, 320
tahini, 176
takeaways, 35
tamarind, 150, 172
tartrazine (E102), 55, 211–15, 218, 220,
    311, 352
tea, 39, 42, 191, 216, 222–3, 226, 229, 330,
    353
tertiary prevention, 279
test food matrix, 100
Th1 and Th2 cells, 6, 7, 27
thaumatin-like proteins, 149
The Anaphylaxis Campaign, 171
The British Society for Allergy and Clinical
    Immunology, 131
theobroma cacao, 226
theobromine, 225, 226
theophylline, 225
thiamine, 121, 130, 196, 207
thioredoxins, 205
titanium dioxide, 47, 48
TLP, 152
TNF-α, 27, 78, 82, 83
tofu, 123, 173

tolerance, 6, 38, 47, 95, 108, 126–9, 131–2, 142, 160, 193–4
tomatoes, 8, 16, 24, 64, 148, 152, 155–6, 158, 218, 222–4, 229, 230, 257, 353
toothpaste, 56, 57, 219, 223
topical antibiotics, 317
topical anti-inflammatory drugs, 305
topical corticosteroids, 319, 320
topical creams, 316, 318
topical immunosuppressants, 320
total parenteral nutrition, 48
toxic protein fractions, 183, 185
trace elements, 257–8
tragacanth gum (E413), 172, 219
translation cards, 272, 274
tree nuts, 9, 13, 15–17, 24, 27, 110, 112, 148–9, 155–6, 158, 160, 166–7, 169, 176–80, 203, 226
trees, 110, 147, 155–6, 160
trialling food avoidances, 67
triggers, 311, 325
triticale, 191, 195
tropomyosin, 109, 138–9, 141
tryptamine, 7, 223
tryptase, 324
tuna, 138–40, 142, 224, 353
Turkish delight, 179
turmeric (E100), 151, 214, 352
turnip, 150, 157
type 1 diabetes mellitus, 187
type I hypersensitivity, 212
type III hypersensitivity, 6
type IV hypersensitivity, 212
tyramine, 7, 75–6, 223–5

umami, 218
una, 137
urine analyses for ASD, 64
urticaria, 6–8, 22–5, 95, 97, 101–2, 119, 128, 140, 156–7, 204, 210–11, 214–19, 224, 226, 228, 291, 317, 320–1, 323–4, 342, 345–6, 348–9, 351, 352, 354
    idiopathic urticaria, 210

vaccines, 131–2
vanilla, 124, 219
vasoactive amines, 34, 77, 107, 219, 223–5, 352–3

Vega testing, 91
vegan, 83, 246, 253, 267–8, 275
vegetables, 14–15, 31, 39–40, 50, 64, 86, 93, 109, 141, 147–9, 151–5, 157–61, 190, 197–8, 222–3, 229, 231, 257, 285, 293–4, 308, 333, 353
    vegetable allergy, 152
    vegetarians and vegans, 83, 131, 174, 180, 251, 253, 268
vertebrate fish, 139
vicilin superfamily, 108, 110, 167, 172, 174, 178
villous atrophy, 185, 186, 188
vinegar, 65, 152, 194, 217
viruses, 110, 149, 279, 281, 287
Vitaceae, 151
vitamins and minerals, 65, 72, 122, 142, 249, 251, 254, 256–8, 283, 293–4, 351
    vitamin A, 72, 121, 247, 251, 285
    vitamin and mineral supplements, 67, 72, 251, 257
    vitamin B_{12}, 196, 247, 251, 350
    vitamin B_6, 65, 72
    vitamin C, 257, 285, 289
    vitamin D, 120, 124, 248, 251, 258, 283, 293
    vitamin E, 130, 212, 251
vodka, 228
vomiting, 24, 74, 78, 102, 119, 128, 139, 185, 227, 317, 323, 333, 344, 346, 349, 350

walnut, 176, 177, 178, 255
water buffalo, 118
watercress, 123, 150
watermelon, 150, 154–5
weaning, 119, 122, 185, 198, 248, 279, 282, 286, 292–5, 346, 350
weed pollens, 147, 154
weeds, 110, 155
weight, 244, 246, 248, 255, 260–1, 317, 327, 350
weight gain, 70
weight loss, 46, 70, 71
wet-wrap therapy, 320
wheal diameter, 87
wheat, 9, 13–17, 24–5, 27, 29, 34, 38–41, 49, 55, 59, 64, 78, 82–3, 92, 100, 107,

111–12, 148, 171–2, 183, 190, 193–5, 197, 203–7, 228, 230–1, 245, 255–6, 266, 268, 270–1, 275, 293–4, 317–18, 333, 338, 350–4
wheat beer, 228
wheat gliadins, 107
wheat substitute, 207
wheat thioredoxin-hB, 34
wheat-dependant, exercise-induced anaphylaxis (WDEIA), 111, 203, 205–6, 230, 351
wheat-free foods, 267
wheeze, 33, 119, 139, 283, 310, 314, 343, 345
whey, 118, 121
whisky, 228
white bread, 123
white wine, 14, 217

wholemeal bread, 123
willow, 221
wine, 8, 34, 74–5, 142, 152, 191, 213, 217, 219, 222–5, 227–9, 311, 353
wolf-fish, 137
Worcestershire sauce, 142, 143, 347
World Health Organization, 68, 292

yeast, 39, 41–2, 64–5, 72, 82, 157, 191, 213, 218, 223–5
yeast extract, 64, 218, 224–5
yeast-free diet for ASD, 64
yellow fever, 131
yellowtail, 137
yoghurt, 64, 117, 121, 128, 191, 214, 216, 268, 337–8

Zingiberaceae, 151

3